Mental Health Practice: A Case-Based Approach

Mental Health Practice: A Case-Based Approach

Edited by Joey Webb

STATES
ACADEMIC PRESS
www.statesacademicpress.com

States Academic Press,
109 South 5th Street,
Brooklyn, NY 11249, USA

Visit us on the World Wide Web at:
www.statesacademicpress.com

ISBN: 978-1-63989-351-5

Cataloging-in-Publication Data

Mental health practice : a case-based approach / edited by Joey Webb.
p. cm.
Includes bibliographical references and index.
ISBN 978-1-63989-351-5
1. Mental health--Case studies. 2. Psychiatric consultation. 3. Psychiatric aides. I. Webb, Joey.
RA790 .M46 2022
616.89--dc23

Table of Contents

Preface

Every book is initially just a concept; it takes months of research and hard work to give it the final shape in which the readers receive it. In its early stages, this book also went through rigorous reviewing. The notable contributions made by experts from across the globe were first molded into patterned chapters and then arranged in a sensibly sequential manner to bring out the best results.

The behavioral, cognitive and emotional well-being of a person falls under mental health. It has a wide range of impacts, affecting physical health, relationships and daily life. The mental health of a person can be negatively affected by conditions such as stress, depression and anxiety. The disorders related to mental health can be categorized as anxiety disorders, mood disorders and schizophrenia disorders. Some of the anxiety disorders are generalized anxiety disorder, panic disorders and phobias. A few types of mood disorders are major depression, bipolar disorder and seasonal affective disorder. The treatment of mental health disorders can be done through various techniques and methods such as psychotherapy, medication and self-help. This book unravels the recent studies in the field of mental health. It consists of contributions made by international experts. This book is a resource guide for experts as well as students.

It has been my immense pleasure to be a part of this project and to contribute my years of learning in such a meaningful form. I would like to take this opportunity to thank all the people who have been associated with the completion of this book at any step.

Editor

1

Art of Recovery: Displacement, Mental Health, and Wellbeing

Emma Rose [1,*], Amanda Bingley [2], Macarena Rioseco [3] and Kirsten Lamb [4]

1 Lancaster Institute for the Contemporary Arts, Lancaster University, Lancaster LA1 4YW, UK
2 Division of Health Research, Lancaster University, Lancaster LA1 4YG, UK; a.bingley@lancaster.ac.uk
3 Lancaster Institute for the Contemporary Arts, Lancaster LA1 4YW, UK; m.riosecocastillo@lancaster.ac.uk
4 Freedom from Torture, Manchester M1 1JU, UK; klamb@freedomfromtorture.org
* Correspondence: e.rose@lancaster.ac.uk

Abstract: *Art of Recovery* explores the potential of a participatory arts engagement with place to contribute toward the recovery and reconnection of refugees who experience trauma. The study responded to the international challenge of refugees' mental health as a global priority as they experience higher prevalence rates of severe mental health disorders in comparison with the general population. The role of participatory arts in contributing toward recovery and reconnection is growing, but policymakers and health professionals are constrained by the lack of research exploring its benefits. We worked with 14 participants in four participatory arts workshops exploring the benefits of artwork focusing on remembered or imagined healing places. A qualitative thematic analysis of the artwork drew on Herman's theory of recovery identifying "remembrance", "mourning", and "reconnection" to assess the elements of potential recovery, including aspects of the participants' experience of transition between their homeland and the United Kingdom (UK), and new social connections. In conclusion, the study suggests that participating in a group making artworks of places associated with safety may contribute to processes of transition and social connectedness, prompting in turn feelings of wellbeing. The study offers insights into arts and health issues of interest to refugee-supporting communities, health professionals and policymakers.

Keywords: refugees; participatory arts; recovery; social reconnection; transition; mental health

---

1. Introduction

Art of Recovery responded to the current global context and the mental health challenge associated with refugees and asylum seekers. Internationally foregrounded by the European Union, the United Nations High Commission for Refugees (UNHCR) and the World Health Organization (WHO), the health of refugees and asylum seekers is now a global priority (UNHCR 2018; WHO 2017). Since May 2017, WHO has shifted its approach on migration from a solely humanitarian-based approach to one based on health systems that strengthen the physical and mental health of refugees (WHO 2017). WHO's premise is that at global and national levels, health policies and strategies to manage the health consequences of migration and displacement have not kept pace with the speed and diversity of modern migration and displacement.

The project was a collaboration with the charity Freedom from Torture, who provided a supportive environment for the research in one of their North of England centres. *Art of Recovery* explores how participatory art contributes to the recovery of refugees who experience trauma.

The project developed from a growing recognition that refugees appear to benefit from engagement in creative arts (Andemicael 2011; Dutton 2017), and participatory arts in particular (Rose and Bingley 2017; Barnes 2009). With the aim of developing an appropriate research design, we first undertook a pilot study, *Migrating Art* (2017), in partnership with the Merseyside Refugee & Asylum Seekers Pre & Postnatal Support Group in Liverpool, United Kingdom (UK). This charity supports women migrants who are victims of rape, trafficking, sexual violence, domestic servitude, and other forms of gender-based violence and human rights abuses. *Art of Recovery* built on this earlier pilot, in particular in relation to working in a safe, therapeutically supportive space. Both projects adhered to strict ethical guidelines provided by the University Ethics Committee and respective ethics committees of the migrant-supporting charities (approved in April 2016 and May 2017).

Freedom from Torture (FfT), as one of the world's largest charities in the field, has provided treatment for more than 57,000 survivors of torture. The charity provides a broad range of support for clients who attend weekly sessions, including psychological and physical therapies, forensic documentation of torture, legal and welfare advice, and creative projects. Their centres employ language interpreters ensuring well-supported communication for clients.

Although organisations supporting refugees through arts projects in the UK have grown over the last decade, there is a need for more research and evaluation of the rehabilitative potential of participatory visual art (Hayhow et al. 2016). While these organisations may reflect on their practice and keep records of outputs and impacts achieved, there is little collation of evaluative material in arts projects, other than in reports to funders (Sonn et al. 2013). Evaluation is required to enable practitioners of participatory visual arts with refugees to establish methods of best practice (Sonn et al. 2013). *Art of Recovery* conducted a qualitative thematic evaluation to ascertain the impact of participatory arts for a small group of refugees, supported by FfT.

In this paper, we first discuss the context for refugees who have been tortured and displaced. We describe the model of recovery on which we explore the participatory arts intervention, and map key theories underpinning the research. The explanation of research methods involves qualitative participatory approaches, the thematic narrative and visual data analysis methods, followed by a section exploring the findings. Finally, an evaluation of the intervention assesses the potential of arts-based approaches to contribute to the recovery and transition of refugees who experience trauma.

1.1. *Displacing Mental Health and Well-being*

According to the United Nations High Commission for Refugees (UNHCR 2018), the world is witnessing the highest levels of human displacement on record. UNHCR estimates there are 65.6 million forcibly displaced people worldwide, of which 22.5 million are refugees and asylum seekers living in exile. In 2016, the number of applications for asylum in the UK, excluding dependents, was 30,747 (Refugee Council 2017). Refugees and asylum seekers often experience traumatic events, before and during displacement (Hargreaves 2002; Hollifield et al. 2002; Nosè et al. 2017), and afterwards. Post-displacement trauma can continue after arrival in the UK, where trauma can occur in relation to imprisonment in detention centres (adults and children), and resettlement stress related to stigma, shame, hostility, racism, and discrimination (Miller et al. 2006). In comparison with the general population, refugees and asylum seekers have been shown to experience higher prevalence rates of a range of mental health disorders, and disorders specifically tied to stress (Fazel et al. 2005; Bogic et al. 2015; Slewa-Younan et al. 2015). The most studied mental health problem in the refugee population remains post-traumatic stress disorder (PTSD), as it is 10 times more likely in refugees and asylum seekers compared to host populations (Fazel et al. 2005; Bogic et al. 2015; Slewa-Younan et al. 2015). Even if the prevalence of PTSD is over-estimated for instrumental purposes to mobilise resources (Fassin and d'Halluin 2007), there is evidence that it is substantially increased in refugees, whether adults or children (Fazel et al. 2012). Research indicates the prevalence of PTSD in survivors of torture is over 90% (Johnson and Thompson 2008; Moisander and Erik 2003; Mollica et al. 1998). FfT (originally known as the Medical Foundation for the Care of Victims of Torture) treats over 1,000 torture survivors each year. Most arrive traumatised, vulnerable, and fearing further persecution. They have a right to rehabilitation under Article 14 of the United Nations Convention against Torture (UNCAT 2012). It is important to provide treatment soon after the events, because early psychosocial support is a decisive factor in limiting the development and severity of PTSD symptoms (Dutton 2017; Wilson and Drožđek 2004). A systematic review undertaken by Robjant et al. (2009) indicates that lengthy asylum processes result in increased risk of psychiatric disorder. Long delays and very slow administrative processes for asylum seekers in the UK means that sometimes individuals are in the system for many months, sometimes years. Many detained indefinitely in immigration centres are destabilised, or retraumatised by the experience having encountered torture in similar conditions (Boyles 2017).

Mental and physical repercussions of torture mean its survivors are particularly susceptible to social isolation and its adverse psychological effects (Acheson 1998; Burnett and Peel 2001; Gorst-Unsworth and Goldenberg 1998). Having left behind their culture and homeland, known way of life, community, work, political life, home, friends, and family, many refugees hope to be reunited with family at a later time (Boyles 2017), but many live on their own in exile, reliant on their inner resources. Migration itself is a potentially traumatic experience (Grinberg and Grinberg 1989), felt by the individual as a discontinuity, a breakage in the self, in the relationship with the environment, and with the individual's past (Le Roy 1994). Reconnection is a significant element in enhancing mental health outcomes (Burnett and Peel 2001), and it is important for migrants to find ways to reconnect with society, and crucial for survivors of torture on their journey of recovery (Herman 1992). Gorst-Unsworth and Goldenberg (1998) examine the health needs of refugees to suggest the importance of establishing informal groups, as a useful way of sharing experiences and ways of coping and making sense of past experiences. They highlight the importance for refugees to develop ongoing links and friendships with people in the host community, as well as making contact with people from their own countries (Epstein 1996); in this way, the best mental health outcomes are achieved (Burnett and Peel 2001).

1.2. The Road to Recovery

Examining the meaning and process of recovery is useful in this context. In this research, we draw on Herman (1992) three-stage model of recovery from trauma, the model recommended by the UK Psychological Trauma Society for use by trauma therapists based in the UK (McFetridge et al. 2017). In this model, Herman identifies the key features as three stages in the process of recovery, namely, safety, remembrance and mourning, and reconnection. She defines recovery as based on the empowerment of the survivor and the creation of new connections (Herman 1992). As (Lamb 2017, p. 56) explains, recovery as defined in the mental health field is the process by which individuals find ways to live a meaningful, ordinary life, even if they continue to experience symptoms. For Lamb, Herman's model is applicable to survivors of torture, even those who experienced prolonged, repeated trauma, and sustained threat to life. She notes, according to WHO (1992), that these individuals may have developed symptoms of PTSD, and enduring personality change resulting from their catastrophic experiences (Lamb 2017, p.57). When recruiting for *Art of Recovery*, therapists at FfT identified potential participants as those able to engage in stage three of Herman's process of recovery: individuals for whom reconnection proceeds or is possible. Most participants had established a relative level of security and safety in their new environment and were incrementally working through key rehabilitation processes used by therapists aimed at recovery, including: stabilisation of trauma symptoms; facing traumatic memories; moving toward integration of the trauma into a new narrative of self and personality (Lamb 2017, p. 57). As Lamb suggests, "the goal is to help survivors connect with the changed person they have become, the trauma more or less integrated into their autobiographical identity" (p. 57). In Herman's terms, participants were in various stages of the ability to move forward to live an ordinary life.

According to Kidd et al. (2016), the inclusion of refugees and asylum seekers in participatory arts has emerged gradually as a recognizable phenomenon in the UK. In 2016, around 200 organisations in the UK provided programmes related to arts and refugees (Hayhow et al. 2016), and the provision is growing as councils, community groups, churches, and charities respond to the increased numbers of displaced people in the UK. There is recognition of the role of participatory arts in healing trauma, as the approach supports individuals in accessing unprocessed traumatic responses and provides an opportunity for creative expression (Dutton 2017, p. 275). Survivors of trauma with limited language or the inability to put ideas into speech are particularly likely to benefit from self-expression through art, music, movement, or play as they provide the means to convey ideas without words (Dutton 2017, p. 271).

The focus of participatory arts is slightly different to that of art therapy. Participatory arts and art therapy are sometimes positioned against one another, with participatory arts set up within a recreational, social, or research context with little or no direct therapeutic focus. However, as Pavlicevic et al. (2014) note, there can be similarities in that artmaking, whether in a participatory or an art therapy context, can both use expressive media and be experienced as therapeutic whether intentional or not. The differences are in the context and intention: art therapy is a psychotherapeutic technique using art as a means to express thoughts and feelings, facilitated either in a group or individual sessions by trained therapists using recognised models of interaction and intervention (Malchiodi 2003). Participatory arts is a means to bring people together to share ideas, events, and experiences using arts media. Although participation is not intended to be directly therapeutic, participants do report indirect benefits of these kinds of arts events and groups, both within community or research contexts (Tsekleves et al. 2018). *Art of Recovery* sought not to provoke the exploration of difficult issues, or traumatic memories, but aimed to provide a space for people to meet, carry out meaningful art activities together, and connect with and share thoughts and feelings about places with positive associations. Refugee-supporting organisations are interested in the use of participatory arts as an adjunct to support clients engaged in therapy and, as Stickley (2010) argues, to better understand the potential for these arts-based approaches to open up possibilities for recovery beyond models focused on mental health.

2. Materials and Methods

The aim of *Art of Recovery* was to explore the potential of a participatory arts engagement with place to contribute toward the recovery and reconnection of refugees who experience trauma. To this end the project set up art workshops where participants could engage in 2D and 3D artmaking: painting with acrylics, drawing with crayon and pencil, and creating collage using a range of tactile materials, including textiles, felt, wool, stones, and feathers. Through these media, participants expressed their experience of safe spaces and places, encountered as safe havens, either recalled from their country of origin, or experienced on their journey toward safety, or an imaginary place. Emphasis in research design on positive memories and associations sought to minimise the potential for re-traumatisation. Artmaking from remembered or imagined safe places was examined in terms of the contribution to the participant's recovery and transition to a new environment. We explored how best to facilitate participants in connecting with a safe place within themselves through imaginary and visual representation. The project was informed by practices in participatory arts, therapeutic therapies, and the theoretical framework of therapeutic landscapes (see Rose 2012 for a detailed discussion of therapeutic landscapes in this context).

There were three phases to the project:

Phase 1. Ethical approval was provided by the authors' university research ethics committee (Ref: FL16211) and by FfT (Ref: R37). Prior to recruitment for workshops, researchers twice met FfT's therapists to discuss research design and to address specific vulnerabilities in the group. A former client serving on their Advisory Board was involved in discussions, as were five language translators to discuss terms and uses of language, and to identify possible cultural differences in interpretation. Therapists' professional knowledge gauged the suitability of participants invited to join the project. Each was at a stage in recovery with the potential to benefit from participatory artmaking, but not regularly attending other activities.

Phase 2. Following recruitment, four participatory arts workshops were delivered over six weeks. Qualitative data collection included demographic data providing a general profile of the participant group, three questionnaires designed to prompt semi-structured individual and group discussions during workshops, end of workshop informal reflections, observations in the form of field notes, and photographs of participants' artwork. Demographic data, questionnaire responses, and discussions together with visual data were collated with written field notes for each workshop. After each workshop, the research team met to debrief with the therapist, the former client, and interpreters. Following the final workshop, the research team had a final debrief with the lead FfT therapist to discuss key data analysis and findings as part of the triangulation process.

A qualitative thematic analysis of written, visual and observational data was completed by the research team, using primary codes based on Herman's theory of recovery: terms of remembrance (images or comments relating to original homeland), mourning (images or comments communicating nostalgia, loss, and grief), and reconnection (images or comments expressing life lived in the present). Secondary coding identified two sub-themes: the participants' experience of transition between their homeland and the UK; and new social connections, including the participation in the workshops, and how this contributed to their sense of well-being. The findings were interpreted by the research team and are discussed below.

Phase 3. Dissemination of findings with an accessible summary of findings produced for FfT, participants, and other interested refugee groups, made available on FfT's website.

Demographic data recorded a total of N = 14 clients, of whom N = 10 were male and N = 4 female, aged between 20 and 40 years, with the majority aged between 20 and 30 years old. Most participants had spent all their lives in their country of origin before exile, a small number (N = 2) having migrated to a country other than the UK at an earlier age. The research element of the project constituted workshops 2, 3, and 4 (W.2, W.3, W.4), producing 33 artworks, recorded as digital photographs. The participants originated from Cameroon, Democratic Republic of Congo, Iran, Iraq, and Sri Lanka. All participants had family remaining in their homeland.

W.1. Facilitated participants in making a collage or painting on any subject with positive associations. Designed as a "warm-up", activities introduced working with art materials, and helped to relax everyone into sharing ideas and artmaking together in this context. Demonstrations in assembling tactile materials emphasised collage as an accessible approach, alongside demonstrations in applying acrylic paints on canvas, mixing colours, and using different brushes for specific effects. Such demonstrations sought to invest participants with a greater means of expression, rather than to achieve a level of expertise.

W.2. Facilitated participants' artmaking on the research theme outlined above. Participants made collage, paintings, or a combination, on A4 or A3 sized canvasses. They continued to explore the subject matter throughout W.3 and W.4. Thoughts about artworks were shared in individual discussions with researchers, and each other. After W.3 and W.4, an exhibition in the space of the artworks enabled everyone to see all the artworks produced, and to discuss their thoughts and reflections. Questionnaires provided toward the end of each workshop enabled individuals to work with their language translator to provide written responses to questions about the experience of being in the workshop, the process of creating artworks, and their subject matter.

3. Findings

3.1. *Artworks*

Of the paintings produced, participants almost entirely chose to depict existing places and objects (N = 33) rather than imagined. Places were predominantly from their homeland (N = 26) and were places with which they had positive associations. Some also represented places from their present life in the UK. Within the total output, landscapes featuring natural elements were most prevalent (N = 49), with the sea, lake, rivers, fields, mountains, gardens, and croplands occurring most frequently. These settings were populated by trees and flowers (N = 10), enhancing places where people gathered, shaded from the sun under a tree, or in a pavilion, park, or garden (see Figure 1).

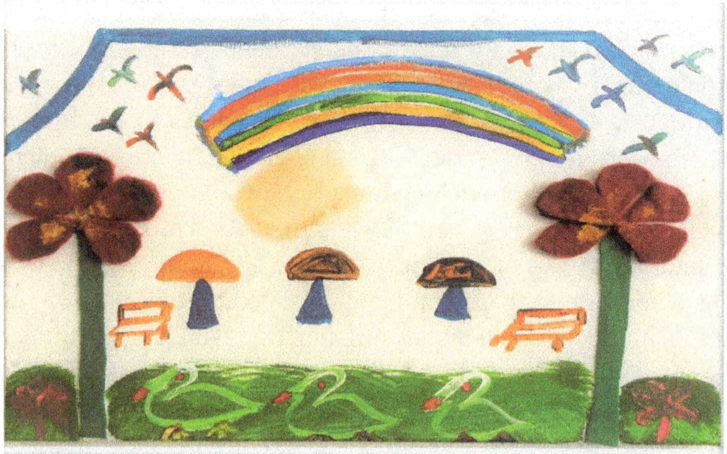

Figure 1. Image by Hiruni* originally from Sri Lanka. ©Photo taken by author. (*all names are pseudonyms).

Natural landscapes frequently depicted weather: sun, rain, and rainbows (N = 9). There were a number of non-natural environments (N = 27) represented by buildings, interiors, cityscapes, a temple, church, house, restaurant, etc. (N = 12), and other depictions, such as roads, cars, trucks, a carpark, a football pitch (N = 8), and ships, boats, and bridges (N = 7). As participants explained, none of their artworks represented journeys undertaken in search of a safe haven. Ships and boats signified previous occupations as fishermen, as did cars and trucks, rather than journeys.

Several images depicted fields and croplands on farms where a participant once lived, and several artworks represented places where they once worked, or their previous occupations (see Figures 2–5 below). Respondents described feeling nostalgic, and both sad and happy while they were engaged in making these artworks. Even though they were pleased to remember places, they mourned their previous occupation, their home, and their family, knowing they were unable to return. Previous occupations were important factors in identity, financial independence, and social and family roles, regarded as positive and valued. Participants experienced conflicting emotions in relation to places they remembered versus their present situation, where loss of occupation was allied with loss of identity, as illustrated by Mahamadou in Figure 2 below.

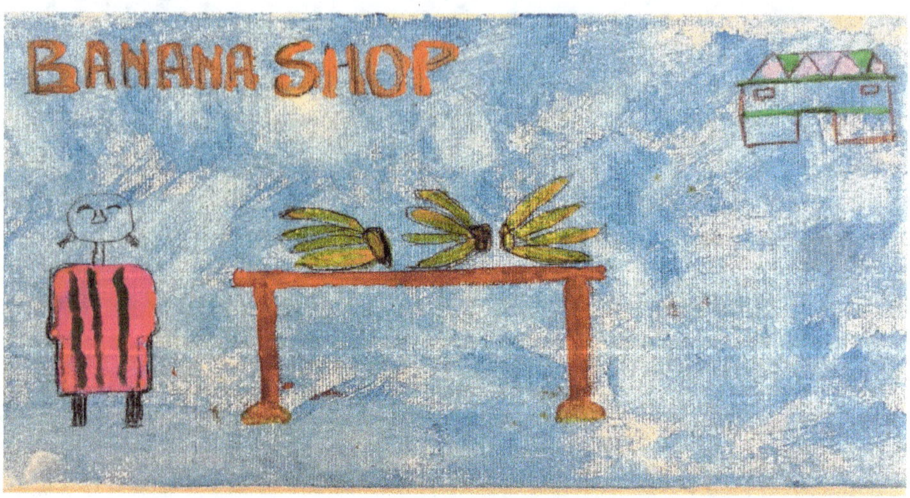

Figure 2. Image by Mahamadou originally from Democratic Republic of Congo. ©Photo taken by author.

One participant articulated this when he declared himself: "Not happy, no joy inside. Speaking English is a joyful language, so I will not speak English. I used to drive a lorry and now I can't", Zain (Iraq).

Participants expressed conflicting emotions regarding the beauty of their homeland against the reasons why they had to leave, and their present situation. As Chathura states, *"I feel nostalgic and I miss my village"*, Chathura (Sri Lanka), and Tharindu (Sri Lanka), *"This is a place in Vanni in Sri Lanka (. . .) where I was a fisherman, fishing with a group of men. It is helpful to remember and I miss this place"*, (see Figure 3).

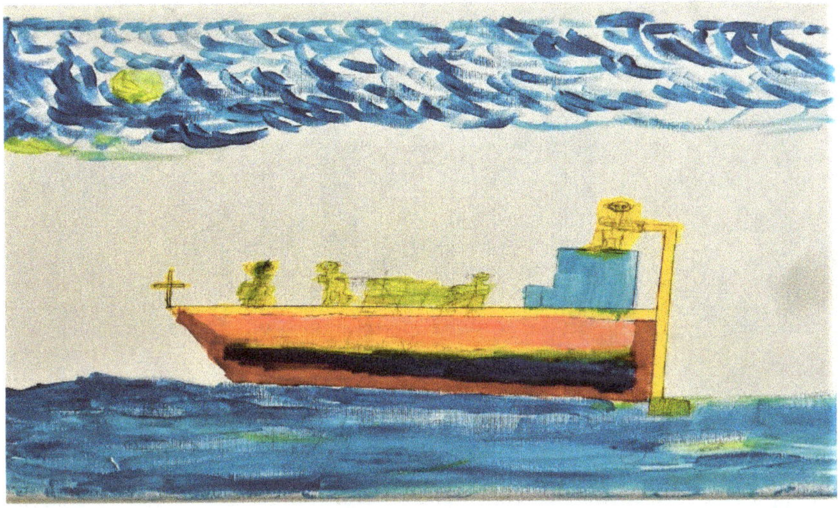

Figure 3. Image by Tharindu originally from Sri Lanka. ©Photo taken by author.

Participants expressed pleasure in reengaging with these places, even while experiencing their loss: "When I draw this, I will see my birthplace and I really miss my birthplace (. . .). It is the most wonderful place ever in my life. Wherever we go, however we live, we still miss this beautiful Island", Hiruni (Sri Lanka). Remembering the place where they lived and worked was a trigger for concern for what has since happened to it, or their remaining family, "This is the paddy (rice) field I worked (. . .) it was very hard because I do not know what happened to that field (. . .) I worry about my family back home", Roshan (Sri Lanka). Participants noted the importance of these remembered places as real, as Roshan comments, "These places are not my imagination, but the place where I lived with my parents and five sisters. I am remembering how we were a happy family. I heard from my wife it had been destroyed by the Sri Lankan army". Roshan explained he now fears for the safety of his family (see Figure 4).

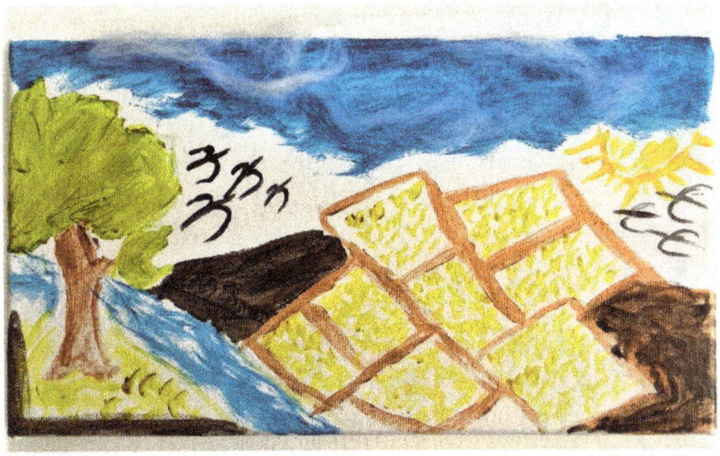

Figure 4. Image by Roshan originally from Sri Lanka. ©Photo taken by author.

Several participants represented buildings inhabited by people, such as a painting marked by a Red Cross entitled *Pharmacy* painted by Divine (Democratic Republic of Congo). The painting depicts the interior of the clinic where a pregnant woman lies on a bed, surrounded by medical drips and stethoscopes, another person, possibly a doctor, sits in a chair, while outside there are other women with their children (see Figure 5).

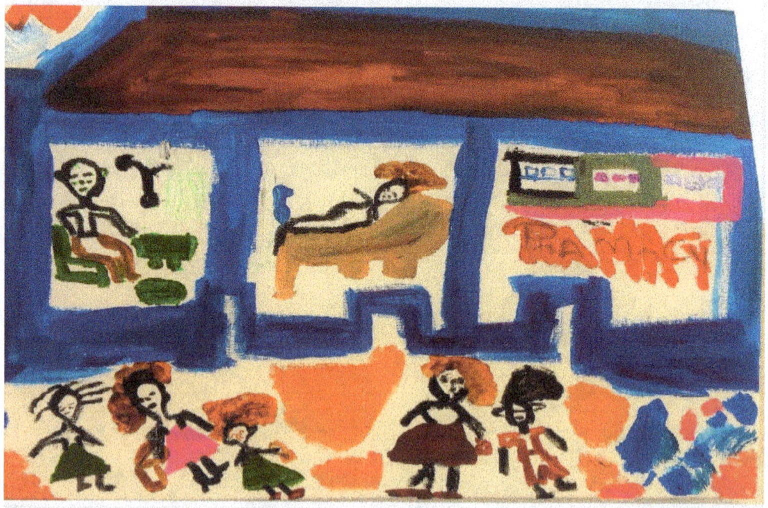

Figure 5. Image by Divine originally from Democratic Republic of Congo. ©Photo taken by author.

Divine also painted her Sunday school, depicting how as children they would go to a smaller annex of the church, while adults prayed in the big church. Both paintings are notable for the thick walls and sturdy rooves of the buildings. Some participants chose to make artworks of objects associated with feelings of safety. Both Alizia and Divine made images of cassava grinding pots using paint with feathers and wool. In a later workshop, Alizia made a bright red painting of her hand, commenting: "*I paint my hand. My hand is special. I burnt my hand. It is special because I cook nice food with my hand for my family; I cook cassava, mixed with palm oil*", Alizia (Democratic Republic of Congo).

3.2. Participation

In analysing respondents' answers to workshop questionnaires asking how they experienced producing artwork in the group setting, researchers made a general assessment regarding clients' engagement with the participatory element of the programme. In terms of the experience of creating artworks, all participants, without exception, gave positive responses, for example, it was a "*very, very good experience*"; "*very, very nice, I don't want it to stop*" Akram (Iraq); "*really useful*" Hiruni (Sri Lanka); "*inspirational*" Mahamadou (Democratic Republic of Congo), "*It is taking my memory back. You give me a space to think for myself and that is better*" Divine (Democratic Republic of Congo).

Participants were confident from the start in the process of creating art. The "warm-up" encouraged participants to adopt an experimental approach on large shared sheets of paper, and to test their own ways of creating collage and painting. Sharing large sheets of paper helped participants overcome anxieties about making mistakes, or lack of expertise. The approach was empowering and participants quickly made artworks they felt were significant. The "warm-up" was successful in generating a sense of community, one in which participants felt supported and safe. Notably, female participants, with one exception, were comfortable with soft fabrics and wools. In contrast, male participants preferred harder collage materials: stone, cork, and drawing with a ruler. In future, it may be useful to provide more building-like materials, such as miniature bricks. In later workshops, participants enjoyed using paints on individual ready-made canvasses. Large canvasses were the most popular, with participants adding collage to paintings. Researchers observed that the contained shape of the canvas appeared to reassure participants and encouraged their creativity. The participants worked alongside others of similar languages with an interpreter, who supported discussion of ideas and meanings of artworks in the group. This arrangement was effective in ensuring good communication between researchers and participants.

When identifying potential participants for recruitment, FfT therapists suggested inviting clients to take part who did not attend many other activities at the centre. Consequently, it was interesting to note several responses in questionnaires where clients clearly valued the participation with others, "*I feel good to do art together with other people. The people inspired me to get out again*", Alizia (Democratic Republic of Congo). Fahad described the experience, "*Positive, helped me feel confident and comfortable among others (...) it is a good distraction, it also helped me to socialize and mix with others*", Fahad (Iran). For some participants working together, sharing ideas and the stories behind their artworks was an important part of the participatory experience. Mahamadou found the experience, "*very motivating, because we exchange ideas*" Mahamadou (Democratic Republic of Congo); similarly Alizia explained, "*We work together, inspire each other and friendly people*" (Democratic Republic of Congo). Errolvie and Chathura made similar points regarding sharing their stories, "*Very motivating as we were sharing stories behind our drawings*", Errolvie (Democratic Republic of Congo). Others echoed these sentiments, "*Very interesting, because we discuss what is very special behind our drawings*", Chathura (Sri Lanka). Many participants were disappointed the programme would not continue for longer, "*We would like more, it is good for us. I make art about my country, my home, my city. I feel sad because of so many bad memories. But I feel good to do art together with other people*" Alizia (Democratic Republic of Congo).

3.3. *Recovery and Reconnection*

In Herman's theory, the three stages of recovery from trauma are not distinct and separate (Lamb 2017, p. 59); their elements might overlap, there are advances and setbacks. Stage two, remembrance and mourning, and stage three, reconnection, are not necessarily linear in progression. An analysis of the data collected by the research team from workshops 2, 3, and 4 indicated all participants (N = 14) explored remembrance of place in their artworks (N = 30), and recorded comments to this effect in questionnaires (N = 22) and in discussion (N = 18). In terms of mourning, it is difficult to gauge from the artworks whether mourning constituted an element of subject matter. However, recorded comments indicated that the activity of making artworks of remembered places provoked feelings of mourning expressed as "nostalgia", "sadness at loss", "grief", "missing family/place/warm sun/flowers/fields" (N = 34). Reconnection was identified by the research team in two ways: artworks depicting lives lived in the present (N = 5), see below, and recorded comments indicating reconnection with the world and with others (N = 4), for example, "making art helped me feel confident and comfortable among others" (Alizia).

The workshop design sought to minimise the possibility of re-traumatisation in the workshops by enabling clients to work at their own pace and by encouraging artworks that drew on the present as well as the past, allowing participants the choice to avoid subject matter that could prompt difficult memories. This process highlighted the points of overlap between these stages of recovery. Interestingly, the artworks based in the present appeared more as signs of reconnection, rather than avoidance of difficult memories. Production of these artworks occurred in W.4. after individuals had already made artworks of remembered places. The subject matter of artworks based in the present represented places encountered in ordinary life, suggestive of the individual reconnecting with the world around them. For example, the participant Mahamadou depicted remembered places in W.1 and W.2: a pick-up lorry he could no longer drive, a banana stall selling fresh bananas he could no longer eat, in a city he could no longer visit. He particularly mourned the fresh bananas. In W.3 and W.4, he depicted places in his present life: a local church where he found solace in prayer and conversations with the priest and a football pitch where he regularly enjoyed playing football. These images of life in the present suggest some degree of integration of the trauma into a new narrative of self and personality. Similarly, Alizia's bright red painting of her hand connects the injury she sustained in the past with the positive activity of cooking cassava for her family in the present. In an early workshop, Akram (Iraq) depicted an idealised image of a beautiful tree, surrounded by sunshine and blue skies, the image decorated with small pink roses, indigenous to his home country of Iraq. In W.4, using a ruler and sharpened pencils, he carefully delineated his psychotherapist's room, where in his present life he received treatment. Every detail meticulously rendered, the clock at the appointed hour, the position of the chairs, his interpreter, the desk, the computer, a cushion, etc., and above the artwork it says "*the best place in my life*". To the question of whether it is useful for Akram to remember this place when stressed, he replies "*sure, all the time in my mind*". To the question of whether the experience of making art has changed him in any way, he says "*Sure, because every time I look at my work on my phone or at the wall I feel happy*" Akram (Iran) (see Figure 6).

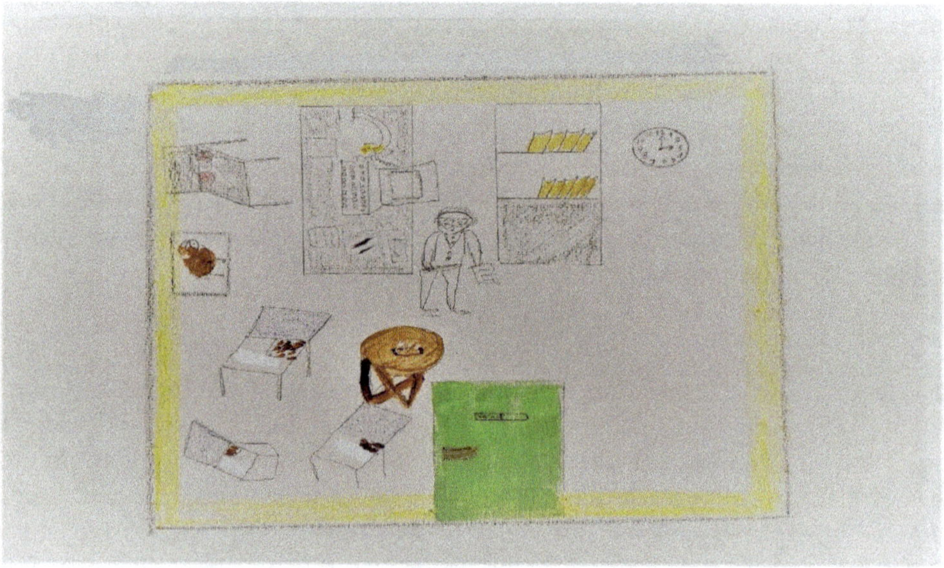

Figure 6. Image by Akram originally from Iraq. ©Photo taken by author.

The research team interpreted artworks of lives lived in the present as representative of the individual reconnecting with the world around them. As such, they correspond to Herman's stage three, reconnection, indicating a level of recovery that enables survivors to connect with the changed person they have become. As described earlier, therapists working with survivors of torture understand this form of reconnection within a process of recovery as one where autobiographical identity integrates the trauma into a new narrative, enabling survivors to live in the present (Lamb 2017, p. 59).

In exploring the potential of engagement with place to contribute toward recovery, we noted some relevant comments made by participants that suggested that the act of creating artworks was an expression of their recovery process. For example, Fahad (Iran) painted a restaurant in the lee of a mountain facing a lake. It is night-time, the sky is dark, and small twinkly lights illuminate some of the way to the summit. Fahad tells us that for a time he could only go out at night, but he has walked to the top, he says it is a beautiful, quiet place (see Figure 7). He says, "*I have been to this place in the past and going there always made me feel happy. Remembering it now makes me feel sad and happy now*". Harnessing conflicting feelings, Fahad was able to explain that making the artwork in a group was "*Good, made me feel better*" and "*I feel relax and comfortable*". In terms of Herman's second and third stages of recovery, Fahad's painting and his comments suggest remembrance, mourning, and reconnection, the components of recovery.

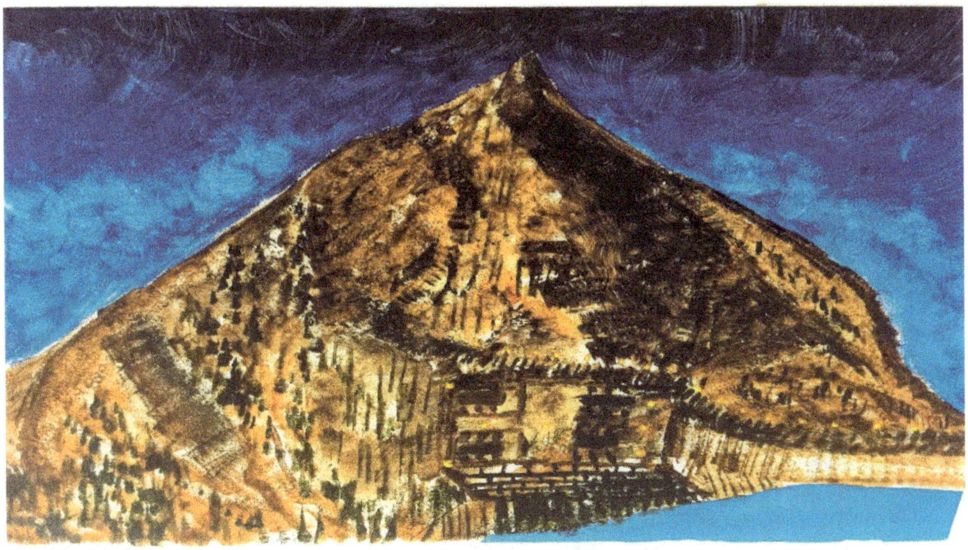

Figure 7. Image by Fahad originally from Iran. ©Photo taken by author.

Many participants commented that it was useful for their recovery to remember places from their country of origin. Data findings from observation, field notes, and photographs indicated that the majority of participants were motivated to represent places precisely, whether this was mixing a specific colour or achieving structural accuracy. For example, Fahad had to have exactly the right black before he would paint the earth and the sky, Akram the right pink for his Iraqi Rose, and Mahamadou, Tharindu, and Akram insisted on using a ruler and sharp pencils to draw their image before they would use colour.

As researchers, we interpreted that the participants' requirement for precision and their great concentration during the artmaking period reflected the personal significance of their images. They cared a lot about how their special place was expressed to themselves and to others, suggesting to us that they closely associated those places with their identity. Remembrance and expression of places connected to personal identity also arose in participants' paintings of villages associated with their family's history, or their childhood home, even if they and family members no longer lived there.

When considering whether these images contributed to recovery, Chathura answered, "*Yes, I feel relieved because I am expressing what I have within me*", Chathura (Sri Lanka). The research team observed that participants' artworks expressed a strong sense of cultural identity and historical rootedness. The project enabled them to connect with a deeper place related to their identity, a safe place, and potentially a healing place within.

4. Conclusions

The research drew upon Herman (1992) three-stage model of recovery from trauma to provide a qualitative thematic analysis of written, visual artwork, and observational data, and its interpretation. Researchers identified primary codes based on Herman's theory of recovery in terms of remembrance, mourning, and reconnection, and were able to interpret that the participants' engagement with these elements supported a trajectory of recovery. Secondary coding identified two sub-themes, namely, the participants' experience of transition between their homeland and the UK, and new social connections. Data analysis of these themes enabled researchers to infer that participating in a group making artworks of places associated with safety may contribute to processes of transition and social connectedness. This combination, we suggest, indicates that this model of participatory art has the potential to contribute toward feelings of well-being and a trajectory of recovery for refugees who experience trauma.

The artworks produced by some participants across the four workshops appeared to provide a visual microcosm of this transition from past into present, from remembrance and mourning, to reconnection. For these individuals, artworks in early workshops were characterised by images of remembered homelands with mixed feelings of nostalgia, loss, and attachment to place. Artworks in later workshops tended to depict images of present places encountered in ordinary life, suggestive of the individual reconnecting with the world around them. Herman's model of recovery would suggest that artworks representing life in the present indicate the individual is integrating trauma sufficiently to be able to envisage the start of a new narrative of self and personality, and able to project that identity to others. For other participants, the focus centred on the remembrance of places from their homeland associated with their identity, and the mixed feelings generated by these memories. These participants may have potentially connected emotions they felt in the present with memories of the past, and this process may also support recovery.

In developing this idea, the project *Art of Recovery* explored how artmaking involving the expression of remembered safe places might contribute not only to early phases of recovery, but also to later stages of transition, to connecting and building a relationship with a new environment. Through processes of remembering a safe place and its visual realisation, participants reconnect with a place, connecting their past with their present, and express their past and present selves to themselves and to others. Conceivably, these artworks serve as physical symbols through which participants connect their past with their present self, prompting self-understanding, and potentially understanding of others.

The study found that the process of creating art in a group was helpful in counteracting a sense of individual isolation, with the potential to enhance feelings of personal growth and supportive of transition to the new environment. In this respect, a particularly useful feature of the research design was to group individuals with others speaking similar languages, enabling a sharing of experiences. Indeed, some participants noted that usually they would not have met and talked with others and that the workshops were important in terms of social interaction. This appears to be an important element in the success of the programme and is underscored by Burnett and Peel's study (Burnett and Peel 2001) highlighting the importance for refugees to make contact with people from their own countries, a significant step in enabling them to better connect with host communities.

Researchers and therapists observed that the workshops appeared to facilitate participants in making artworks that they felt had significance in terms of their experience. They seemed to enjoy the opportunity to create and express themselves in artmaking, particularly for those with, as yet, little or no English. Such findings prompted researchers to understand the significance of participatory art in revealing memories and emotions not always easily accessible or readily articulated into words, but conducive to therapeutic processes.

Through imagining place and its physical representation in art, the project explored the facilitation of participants in connecting with a safe place within themselves, held in mind in times of stress, a process that may contribute toward their recovery. Participants were seen to exercise considerable attention to detail with specific elements of their artwork, reflecting a strong mental image they sought to express. The artistic process appeared to reinforce the presence of a healing place within participants, both as a positive mental image and as external expression. As Akram said, he could now look at the photo on his phone and on the wall, and this made him happy.

A limitation of the programme was its brevity. Many participants requested sessions for a longer period and expressed disappointment when the programme finished. This also meant there was no time to follow up or reflect with the participants on the wider long-term impact of the intervention or evaluation of the benefits and challenges of participation. Psychotherapists working at FfT after the workshops finished were able to continue a discussion of the artworks, and the safe places visualized, with individuals and groups, and many of the artworks are exhibited on the walls of the centre. These strategies helped participants to keep these safe places in mind following the end of the project. However, limitations of the project will be addressed as we have now further funding to support a longer programme of participatory arts workshops to assess longer term impacts. Further research is designed to foster greater creative development, exploration of participants' cultural differences, and deeper exploration of personal stories. Potentially, we aim to explore more profound, longer-lasting benefits and challenges of this kind of participatory arts intervention.

FfT was able to provide a safe containing space with which participants were familiar, they ensured clients taking part would find artmaking suitable at their stage of recovery, and they provided experienced therapists and interpreters throughout the workshops, all of which provided invaluable support, as did prior meetings between researchers and professionals during the design stage of the project. A reported benefit of these participatory arts workshops was their use as an adjunct to the therapeutic work of FfT. An important feature of participatory arts is its capacity to contribute to recovery in a large group, within a designated period. For example, participatory arts programmes can support less formal social interaction within the context of a shared activity, an aspect that is not part of one-to-one therapy sessions or purely social meetings. Thus, the workshops provided an opportunity for refugee participants to meet others, in the context of shared artmaking, who understood their situation, and this has potential to counter some social and emotional isolation. With its focus on remembrance of place, the programme fostered the sharing of stories and experiences visually and verbally, in ways that were creative and rewarding. In this way, the artmaking process provides some of the elements necessary to effect positive change in self and the production of a new narrative, necessary for reconnection and recovery.

Author Contributions: Conceptualization, methodology, analysis: E.R. and A.B. Investigation and data curation: E.R., A.B., and M.R. Writing—original draft preparation and writing—review and editing: E.R. and A.B. Fieldwork support: Kirsten Lamb.

References

Acheson, Donald. 1998. *Independent Inquiry into Inequalities in Health: Report*. London: HM Stationery Office.

Andemicael, Awet. 2011. *Positive Energy: A Review of the Role of Artistic Activities in Refugee Camps*. Geneva: UNHCR.

Barnes, Stella. 2009. Drawing a line: A discussion of ethics in participatory arts with young refugees. In *Participatory Arts with Young Refugees*. London: Oval House Theatre, pp. 33–39.

Bogic, Marija, Anthony Njoku, and Stefan Priebe. 2015. Long-term mental health of war-refugees: A systematic literature review. *BMC International Health and Human Rights* 15: 29. [CrossRef] [PubMed]

Boyles, Jude. 2017. Assessing survivors of torture for psychological therapy. In *Psychological Therapies for Survivors of Torture: A Human-Rights Approach with People Seeking Asylum*. Edited by Jude Boyles. Ross-on-Wye: PCCS Books Ltd., pp. 11–35.

Burnett, Angela, and Michael Peel. 2001. Asylum seekers and refugees in Britain: Health needs of asylum seekers and refugees. *BMJ: British Medical Journal* 322: 544. [CrossRef] [PubMed]

Dutton, Carl. 2017. Creating a safe haven: A community-based, creative approach to working with refugee and asylum-seeking families and young people affected by torture. In *Psychological Therapies for Survivors of Torture: A Human-Rights Approach with People Seeking Asylum*. Edited by Jude Boyles. Ross-on-Wye: PCCS Books Ltd., pp. 271–88.

Epstein, H. 1996. A life in the day of Perico Rodriguez. *Sunday Times*, February 18.

Fassin, Didier, and Estelle d'Halluin. 2007. Critical evidence: The politics of trauma in French asylum policies. *Ethos* 35: 300–29. [CrossRef]

Fazel, Mina, Jeremy Wheeler, and John Danesh. 2005. Prevalence of serious mental disorder in 7000 refugees resettled in western countries: A systematic review. *The Lancet* 365: 1309–14. [CrossRef]

Fazel, Mina, Ruth V. Reed, Catherine Panter-Brick, and Alan Stein. 2012. Mental health of displaced and refugee children resettled in high-income countries: Risk and protective factors. *The Lancet* 379: 266–82. [CrossRef]

Gorst-Unsworth, Caroline, and Eva Goldenberg. 1998. Psychological sequelae of torture and organised violence suffered by refugees from Iraq: Trauma-related factors compared with social factors in exile. *The British Journal of Psychiatry* 172: 90–94. [CrossRef] [PubMed]

Grinberg, Leon, and Rebeca Grinberg. 1989. *Psychoanalytic Perspectives on Migration and Exile*. New Haven: Yale University Press.

Hargreaves, Sally. 2002. A body of evidence: Torture among asylum seekers to the West. *The Lancet* 359: 793–94. [CrossRef]

Hayhow, Christina, Maani May, Salarzai Naqibullah, and Womack Leslye. 2016. Participatory Arts with Young Refugees. Participedia, Australia. Available online: https://participedia.net/en/cases/participatory-arts-young-refugees (accessed on 6 February 2018).

Herman, Judith L. 1992. *Trauma and Recovery: The Aftermath of Violence*. New York: Basic books, p. 290.

Hollifield, Michael, Teddy D. Warner, Nityamo Lian, Barry Krakow, Janis H. Jenkins, James Kesler, Jayne Stevenson, and Joseph Westermeyer. 2002. Measuring trauma and health status in refugees: A critical review. *JAMA* 288: 611–21. [CrossRef] [PubMed]

Johnson, Howard, and Andrew Thompson. 2008. The development and maintenance of post-traumatic stress disorder (PTSD) in civilian adult survivors of war trauma and torture: A review. *Clinical Psychology Review* 28: 36–47. [CrossRef] [PubMed]

Kidd, Belinda, Samina Zahir, and Sabra Khan. 2016. *Arts and Refugees: History, Impact and Future*. London: Baring Foundation.

Lamb, Kirsten. 2017. Recovery and reconnection. In *Psychological Therapies for Survivors of Torture: A Human-Rights Approach with People Seeking Asylum*. Edited by Jude Boyles. Ross-on-Wye: PCCS Books Ltd., pp. 56–76.

Le Roy, Jaak. 1994. Group analysis and culture. In *The Psyche and the Social World*. London: Jessica Kingsley Publishers, pp. 180–201.

Malchiodi, Cathy. 2003. *Hand Book of art Therapy New York*. New York: Guilford Press.

McFetridge, Mark, Swan Alison, Heke Sarah, Karatzias Thanos, Greenberg Neil, Kitchiner Neil, and Morley Rachel. 2017. *UK Psychological Trauma Society (UKPTS), Guideline for the Treatment and Planning of Services for Complex Post-Traumatic Stress Disorder in Adults*. London: UK Psychological Trauma Society (UKPTS). [CrossRef]

Miller, Kenneth E., Madhur Kulkarni, and Hallie Kushner. 2006. Beyond trauma-focused psychiatric epidemiology: Bridging research and practice with war-affected populations. *American Journal of Orthopsychiatry* 76: 409–22. [CrossRef] [PubMed]

Moisander, Pia, and Edston Erik. 2003. Torture and its sequel—A comparison between victims from six countries. *Forensic science international* 137: 133–40. [CrossRef] [PubMed]

Mollica, Richard F., Keith McInnes, Charles Pool, and Svang Tor. 1998. Dose-effect relationships of trauma to symptoms of depression and post-traumatic stress disorder among Cambodian survivors of mass violence. *The British journal of psychiatry* 173: 482–88. [CrossRef]

Nosè, Michela, Francesca Ballette, Irene Bighelli, Giulia Turrini, Marianna Purgato, Wietse Tol, Stefan Priebe, and Corrado Barbui. 2017. Psychosocial interventions for post-traumatic stress disorder in refugees and asylum seekers resettled in high-income countries: Systematic review and meta-analysis. *PLoS ONE* 12: e0171030. [CrossRef] [PubMed]

Pavlicevic, Mercedes, Giorgos Tsiris, and Camilla Farrant. 2014. *A Guide to Evaluation for Arts Therapists and Arts & Health Practitioners*. London: Jessica Kingsley Publishers.

Refugee Council. 2017. Refugee Asylum Statistics Annual Trends. Refugee Council Information. Available online: https://www.refugeecouncil.org.uk/stats (accessed on 5 February 2018).

Robjant, Katy, Rita Hassan, and Cornelius Katona. 2009. Mental health implications of detaining asylum seekers: Systematic review. *The British Journal of Psychiatry* 194: 306–12. [CrossRef] [PubMed]

Rose, Emma. 2012. Encountering place: A psychoanalytic approach for understanding how therapeutic landscapes benefit health and wellbeing. *Health & Place* 18: 1381–87.

Rose, Emma, and Amanda Bingley. 2017. Migrating art: A research design to support refugees' recovery from trauma—A pilot study. *Design for Health* 1: 152–69. [CrossRef]

Slewa-Younan, Shameran, Maria Gabriela Uribe Guajardo, Andreea Heriseanu, and Tasnim Hasan. 2015. A systematic review of post-traumatic stress disorder and depression amongst Iraqi refugees located in western countries. *Journal of Immigrant and Minority Health* 17: 1231–39. [CrossRef] [PubMed]

Sonn, Christopher C., Michele Grossman, and Angela Utomo. 2013. Reflections on a participatory research project: Young people of refugee background in an arts-based program. *Journal for Social Action in Counseling & Psychology* 5: 95–110.

Stickley, Theo. 2010. Does prescribing participation in arts help to promote recovery for mental health clients. *Nursing Times* 106: 18–20. [PubMed]

Tsekleves, Emmanuel, Amanda F. Bingley, Maria A. Luján Escalante, and Adrian Gradinar. 2018. Engaging people with dementia in designing playful and creative practices: Co-design or co-creation? *Dementia*. [CrossRef] [PubMed]

UNCAT. 2012. *Convention against Torture and Other Cruel, Inhuman or Degrading Treatment or Punishment*. New York: United Nations Publication.

UNHCR. 2018. Health. Available online: http://www.unhcr.org/uk/health.html (accessed on 12 February 2018).

WHO. 1992. *The ICD-10 Classification of Mental and Behavioural Disorders: Clinical Descriptions and Diagnostic Guidelines*. Geneva: WHO.

WHO. 2017. Promoting the Health of Refugees and Migrants Seventieth World Health Assembly. Available online: http://www.who.int/migrants/news-events/A70_24-en.pdf (accessed on 5 February 2018).

Wilson, John P., and Boris Drožđek. 2004. *Broken Spirits: The Treatment of Traumatized Asylum Seekers, Refugees and War and Torture Victims*. Abingdon-on-Thames: Routledge.

2

The Global Problem of Insufficient Sleep and its Serious Public Health Implications

Vijay Kumar Chattu [1,*], Md. Dilshad Manzar [2], Soosanna Kumary [1], Deepa Burman [3], David Warren Spence [4] and Seithikurippu R. Pandi-Perumal [5]

1 Faculty of Medical Sciences, The University of the West Indies, St. Augustine, Trinidad and Tobago; susanna.poul@gmail.com
2 Department of Nursing, College of Applied Medical Sciences, Majmaah University, Majmaah 11952, Saudi Arabia; m.manzar@mu.edu.sa
3 School of Medicine, University of Pittsburgh, 4200 Fifth Ave, Pittsburgh, PA 15260, USA; dr.deepa.burman@gmail.com
4 Independent Researcher, 652 Dufferin Street, Toronto, ON M6K 2B4, Canada; dwspence@fastmail.fm
5 Somnogen Canada Inc., College Street, Toronto, ON M1H 1C5, Canada; pandiperumal2019@gmail.com
* Correspondence: Vijay.chattu@sta.uwi.edu or drvkumar.ch@gmail.com;

Abstract: Good sleep is necessary for good physical and mental health and a good quality of life. Insufficient sleep is a pervasive and prominent problem in the modern 24-h society. A considerable body of evidence suggests that insufficient sleep causes hosts of adverse medical and mental dysfunctions. An extensive literature search was done in all the major databases for "insufficient sleep" and "public health implications" in this review. Globally, insufficient sleep is prevalent across various age groups, considered to be a public health epidemic that is often unrecognized, under-reported, and that has rather high economic costs. This paper addresses a brief overview on insufficient sleep, causes, and consequences, and how it adds to the existing burden of diseases. Insufficient sleep leads to the derailment of body systems, leading to increased incidences of cardiovascular morbidity, increased chances of diabetes mellitus, obesity, derailment of cognitive functions, vehicular accidents, and increased accidents at workplaces. The increased usage of smart phones and electronic devices is worsening the epidemic. Adolescents with insufficient sleep are likely to be overweight and may suffer from depressive symptoms. The paper concludes by emphasizing sleep quality assessments as an important early risk indicator, thereby reducing the incidence of a wide spectrum of morbidities.

Keywords: insufficient sleep; insomnia; sleep disorders; sleep apnoea; cardiometabolic diseases

1. Introduction

Insufficient sleep is associated with a range of negative health and social outcomes, including an adverse performance at school and in the labor market. Reduced sleep duration has been linked to 7 of the 15 leading causes of death in the U.S., including cardiovascular disease, malignant neoplasm, cerebrovascular disease, accidents, diabetes, septicemia, and hypertension [1]. The evidence suggests that the link between inadequate sleep and negative outcomes is more direct, whereas the link between excessive sleep and negative outcomes seems to be more indirect (i.e., excessive sleep is driven by underlying chronic health conditions and not vice versa). Hence, the impact of insufficient sleep appears to be the more salient issue in our society and, because of its broad-ranging effects, represents a major public health concern. In this review, we note some of the more serious consequences of insufficient sleep, and additionally consider how these might be best addressed by changes in individual behavior, actions by employers, and by public policy measures [2].

According to the International Classification of Sleep Disorders (ICSD-3), insufficient sleep is defined as a curtailed sleep pattern that has persisted for at least three months for most days of the week, along with complaints of sleepiness during the day. Further, a resolution of sleepiness complaints is shown to follow an extension of total sleep time. Frequently occurring episodes of insufficient sleep are associated with the experience of unfavorable mental and physical well-being [3]. Sleep insufficiency is sometimes confused with insomnia, but the opportunity to sleep differs in the two disorders (with insomnia sufferers typically being unable to sleep despite having opportunities to do so).

2. Materials and Methods

An extensive literature search was done, and relevant articles were identified through online searches of electronic databases (i.e., the PubMed, Medline, PsycINFO, Web of Science, Scopus, and Global Health databases). Relevant keywords relating to "insufficient sleep", in combination with (and/or) public health impact were searched, around 3626 articles were screened for duplication and relevance to fit the inclusion criteria, and finally 111 articles with full texts were included in this review, as shown in the flow chart below (Figure 1). Articles on cardiometabolic disorders, mental health, accidents and trauma, sleep apnoea, obesity, adolescents, meta-analysis, randomized control trials, longitudinal studies, and cross-sectional studies were included (that reflected the public health impacts of insufficient sleep). Additional publications were identified from references cited in the original articles. The major findings were classified into different categories and are presented in the tables, figures, and narrative description below.

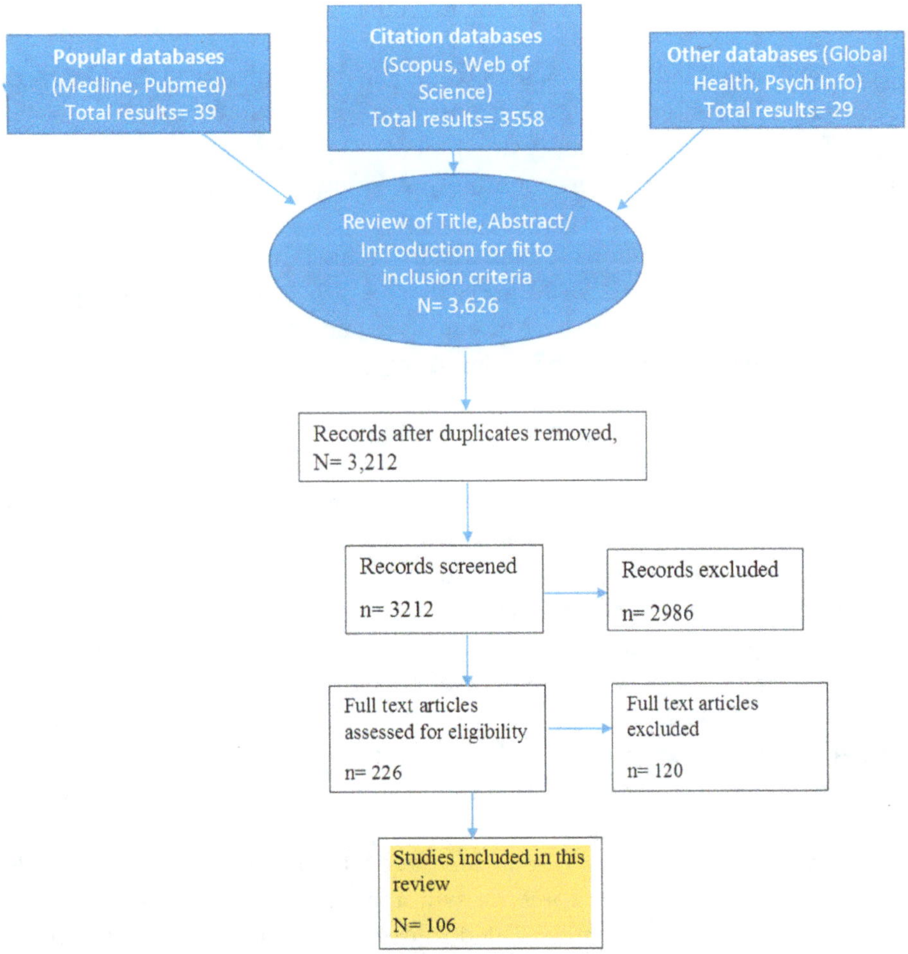

Figure 1. Flow chart of literature search.

2.1. Epidemiology

A recent study of the prevalence of sleep disorders investigated over 20,000 patients in the Netherlands who were aged 12 years old or older. The study found an alarming prevalence rate of 27.3%, with 21.2% of the males and 33.2% of the females reporting that they had some type of sleep disorder [4]. A national quasirandom sample study of sleep disorders in 12 provinces of the Netherlands showed a prevalence of 23.5% [5], while a similar nationally representative sample of individuals in the age group of 18–70 years also showed high prevalence rates. Polling based on a validated questionnaire of ICSD revealed that, among the total sample, 32% complained of experiencing general sleep disturbances while 43.2% said they suffered from insufficient sleep [6]. Other surveys by Hublin et al. [7] and Ursin et al. [8] found the prevalence rates for disturbed sleep to be, respectively, 20.4% and 20%. Discrepancies in the prevalence rates found by the various surveys were possibly due to the separate questionnaires that were used, differences in sampling techniques, or other possible methodological differences. Nevertheless, the findings were in concordance in showing that poor-quality sleep is a problem for a major segment of the samples that were surveyed.

Although the need for sleep among adolescents has been determined to be about 9.25 h per day [9], there are still many adolescents who obtain less sleep than they actually need [10], thus creating a chronic sleep debt. A study conducted in Norway among 1285 high school students (aged 16–19 years) showed an estimated 10.4% prevalence of behaviorally induced insufficient sleep syndrome (i.e., the condition was due to individual choices regarding bedtimes rather than being the consequence of a medical condition) [11]. Among a sample of 2738 soldiers who were surveyed about their sleep behavior and perceived feelings of sleepiness, the average reported sleep duration was found to be 5.8 ± 1.2 h, with 1959 soldiers, or 72% of the sample, reporting that they slept less than 6 h [12].

Sleep needs vary among individuals based on age, and even response to sleep restriction changes with age. According to a Centers for Disease Control and Prevention (CDC) state-based survey in 2014, only 65% of adults reported a healthy duration of sleep. In a recent survey, an estimated 83.6 million adults in the United States were reportedly sleeping <7 h in 24 h [13]. The prevalence of continuous insufficient sleep among American Indians and Alaska Natives (AI/AN) has not been formally surveyed, but anecdotal reports suggest that the figure is high in these minority groups. It has been suggested that the rates of mental disturbance that are also known to be elevated in these groups may possibly be, in part, attributable to insufficient sleep, and thus that public health and education efforts to address these problems should be undertaken [14].

Magee et al. [15], for instance, explored the determinants of sleep duration among a cohort of Australian adults aged 18 to 64 years. Using multivariate statistical analysis, the study found that short sleep durations were associated with longer working hours, lower education levels, being single rather than married, being a current cigarette smoker, or with showing high levels of alcohol consumption, obesity, or depression or anxiety, as shown in Figure 2 below. Krueger and Friedman [16] found that factors such as low levels of education and cardiovascular disease were associated with both short and long sleep (e.g., more than nine hours). Short sleep was associated with being in an older age group, being a frequent smoker or consumer of alcohol, being overweight or obese, as well as with having young children. A study from Finland by Kronholm et al. [17] reported that gender, as well as marital status, occupation, and physical activity, were major drivers of short sleep duration. According to the study, men were more likely to be short sleepers than women. A study of the effects of workplace-related factors found that job stress factors such as quantitative workload and interpersonal conflict led to short sleep duration among male Japanese manufacturing workers [18]. Psychosocial factors such as tension or anxiety and depressive symptoms have also been associated with reduced sleep. In addition, organizational factors related to discrimination, work-life balance, high work demands, and job insecurity were associated with an increased prevalence of sleep problems [19,20].

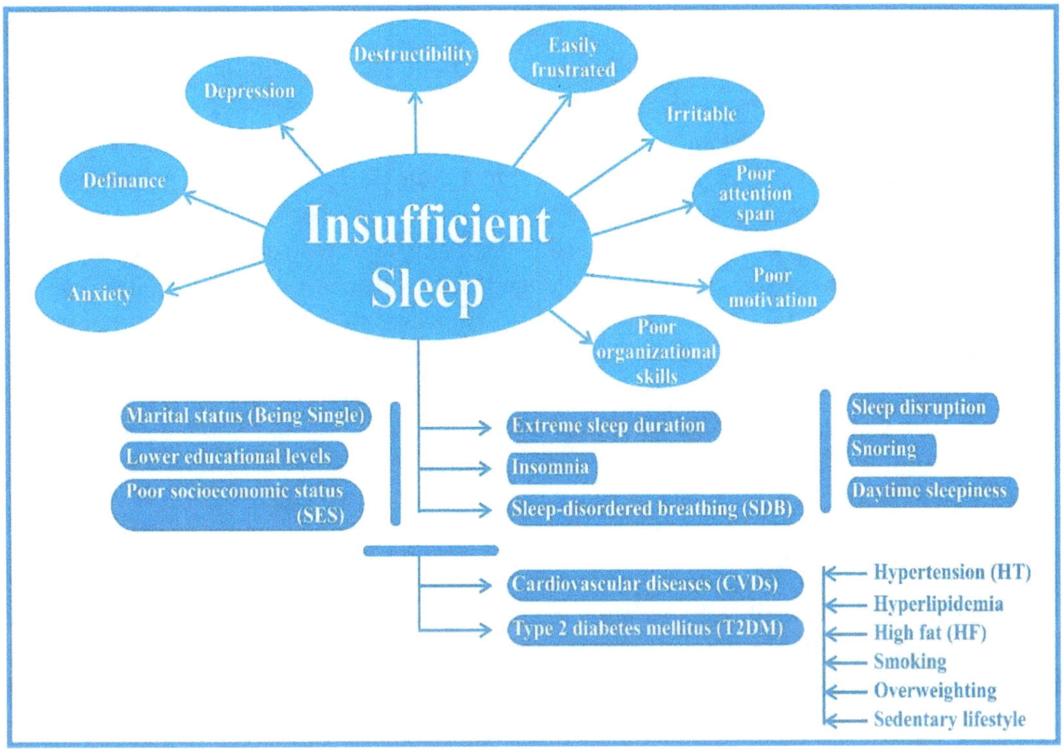

Figure 2. Insufficient sleep and its impact on the pathophysiology of the human body.

Lack of sleep has been shown to increase the risk of premature mortality. In a recent review of various surveys, it was concluded that individuals who slept for less than six hours each night had a tenfold greater risk of premature mortality than those who obtained seven to nine hours of sleep [21]. Given the potential antagonistic impacts of inadequate mull or consideration over well-being, prosperity, and profitability, the outcomes of lack of sleep have expensive financial results. Insufficient sleep is a global problem that is becoming increasingly common in today's society. Compared to a few decades ago, significant changes in sleep culture have been observed worldwide. This global trend has produced massive social and economic shifts, and additionally has had marked public health consequences, and foremost among these is the significant reduction in total sleeping hours that have occurred in both adults and children [22].

2.2. *All-Cause Mortality*

Epidemiological evidence suggests that sleep duration and poor sleep are associated with premature mortality, as well as with an extensive variety of adverse health outcomes [23]. The Sleep Heart Study was done to determine the association between insufficient sleep conditions, including insomnia or poor-quality sleep and objectively measured short duration sleep, and the incidence of cardiovascular disease (CVD) and mortality in the general population. The study found that there was a 29% higher risk of CVD in study subjects who had insomnia or poor sleep with short sleep when compared to a reference group, thus supporting the conclusion that poor sleep with objectively measured short sleep was associated with a higher risk of CVD development [24].

2.3. *Sleep Duration Recommendations by Age*

The American Academy of Sleep Medicine (AASM) and the Sleep Research Society (SRS) have recommended that adults aged 18 to 60 years should sleep seven or more hours per night on a regular basis for ideal sleep health. Additionally, the National Sleep Foundation (NSF) consensus report has stated that seven to nine hours is recommended for adults aged 18 to 64 years, while seven to eight hours is suggested for those 65 years of age and older [25].

2.4. *Pathophysiology*

There are specific biomarkers that are released throughout insufficient sleep. Experimental studies with human subjects have demonstrated that proinflammatory markers undergo changes following laboratory-induced sleep loss. Markers that have been found to be dysregulated in acute sleep deficiency include IL-6 [26], IL1 receptor antagonist [27], and salivary amylase. However, there are biomarkers needed for the prediction of sleepiness and other consequences of sleep deprivation. Another study used NMR measures of metabolism to determine how the pathways involved in cholesterol metabolism and inflammatory responses changed due to prolonged sleep restriction. The investigation found that, compared to normal, sleep-restricted subjects showed decreases in levels of low-density lipoprotein (LDL), whereas there were no significant changes in high-density lipoprotein (HDL) levels. In a comparison group of subjects who reported that they suffered from subjective sleep insufficiency, HDL levels were decreased, but LDL levels did not differ from those of the restricted group [28]. In an analysis of data from 1024 adults surveyed in the Wisconsin Sleep Cohort Study, it was found that short sleep durations were associated with lower leptin and higher ghrelin levels [29].

2.5. *Contributing Factors*

Studies have observed that sleep duration and daytime sleepiness varies by gender and marital status. The presence of children in a family often contributes to insufficient rest or sleep among the adults with whom they live [14]. Insufficient sleep is typically a long-standing condition, often linked to biological or circadian disruption factors. Reviews of studies of possible causal factors have additionally suggested that genetic influences may account for possibly as much as one-third of cases of insufficient sleep [7]. Insufficient sleep duration is associated with an elevated intake of soda via excessive consumption of salt or carbonated beverages, and less frequent vegetable consumption [30]. Various types of stress also contribute. Housing insecurity and food uncertainty are psychological stressors associated with insufficient sleep [31]. Social and behavioral predictors of health exclusively add to the explosion of insufficient sleep [32]. Active smoking, smokeless tobacco, and secondhand smoke exposure have been additionally associated with insufficient sleep [33]. An increasing number of studies have shown that insufficient sleep and behavioral or emotional problems have reciprocal and mutually facilitating effects. It is known, for instance, that mood disorders are frequently associated with severe sleep problems and that the problems that are linked to inadequate sleep, such as reduced impulse control, reductions in attention span, and memory impairments, may further exacerbate a pre-existing mood disorder [34].

3. Results: Manifestations of Insufficient Sleep

3.1. *Cognitive Effects*

Insufficient sleep can contribute to aberrant behavior. Subjects who are chronically sleep-restricted may exhibit increased risk-taking behavior, or subjectively may show deficiencies in reasoning that result from seeking premature conclusions without considering all aspects of a problem. This type of impulsivity may manifest also as increased but unnoticed risk-seeking [35]. Insufficient sleep that occurs in children in the preschool and early school years is associated with poorer mother- and teacher-reported neurobehavioral processes, which particularly manifest in mid-childhood [36].

3.2. *Mood and Judgment*

Chronic sleep restriction among adolescents may increase suicidal risk [37]. Sleep loss can have adverse effects on the control of mood and behavior. Irritability, moodiness, and poor frustration tolerance are the most frequently described symptoms in subjects who are suffering from sleep restriction [34]. One study investigated the behavioral and psychological consequences of chronic sleep deprivation in different age or social groups. Among all groups, sleep restriction had generally adverse effects, but some subgroup differences were noted. Adolescents complained of tiredness upon awakening (46%), nervousness, and general weakness; university students reported experiencing excessive drowsiness (50%), tension, and nervousness; and working adults suffered mostly from negative moods, such as tension (49%), nervousness, and irritability [38].

3.3. *Sleepiness and Microsleep*

Daytime sleepiness is the most direct result of sleep loss reported by adolescents and manifests most significantly as difficulty in getting up in the morning. Sleepiness is also connected to a strong tendency toward brief mental lapses (or microsleep episodes), occurrences that significantly increase the risk of motor vehicle and other accidents [34]. A study based on the monitoring of microsleep episodes was carried out to investigate the consequences of sleep restriction (SR) on the maintenance of wakefulness and diurnal sleepiness. The investigators found that during sleep restriction, daytime microsleeping correlated with the Karolinska Sleepiness Scale (KSS) but not with the Maintenance of Wakefulness Test (MWT). The study also concluded that the frequency of microsleeping is an objective marker of diurnal sleep pressure [39].

3.4. *Effects on Respiratory Physiology*

There is growing interest in the impact of sleep and its disorders on the regulation of inflammatory processes and tissue morbidities, particularly in the context of metabolic and cardiovascular diseases. Obstructive sleep apnea syndrome (OSAS) is commonly seen in conjunction with insufficient sleep [40].

The condition of narcolepsy-cataplexy is characterized by disrupted nocturnal sleep as one of its most noticeable features, which in turn contributes to excessive daytime sleepiness in affected patients. Another feature of the condition is the lack of adequate non-rapid eye movement (NREM) sleep, which is related to nonconsolidated nocturnal sleep in narcolepsy-cataplexy, which also occurs in this patient group [41].

3.5. *Wakefulness and Vigilance*

Chronic insufficient sleep duration equivalent to an average of 5.6 h of sleep during a 24-h period has been found to double neurobehavioral reaction time performance and to increase lapses of attention fivefold. Impairments in neurobehavioral performance were worsened during the circadian night and did not recover during the circadian day, thus indicating that the deleterious effect from the homeostatic buildup of chronic sleep restriction (CSR) is expressed even during the circadian promotion of daytime arousal [42].

3.6. *Tiredness and Fatigue*

There is evidence that sleep loss can impair active cognitive processes such as planning, coping, and problem-solving. In sleep-impaired individuals, these deficits may particularly manifest in behaviors that require creative solutions to problems that are either complex or are lacking in sufficient information. The energy that is required to analyze unfamiliar environmental challenges or to sustain an extended chain of logical thought is especially reduced in sleep-deprived subjects. This internal state cognitive impairment may thus affect their ability to initiate behaviors related to long-term or abstract goals, and, as a result, may decrease their motivation to work toward those goals [34].

3.7. *Effects on Mental Health*

Chronic sleep loss and associated sleepiness and daytime impairments in adolescence are a genuine impediment to the achievement of academic success, health (for example depression, increased obesity risk), and safety (such as driving accidents) [43]. Emotional excitement and pain can cause difficulties with either sleep initiation or sleep maintenance. Behavioral issues and family conflict can contribute to even later bedtimes and to sleep schedules that are particularly at variance with daily schedules [34]. Further, a number of studies have shown that inadequate sleep increases the likelihood of daytime accidents and critical mistakes in the workplace.

3.8. Increased Incidence of Cardiovascular Morbidity

Insufficient sleep is associated with cardiovascular disease, and has been studied in numerous racial and ethnic groups. Similarly, the association between insufficient sleep and diabetes mellitus has been demonstrated to occur in a number of racial and ethnic minorities, with the exception of non-Hispanic blacks [44]. Insufficient sleep is also associated with cardiometabolic risk and neurocognitive impairment. Determinants of insufficient sleep include many social and environmental factors. Surveys have shown that the incidence of inadequate sleep is not consistent across all areas of the United States. Respondents in a few areas, and particularly in Appalachia, have reported excessively high levels of inadequate rest [45]. Insufficient sleep has also been shown to be linked to an increased risk of acute myocardial infarction [46]. It has been reported by Curtis [47] that more than one-half of racial differences in cardiometabolic risk can actually be explained by sleep patterns, and, more specifically, that, compared to Caucasian American adults, the reduced total sleep time and lower sleep efficiency of African-Americans is largely attributable to lifestyle or personal choice factors rather than racial or genetic influences. The study found that, compared to Caucasian Americans, African Americans obtained less sleep (341 vs. 381 min) and had lower sleep efficiency (72.3 vs. 82.2%) (P-value < 0.001). Further, 41% and 58% of the racial difference in cardiometabolic risk was explained by sleep time and sleep efficiency, respectively.

3.9. Effects on the Immune System

Sleep loss can adversely affect components of the immune system critical to host resistance to infectious illness. Furthermore, short sleep duration and sleep disturbances prospectively predict increased susceptibility to upper respiratory tract infection after an experimental viral challenge [48]. Additional findings are listed in Table 1.

3.10. Obesity and Metabolism

Sleep plays a pivotal role in energy metabolism. Both sufficient sleep and high-quality diets are vital for the prevention of obesity [49]. Various studies have shown linkages between insufficient sleep and obesity. Increased food intake during insufficient sleep is a physiological adaptation to provide the energy needed to sustain additional wakefulness, yet when food is easily accessible, intake often exceeds that which is required [50]. There is reliable evidence supporting the conclusion that sleep restriction increases food intake, and further that this association is due to increased production of the appetitive hormone ghrelin [29,51]. As a consequence, insufficient sleep is associated with increases in body mass index (BMI). Sleep loss can alter energy intake and expenditure. The amount of human sleep contributes to the maintenance of fat-free body mass at times of decreased energy intake. Lack of sufficient sleep may compromise dietary interventions for weight loss and related metabolic risk reduction [52]. Chronic sleep restriction is a potential risk factor for the maintenance of metabolic health. There is an association between insufficient sleep and an increased incidence of obesity and related morbidities. Thus, overweight and obese individuals attempting to reduce their caloric intake and maintain increased physical activity should obtain adequate sleep and, if needed, seek effective treatment for any coexisting sleep disorders [53].

3.11. Increased Risk for Diabetes Mellitus

Insufficient sleep, or more precisely the suppression of slow wave sleep and rapid eye movement sleep, has been associated with insulin resistance [54]. There is a high prevalence of insufficient sleep in young patients with diabetes mellitus type 1 (type 1 diabetes) and their relatives [55]. Inadequate sleep is also associated with an increased risk of hypertension, cardiovascular disease, and mortality. Lower scores on a scale of self-rated health (SRH), which are also linked to insufficient sleep, have been shown to indicate an elevated risk of CVD and death [56].

3.12. Migraine

The prevalence of insufficient sleep is significantly higher in patients with migraines when compared to those in nonmigraine headache or nonheadache groups [57]. The Chronic Migraine Epidemiology and Outcomes (CaMEO) Study, which assessed the relationship between sleep disturbances, including sleep apnea, and episodic or chronic migraines, concluded that the conditions were associated, and that the risk was enhanced in the elderly and in those with a higher BMI [58].

3.13. Clinical Burnout

In one study, it was found that insufficient sleep, preoccupation with thoughts of work during leisure time, and high work demands were risk factors for consequent clinical burnout [59]. It has also been found that sleep problems tend to precede symptoms of low back pain (LBP) and burnout in working individuals. It has therefore been suggested that health promotion initiatives should emphasize assessments of sleep quality as an important early risk indicator, and, further, that interventions should focus on promoting a better quality of sleep, in an attempt to reduce the incidence of LBP and burnout [60].

3.14. Increased Risk of Cancers

Insufficient sleep, including short sleep duration and sleep disruption, might be related to an increased risk of cancerous tumor formation [61]. Sleep disturbance increases the risk of breast cancer. It has been suggested that melatonin is involved in the relationship between sleep and breast cancer, in as much as exogenously applied melatonin provides an antiproliferative effect on breast cancer cells [62].

3.15. Sleep-Wake Disturbances in Shift Workers

Self-reported bruxism may indicate sleep problems and associated fatigue in daytime waking hours in nonpatient populations. It may be more prevalent among people who do shift work schedules or who work in jobs with irregular hours [63]. Laboratory studies have indicated that cardiometabolic stress and cognitive impairments are increased by shift work, as well as by insufficient sleep. A recent study by Kervezee [64] found that four days of simulated night shifts was associated with a loss in temporal coordination between internal circadian rhythmicity and the external environment, which in turn produced broader associated adverse health effects, which are commonly seen in night shift workers. A recent review [65] based on 38 meta-analyses and 24 systematic reviews summarized the linkages between shift work and adverse consequences, such as insufficient sleep, cardiovascular diseases, and accidents. The meta-analysis showed that shift work was closely linked to cardiometabolic diseases and accidents and that these associations tended to mimic those seen in persons with insufficient sleep. All these impairments because of insufficient sleep are described in Table 1 below.

Table 1. Sleep deprivation, which has been recognized as a "public health epidemic" linked to a range of medical and mental health issues.

Health Issues and Impairments Associated with Sleep Deprivation	Comments	References
Hypertension	Sleep deprivation is linked to an increased risk of hypertension	Schlafer et al., 2014 [66]
Cardiovascular incidents	Sleep-deprived people are at greater risk for coronary heart disease	Ayas et al., 2003 [67]
	Increased heart attacks	Janszky and Ljung, 2008 [68]
Type 2 diabetes mellitus (T2DM)	Sleep deprivation is linked to an increased risk of hypertension	Schlafer et al., 2014 [66]

Table 1. *Cont.*

Health Issues and Impairments Associated with Sleep Deprivation	Comments	References
Depression	Increases the risk of developing depression	Chen et al., 2012 [69]
	Increases the relapse of depression	Howland, 2011 [70]; Okun et al., 2011 [71]
	High reporting of depressive symptoms among students	O'Brien, 2005 [72]; Catrett, 2009 [73]
	Anxiety, depression, and withdrawal increased depression among adolescents	Coulombe et al., 2010 [74]; Pallesen et al.,2011 [11]; Lund et al., 2010 [75]; Roberts et al., 2009 [76]
Obesity	Sleep deprivation is linked to an increased risk of obesity	Schlafer et al., 2014 [66]
	Suffer more obesity	Taheri et al., 2004 [29]
	Increased obesity among adolescents by 80%	Gupta et al., 2002 [77]
Cancer	Linked to an increased risk of cancer	Markt S.C. et al., 2015 [61]; Lehrer S. et al., 2013 [62]
Mortality risks	Die at an early age	Kripe et al., 2002 [78]
Cognitive performance	Impairs visuomotor performance	Paula Alhola and Paivi Kantola, 2007 [79]
	Impairment in saccadic eye movements	Bocca and Denise, 2006 [80]
	Increases rigid thinking, perseveration errors, and difficulties in utilizing new information in complex tasks	Harrison and Horne, 1999 [81]
	Affects high-level cognitive executive functions	Beebe, 2011 [82]
Memory	Impaired performance in probed force memory recall and memory search	Wright and Badia, 1999 [83] McCarthy and Waters, 1997 [84]
	Deterioration of temporal memory for recall of faces after 36 h of sleep deprivation	Harrison and Horne, 2000 [85]
Mood	Suffer negative moods	Dinges et al., 1997 [86]
Thinking	Sleep loss produces temporary changes in cerebral metabolism, cognition, emotion, and behavior consistent with mild prefrontal lobe dysfunction	Killgore et al., 2008 [87]
Learning and academic performance	Poor declarative and procedural learning in students, but once sleep was optimized, improvement in academic performance noted	Curcio et al., 2006 [88]
Vigilance	Feedback blunting could be caused by general, downstream impairments from loss of vigilant attention due to sleep deprivation	Lim and Dinges, 2010 [89]
Reaction time	Greater subjective reliance on avoidance as a coping strategy was associated with greater deterioration in performance	Saadat et al., 2017 [90]
Personal injury	Decreased duration led to increased work-related injury	Lombardi et al., 2010 [91]
Traffic accidents	Increased risk of traffic accidents	de Mello et al., 2013 [92]; Pandi-Perumal et al., 2006 [93]
	Increased traffic accidents among doctors under study	Steele et al., 1999 [94]; Schlafer et al., 2014 [66]
	More likely to be involved in vehicular crashes	Drake et al., 2010 [95]
	Increased auto accidents	Coren, 1996 [96]
	Increased car accidents among adolescents	National sleep foundation, 2006 [97]

Table 1. *Cont.*

Health Issues and Impairments Associated with Sleep Deprivation	Comments	References
Industrial accidents	Increased workplace injuries	Barnes and Wagner, 2009 [98]; Lahti et al., 2006 [99]; Kantermann et al., 2007 [100]
Medical errors	Sleep disturbances and internship-enforced short sleep increased risk of depression development and chronicity and medical errors	Kalmbach et al. 2017 [101]
Decision making	Deterioration in decision-making	Linde et.al., 1999 [102]
	Less effective in making decisions	Killgore et al., 2006 [103]
	Affects decision-making	Harrison, 2000 [85]
Moral judgement	Moral reasoning was severely impaired during partial sleep deprivation	Olsen et. al., 2010 [104]
	Lack of sleep is associated with low moral awareness	Christopher Barnes et al., 2014 [105]

4. Discussion

The general public often devalues the seriousness of insufficient sleep and may have a more general attitude that, in the larger scheme of life's difficulties, "not getting enough sleep" occupies a fairly low rung on the stepladder of personal health concerns. As a consequence, sleep insufficiency often goes unreported by patients in medical interviews. Some senior specialists skillfully and intentionally deal with the issue of their patients' sleeping habits, but, as the evidence of the studies reviewed here show, the significance of sleep to health status deserves particular and earnest attention.

To ensure that they obtain sufficient sleep, patients should set predictable wake-up times, refrain from using electronic devices prior to their normal sleep time, and obtain adequate physical exercise [21]. Employers need to be made aware of the significance of rest for overall health and the responsibility of businesses to provide a work environment and conditions that will not interfere with an employee's right to adequate sleep. Business management needs to plan for and create brighter workspaces. Business managers should also strive to discourage conflict in the workplace and discourage the use of electronic devices. Further, school officials should consider establishing later school start times to avoid interference with students' critical need for sleep, which exists during the adolescent years [21].

Policymakers should encourage educational efforts to raise awareness about the importance of sleep, and especially emphasize the contribution that employers can make to ensuring that work assignments do not adversely interfere with sleep schedules. It has been found that adolescents who do not obtain sufficient sleep are likely to be overweight due to lack of engagement in daily physical activity, may suffer from depressive symptoms, may engage in risky behaviors (drinking, smoking tobacco, and using illicit drugs), and may perform inadequately in school [106].

5. Conclusions

Insufficient sleep and its health consequences may go unrecognized by clinicians inasmuch as many medical school curriculums do not emphasize the importance of sleep to overall health. The causes of common patient complaints of daytime weakness, tiredness, sluggishness, languid driving, and intellectual troubles may often be misattributed to life stresses such as family or social problems rather than to the more basic cause of inadequate rest. There is a clear need for medical professionals to ensure that their patients are made aware of common contributors to sleep disruption such as jet lag or shift work. However, more fundamentally, patient attitudes about the adverse effects of inadequate sleep for health need to be addressed.

Author Contributions: Conceptualization, V.K.C. and S.R.P.-P.; methodology, V.K.C., S.R.P.-P., M.D.M. and S.K.; formal analysis, V.K.C. and S.R.P.-P.; resources, D.B. and D.W.S.; data curation, D.W.S.; writing—original draft preparation, S.R.P.-P.; writing—review and editing, V.K.C., M.D.M., S.K. and D.B.; supervision, S.R.P.-P. All authors read and approved the final version of the manuscript.

References

1. Kochanek, K.D.; Murphy, S.L.; Xu, J.; Arias, E. Mortality in the United States, 2013. *NCHS Data BriefS* **2014**, *178*, 1–8.
2. Grandner, M.A.; Hale, L.; Moore, M.; Patel, N.P. Mortality associated withshort sleep duration: The evidence, the possible mechanisms, and the future. *Sleep Med. Rev.* **2010**, *14*, 191–203. [CrossRef] [PubMed]
3. Chapman, D.P.; Croft, J.B.; Liu, Y.; Perry, G.S.; Presley-Cantrell, L.R.; Ford, E.S. Excess frequent insufficient sleep in American Indians/Alaska natives. *J. Environ. Public Health* **2013**, *2013*, 259645. [CrossRef] [PubMed]
4. Nielen, M.M.J.; Spronk, I.; Davids, R.; Zwaanswijk, M.; Verheij, R.A.; Korevaar, J.C. Incidentie en Prevalentie van Gezondheids Problemen in de Nederlandse Huisartsenpraktijk in 2012. NIVEL Zorgregistraties eerste lijn. Available online: https://www.nivel.nl/nl/nzr/zorgregistraties-eerstelijn (accessed on 19 December 2018).
5. Spoormaker, V.I.; van den Bout, J. The prevalence of sleep disorders; relations with depression and anxiety e a pilot study. *NSWO* **2005**, *16*, 155–158.
6. Kerkhof, G.A. Epidemiology of sleep and sleep disorders in The Netherlands. *Sleep Med.* **2017**, *30*, 229–239. [CrossRef] [PubMed]
7. Hublin, C.; Kaprio, J.; Partinen, M.; Koskenvuo, M. Insufficient sleep—A population-based study in adults. *Sleep* **2001**, *24*, 392–400. [CrossRef] [PubMed]
8. Ursin, R.; Bjorvatn, B.; Holsten, F. Sleep duration, subjective sleep need, and sleep habits of 40-to 45- year-olds in the Hordaland Health Study. *Sleep* **2005**, *28*, 1260. [CrossRef] [PubMed]
9. Carskadon, M.A.; Harvey, K.; Duke, P.; Anders, T.F.; Litt, I.F.; Dement, W.C. Pubertal changes in daytime sleepiness. *Sleep* **1980**, *2*, 453–460. [PubMed]
10. Loessl, B.; Valerius, G.; Kopasz, M.; Hornyak, M.; Riemann, D.; Voderholzer, U. Are adolescents chronically sleep-deprived? An investigation of sleep habits of adolescents in the Southwest of Germany. *Child Care Health Dev.* **2008**, *34*, 549–556. [CrossRef]
11. Pallesen, S.; Saxvig, I.W.; Molde, H.; Sørensen, E.; Wilhelmsen-Langeland, A.; Bjorvatn, B. Brief report: Behaviorally induced insufficient sleep syndrome in older adolescents: Prevalence and correlates. *J. Adolesc.* **2011**, *34*, 391–395. [CrossRef]
12. Luxton, D.D.; Greenburg, D.; Ryan, J.; Niven, A.; Wheeler, G.; Mysliwiec, V. Prevalence and impact of short sleep duration in redeployed OIF soldiers. *Sleep* **2011**, *34*, 1189–1195. [CrossRef]
13. Watson, N.F.; Badr, M.S.; Belenky, G.; Bliwise, D.L.; Buxton, O.M.; Buysse, D.; Dinges, D.F.; Gangwisch, J.; Grandner, M.A.; Kushida, C.; et al. Joint consensus statement of the American academy of sleep medicine and sleep research society on the recommended amount of sleep for a healthy adult: Methodology and discussion. *Sleep* **2015**, *38*, 1161–1183. [CrossRef] [PubMed]
14. Chapman, D.P.; Wheaton, A.G.; Perry, G.S.; Sturgis, S.L.; Strine, T.W.; Croft, J.B. Household demographics and perceived insufficient sleep among US adults. *J. Community Health* **2012**, *37*, 344–349. [CrossRef]
15. Magee, C.A.; Iverson, D.C.; Caputi, P. Factors associated with short and long sleep. *Prev. Med.* **2009**, *49*, 461–467. [CrossRef] [PubMed]
16. Krueger, P.M.; Friedman, E.M. Sleep duration in the United States: A cross-sectional population-based study. *Am. J. Epidemiol.* **2009**, *169*, 1052–1063. [CrossRef] [PubMed]
17. Kronholm, E.; Härmä, M.; Hublin, C.; Aro, A.R.; Partonen, T. Self-reported sleep duration in Finnish general population. *J. Sleep Res.* **2006**, *15*, 276–290. [CrossRef]
18. Nishitani, N.; Sakakibara, H.; Akiyama, I. Short sleeping time and job stress in Japanese white-collar workers. *Open Sleep J.* **2013**, *6*, 104–109. [CrossRef]

19. Heo, Y.-S.; Chang, S.-J.; Park, S.-G.; Leem, J.-H.; Jeon, S.-H.; Lee, B.-J.; Kim, H.-C. Association between workplace risk factor exposure and sleep disturbance: Analysis of the 2nd Korean working conditions survey. *Ann. Occup. Environ. Med.* **2013**, *25*, 41. [CrossRef] [PubMed]
20. Park, J.B.; Nakata, A.; Swanson, N.G.; Chun, H. Organizational factors associated with work-related sleep problems in a nationally representative sample of Korean workers. *Int. Arch. Occup. Environ. Health* **2013**, *86*, 211–222. [CrossRef] [PubMed]
21. Hafner, M.; Stepanek, M.; Taylor, J.; Troxel, W.M.; van Stolk, C. *Why Sleep Matters—The Economic Costs of Insufficient Sleep: A Comparative Cross-Country Analysis*; RAND Corporation: Santa Monica, CA, USA, 2016.
22. Chattu, V.K.; Sakhamuri, S.; Kumar, R.; BaHammam, A.; Perumal, P. Insufficient sleep: Is it time to recognize it as a major non-communicable disease? *Sleep Sci.* **2018**, *11*, 56–64. [CrossRef]
23. Silva-Costa, A.; Griep, R.H.; Rotenberg, L. Associations of a short sleep duration, insufficient sleep, and insomnia with self-rated health among nurses. *PLoS ONE* **2015**, *10*, e0126844. [CrossRef] [PubMed]
24. Bertisch, S.M.; Pollock, B.D.; Mittleman, M.A.; Buysse, D.J.; Bazzano, L.A.; Gottlieb, D.J.; Redline, S. Insomnia with objective short sleep duration and risk of incident cardiovascular disease and all-cause mortality: Sleep Heart Health Study. *Sleep* **2018**, *41*, zsy047. [CrossRef] [PubMed]
25. Cirelli, C.; Benca, R.; Eichler, A.F. Insufficient Sleep: Definition, Epidemiology, and Adverse Outcomes. 2017. Available online: https://www.uptodate.com/contents/insufficient-sleep-definition-epidemiology-and-adverse-outcomes (accessed on 21 November 2018).
26. Shearer, W.T.; Reuben, J.M.; Mullington, J.M.; Price, N.J.; Lee, B.N.; Smith, E.O.; Szuba, M.P.; Van Dongen, H.P.; Dinges, D.F. Soluble TNF-alpha receptor 1 and IL-6 plasma levels in humans subjected to the sleep deprivation model of spaceflight. *J. Allergy Clin. Immunol.* **2001**, *107*, 165–170. [CrossRef] [PubMed]
27. Dinges, D.F.; Douglas, S.D.; Hamarman, S.; Zaugg, L.; Kapoor, S. Sleep deprivation and human immune function. *Adv. Neuroimmunol.* **1995**, *5*, 97–110. [CrossRef]
28. Aho, V.; Ollila, H.M.; Kronholm, E.; Bondia-Pons, I.; Soininen, P.; Kangas, A.J.; Hilvo, M.; Seppälä, I.; Kettunen, J.; Oikonen, M.; et al. Prolonged sleep restriction induces changes in pathways involved in cholesterol metabolism and inflammatory responses. *Sci. Rep.* **2016**, *6*, 24828. [CrossRef] [PubMed]
29. Taheri, S.; Lin, L.; Austin, D.; Young, T.; Mignot, E. Short sleep duration is associated with reduced leptin, elevated ghrelin, and increased body mass index. *PLoS Med.* **2004**, *1*, 210–217. [CrossRef] [PubMed]
30. Franckle, R.L.; Falbe, J.; Gortmaker, S.; Ganter, C.; Taveras, E.M.; Land, T.; Davison, K.K. Insufficient sleep among elementary and middle school students is linked with elevated soda consumption and other unhealthy dietary behaviors. *Prev. Med.* **2015**, *74*, 36–41. [CrossRef] [PubMed]
31. Liu, Y.; Njai, R.S.; Greenlund, K.J.; Chapman, D.P.; Croft, J.B. Relationships between housing and food insecurity, frequent mental distress, and insufficient sleep among adults in 12 US States, 2009. *Prev. Chronic Dis.* **2014**, *11*, E37. [CrossRef]
32. Williams, N.J.; Grandner, M.A.; Wallace, D.M.; Cuffee, Y.; Airhihenbuwa, C.; Okuyemi, K.; Ogedegbe, G.; Jean-Louis, G. Social and behavioral predictors of insufficient sleep among African Americans and Caucasians. *Sleep Med.* **2016**, *18*, 103–107. [CrossRef]
33. Sabanayagam, C.; Shankar, A. The association between active smoking, smokeless tobacco, second-hand smoke exposure and insufficient sleep. *Sleep Med.* **2011**, *12*, 7–11. [CrossRef]
34. Dahl, R.E. The consequences of insufficient sleep for adolescents: Links between sleep and emotional regulation. *Phi Delta Kappan* **1999**, *80*, 354–359.
35. Maric, A.; Montvai, E.; Werth, E.; Storz, M.; Leemann, J.; Weissengruber, S.; Ruff, C.C.; Huber, R.; Poryazova, R.; Baumann, C.R. Insufficient sleep: Enhanced risk-seeking relates to low local sleep intensity. *Ann. Neurol.* **2017**, *82*, 409–418. [CrossRef] [PubMed]
36. Taveras, E.M.; Rifas-Shiman, S.L.; Bub, K.L.; Gillman, M.W.; Oken, E. Prospective study of insufficient sleep and neurobehavioral functioning among school-age children. *Acad. Pediatr.* **2017**, *17*, 625–632. [CrossRef] [PubMed]
37. Lee, Y.J.; Cho, S.J.; Cho, I.H.; Kim, S.J. Insufficient sleep and suicidality in adolescents. *Sleep* **2012**, *35*, 455–460. [CrossRef] [PubMed]
38. Oginska, H.; Pokorski, J. Fatigue and mood correlates of sleep length in three age-social groups: School children, students, and employees. *Chronobiol. Int.* **2006**, *23*, 1317–1328. [CrossRef]

39. Bougard, C.; Gomez-Merino, D.; Rabat, A.; Arnal, P.; Van Beers, P.; Guillard, M.; Léger, D.; Sauvet, F.; Chennaoui, M. Daytime microsleeps during 7 days of sleep restriction followed by 13 days of sleep recovery in healthy young adults. *Conscious. Cogn.* **2018**, *61*, 1–2. [CrossRef] [PubMed]
40. Kim, J.; Hakim, F.; Kheirandish-Gozal, L.; Gozal, D. Inflammatory pathways in children with insufficient or disordered sleep. *Respir. Physiol. Neurobiol.* **2011**, *178*, 465–474. [CrossRef]
41. Khatami, R.; Landolt, H.P.; Achermann, P.; Rétey, J.V.; Werth, E.; Mathis, J.; Bassetti, C.L. Insufficient non-REM sleep intensity in narcolepsy-cataplexy. *Sleep* **2007**, *30*, 980–989. [CrossRef]
42. McHill, A.W.; Hull, J.T.; Wang, W.; Czeisler, C.A.; Klerman, E.B. Chronic sleep curtailment, even without extended (>16-h) wakefulness, degrades human vigilance performance. *Proc. Natl. Acad. Sci. USA* **2018**, *115*, 6070–6075. [CrossRef]
43. Owens, J.; Au, R.; Carskadon, M.; Millman, R.; Wolfson, A.; Braverman, P.K.; Adelman, W.P.; Breuner, C.C.; Levine, D.A.; Marcell, A.V.; et al. Insufficient sleep in adolescents and young adults: An update on causes and consequences. *Pediatrics* **2014**, *134*, e921–e932. [CrossRef]
44. Vishnu, A.; Shankar, A.; Kalidindi, S. Examination of the association between insufficient sleep and cardiovascular disease and diabetes by race/ethnicity. *Int. J. Endocrinol.* **2011**, *2011*, 789358. [CrossRef] [PubMed]
45. Grandner, M.A.; Smith, T.E.; Jackson, N.; Jackson, T.; Burgard, S.; Branas, C. Geographic distribution of insufficient sleep across the United States: A county-level hotspot analysis. *Sleep Health* **2015**, *1*, 158–165. [CrossRef] [PubMed]
46. Liu, Y.; Tanaka, H.; Fukuoka Heart Study Group. Overtime work, insufficient sleep, and risk of non-fatal acute myocardial infarction in Japanese men. *Occup. Environ. Med.* **2002**, *59*, 447–451. [CrossRef] [PubMed]
47. Curtis, D.S.; Fuller-Rowell, T.E.; El-Sheikh, M.; Carnethon, M.R.; Ryff, C.D. Habitual sleep as a contributor to racial differences in cardiometabolic risk. *Proc. Natl. Acad. Sci. USA* **2017**, *114*, 8889–8894. [CrossRef] [PubMed]
48. Prather, A.A.; Leung, C.W. Association of insufficient sleep with respiratory infection among adults in the United States. *JAMA Intern. Med.* **2016**, *176*, 850–852. [CrossRef] [PubMed]
49. Cespedes, E.M.; Hu, F.B.; Redline, S.; Rosner, B.; Gillman, M.W.; Rifas-Shiman, S.L.; Taveras, E.M. Chronic insufficient sleep and diet quality: Contributors to childhood obesity. *Obesity* **2016**, *24*, 184–190. [CrossRef] [PubMed]
50. Markwald, R.R.; Melanson, E.L.; Smith, M.R.; Higgins, J.; Perreault, L.; Eckel, R.H.; Wright, K.P., Jr. Impact of insufficient sleep on total daily energy expenditure, food intake, and weight gain. *Proc. Natl. Acad. Sci. USA* **2013**, *110*, 5695–5700. [CrossRef] [PubMed]
51. Chaput, J.P.; St-Onge, M.P. Increased food intake by insufficient sleep in humans: Are we jumping the gun on the hormonal explanation? *Front. Endocrinol.* **2014**, *5*, 116. [CrossRef] [PubMed]
52. Nedeltcheva, A.V.; Kilkus, J.M.; Imperial, J.; Schoeller, D.A.; Penev, P.D. Insufficient sleep undermines dietary efforts to reduce adiposity. *Ann. Intern. Med.* **2010**, *153*, 435–441. [CrossRef]
53. Penev, P.D. Update on energy homeostasis and insufficient sleep. *J. Clin. Endocrinol. Metab.* **2012**, *97*, 1792–1801. [CrossRef]
54. Dutil, C.; Chaput, J.P. Inadequate sleep as a contributor to type 2 diabetes in children and adolescents. *Nutr. Diabetes* **2017**, *7*, e266. [CrossRef] [PubMed]
55. Estrada, C.L.; Danielson, K.K.; Drum, M.L.; Lipton, R.B. Insufficient sleep in young patients with diabetes and their families. *Biol. Res. Nurs.* **2012**, *14*, 48–54. [CrossRef] [PubMed]
56. Geiger, S.D.; Sabanayagam, C.; Shankar, A. The relationship between insufficient sleep and self-rated health in a nationally representative sample. *J. Environ. Public Health* **2012**, *2012*, 518263. [CrossRef] [PubMed]
57. Kim, J.; Cho, S.J.; Kim, W.J.; Yang, K.I.; Yun, C.H.; Chu, M.K. Insufficient sleep is prevalent among migraineurs: A population-based study. *J. Headache Pain* **2017**, *18*, 50. [CrossRef] [PubMed]
58. Buse, D.C.; Rains, J.C.; Fanning, K.M.; Reed, M.L.; Adams, A.M.; Pavlovic, J.M.; Lipton, R. The relationship between sleep disorders and migraine: Results from the chronic migraine epidemiology and outcomes (CaMEO) study. *Neurology* **2018**, *90* (Suppl. 15), S43.007.
59. Söderström, M.; Jeding, K.; Ekstedt, M.; Perski, A.; Akerstedt, T. Insufficient sleep predicts clinical burnout. *J. Occup. Health Psychol.* **2012**, *17*, 175–183. [CrossRef] [PubMed]

60. Elfering, A.; Kottwitz, M.U.; Tamcan, Ö.; Müller, U.; Mannion, A.F. Impaired sleep predicts onset of low back pain and burnout symptoms: Evidence from a three-wave study. *Psychol. Health Med.* **2018**, *24*, 1–15. [CrossRef] [PubMed]
61. Markt, S.C.; Grotta, A.; Nyren, O.; Adami, H.O.; Mucci, L.A.; Valdimarsdottir, U.A.; Stattin, P.; Bellocco, R.; Lagerros, Y.T. Insufficient sleep and risk of prostate cancer in a large Swedish cohort. *Sleep* **2015**, *38*, 1405–1410. [CrossRef]
62. Lehrer, S.; Green, S.; Ramanathan, L.; Rosenzweig, K.E. Insufficient sleep associated with increased breast cancer mortality. *Sleep Med.* **2013**, *14*, 469. [CrossRef]
63. Ahlberg, K.; Jahkola, A.; Savolainen, A.; Könönen, M.; Partinen, M.; Hublin, C.; Sinisalo, J.; Lindholm, H.; Sarna, S.; Ahlberg, J. Associations of reported bruxism with insomnia and insufficient sleep symptoms among media personnel with or without irregular shift work. *Head Face Med.* **2008**, *4*, 4. [CrossRef]
64. Kervezee, L.; Cuesta, M.; Cermakian, N.; Boivin, D.B. Simulated night shift work induces circadian misalignment of the human peripheral blood mononuclear cell transcriptome. *Proc. Natl. Acad. Sci. USA* **2018**, *115*, 5540–5545. [CrossRef] [PubMed]
65. Kecklund, G.; Axelsson, J. Health consequences of shift work and insufficient sleep. *BMJ* **2016**, *355*, i5210. [CrossRef] [PubMed]
66. Schlafer, O.; Wenzel, V.; Högl, B. Sleep disorders among physicians on shift work. *Anaesthesist* **2014**, *63*, 844–851. [CrossRef] [PubMed]
67. Ayas, N.T.; White, D.P.; Manson, J.E.; Stampfer, M.J.; Speizer, F.E.; Malhotra, A.; Hu, F.B. A prospective study of sleep duration and coronary heart disease in women. *Arch. Intern. Med.* **2003**, *163*, 205–209. [CrossRef] [PubMed]
68. Janszky, I.; Ljung, R. Shifts to and from daylight saving time and incidence of myocardial infarction. *N. Engl. J. Med.* **2008**, *359*, 1966–1968. [CrossRef] [PubMed]
69. Chen, M.C.; Burley, H.W.; Gotlib, I.H. Reduced sleep quality in healthy girls at risk for depression. *J. Sleep Res.* **2012**, *21*, 68–72. [CrossRef] [PubMed]
70. Howland, R.H. Sleep interventions for the treatment of depression. *J. Psychosoc. Nurs. Ment. Health Serv.* **2011**, *49*, 17–20. [CrossRef]
71. Okun, M.L.; Luther, J.; Prather, A.A.; Perel, J.M.; Wisniewski, S.; Wisner, K.L. Changes in sleep quality, but not hormones predict time to postpartum depression recurrence. *J. Affect. Disord.* **2011**, *130*, 378–384. [CrossRef]
72. O'Brien, E.M.; Mindell, J.A. Sleep and risk-taking behavior in adolescents. *Behav. Sleep Med.* **2005**, *3*, 113–133. [CrossRef]
73. Catrett, C.D.; Gaultney, J.F. Possible insomnia predicts some risky behaviors among adolescents when controlling for depressive symptoms. *J. Genet. Psychol.* **2009**, *170*, 287–309. [CrossRef]
74. Coulombe, J.A.; Reid, G.J.; Boyle, M.H.; Racine, Y. Concurrent associations among sleep problems, indicators of inadequate sleep, psychopathology, and shared risk factors in a population-based sample of healthy Ontario children. *J. Pediatr. Psychol.* **2010**, *35*, 790–799. [CrossRef] [PubMed]
75. Lund, H.G.; Reider, B.D.; Whiting, A.B.; Prichard, J.R. Sleep patterns and predictors of disturbed sleep in a large population of college students. *J. Adolesc. Health* **2010**, *46*, 124–132. [CrossRef]
76. Roberts, R.E.; Roberts, C.R.; Duong, H.T. Sleepless in adolescence: Prospective data on sleep deprivation, health and functioning. *J. Adolesc.* **2009**, *32*, 1045–1057. [CrossRef] [PubMed]
77. Gupta, N.K.; Mueller, W.H.; Chan, W.; Meininger, J.C. Is obesity associated with poor sleep quality in adolescents? *Am. J. Hum. Biol.* **2002**, *14*, 762–768. [CrossRef]
78. Kripke, D.F.; Garfinkel, L.; Wingard, D.L.; Klauber, M.R.; Marler, M.R. Mortality associated with sleep duration and insomnia. *Arch. Gen. Psychiatry* **2002**, *59*, 131–136. [CrossRef] [PubMed]
79. Alhola, P.; Polo-Kantola, P. Sleep deprivation: Impact on cognitive performance. *Neuropsychiatr. Dis. Treat.* **2007**, *3*, 553–567.
80. Bocca, M.L.; Denise, P. Total sleep deprivation effect on disengagement of spatial attention as assessed by saccadic eye movements. *Clin. Neurophysiol.* **2006**, *117*, 894–899. [CrossRef]
81. Harrison, Y.; Horne, J.A. One night of sleep loss impairs innovative thinking and flexible decision making. *Organ. Behav. Hum. Decis. Process.* **1999**, *78*, 128–145. [CrossRef]
82. Beebe, D.W. Cognitive, behavioral, and functional consequences of inadequate sleep in children and adolescents. *Pediatr. Clin. N. Am.* **2011**, *58*, 649–665. [CrossRef]

83. Wright, K.P., Jr.; Badia, P. Effects of menstrual cycle phase and oral contraceptives on alertness, cognitive performance, and circadian rhythms during sleep deprivation. *Behav. Brain Res.* **1999**, *103*, 185–194. [CrossRef]
84. McCarthy, M.E.; Waters, W.F. Decreased attentional responsivity during sleep deprivation: Orienting response latency, amplitude, and habituation. *Sleep* **1997**, *20*, 115–123. [CrossRef] [PubMed]
85. Harrison, Y.; Horne, J.A. Sleep loss and temporal memory. *Q. J. Exp. Psychol. A* **2000**, *53*, 271–279. [CrossRef] [PubMed]
86. Dinges, D.F.; Pack, F.; Williams, K.; Gillen, K.A.; Powell, J.W.; Ott, G.E.; Aptowicz, C.; Pack, A.I. Cumulative sleepiness, mood disturbance, and psychomotor vigilance performance decrements during a week of sleep restricted to 4–5 hours per night. *Sleep* **1997**, *20*, 267–277. [PubMed]
87. Killgore, W.D.; Balkin, T.J.; Wesensten, N.J. Impaired decision making following 49 h of sleep deprivation. *J. Sleep Res.* **2006**, *15*, 7–13. [CrossRef] [PubMed]
88. Curcio, G.; Ferrara, M.; De Gennaro, L. Sleep loss, learning capacity and academic performance. *Sleep Med. Rev.* **2006**, *10*, 323–337. [CrossRef] [PubMed]
89. Lim, J.; Dinges, D.F. A meta-analysis of the impact of short-term sleep deprivation on cognitive variables. *Psychol Bull.* **2010**, *136*, 375–389. [CrossRef] [PubMed]
90. Saadat, H.; Bissonnette, B.; Tumin, D.; Raman, V.; Rice, J.; Barry, N.; Tobias, J. Effects of partial sleep deprivation on reaction time in anesthesiologists. *Paediatr. Anaesth.* **2017**, *27*, 358–362. [CrossRef]
91. Lombardi, D.A.; Folkard, S.; Willetts, J.L.; Smith, G.S. Daily sleep, weekly working hours, and risk of work-related injury: US National Health Interview Survey (2004–2008). *Chronobiol. Int.* **2010**, *27*, 1013–1030. [CrossRef]
92. De Mello, M.T.; Narciso, F.V.; Tufik, S.; Paiva, T.; Spence, D.W.; BaHammam, A.S.; Verster, J.C.; Pandi-Perumal, S.R. Sleep disorders as a cause of motor vehicle collisions. *Int. J. Prev. Med.* **2013**, *4*, 246.
93. Pandi-Perumal, S.R.; Verster, J.C.; Kayumov, L.; Lowe, A.D.; Santana, M.G.; Pires, M.L.; Tufik, S.; Mello, M.T. Sleep disorders, sleepiness and traffic safety: A public health menace. *Braz. J. Med. Biol. Res.* **2006**, *39*, 863–871. [CrossRef]
94. Steele, M.T.; Ma, O.J.; Watson, W.A.; Thomas, H.A., Jr.; Muelleman, R.L. The occupational risk of motor vehicle collisions for emergency medicine residents. *Acad. Emerg. Med.* **1999**, *6*, 1050–1053. [CrossRef] [PubMed]
95. Drake, C.; Roehrs, T.; Breslau, N.; Johnson, E.; Jefferson, C.; Scofield, H.; Roth, T. The 10-year risk of verified motor vehicle crashes in relation to physiologic sleepiness. *Sleep* **2010**, *33*, 745–752. [CrossRef] [PubMed]
96. Coren, S. Daylight saving time and traffic accidents. *N. Engl. J. Med.* **1996**, *334*, 924–925. [CrossRef] [PubMed]
97. National Sleep Foundation. *2006 Teens and sleep. Sleep in America Polls*; National Sleep Foundation: Washington, DC, USA, 2006; Available online: www.sleepfoundation.org/article/sleep-america-polls/2006-teens-and-sleep (accessed on 22 April 2018).
98. Barnes, C.M.; Wagner, D.T. Changing to daylight saving time cuts into sleep and increases workplace injuries. *J. Appl. Psychol.* **2009**, *94*, 1305–1317. [CrossRef] [PubMed]
99. Lahti, T.A.; Leppämäki, S.; Lönnqvist, J.; Partonen, T. Transition to daylight saving time reduces sleep duration plus sleep efficiency of the deprived sleep. *Neurosci. Lett.* **2006**, *406*, 174–177. [CrossRef] [PubMed]
100. Kantermann, T.; Juda, M.; Merrow, M.; Roenneberg, T. The human circadian clock's seasonal adjustment is disrupted by daylight saving time. *Curr. Biol.* **2007**, *17*, 1996–2000. [CrossRef] [PubMed]
101. Kalmbach, D.A.; Arnedt, J.T.; Song, P.X.; Guille, C.; Sen, S. Sleep Disturbance and Short Sleep as Risk Factors for Depression and Perceived Medical Errors in First-Year Residents. *Sleep* **2017**, *40*. [CrossRef]
102. Linde, L.; Edland, A.; Bergström, M. Auditory attention and multiattribute decision-making during a 33 h sleep-deprivation period: Mean performance and between-subject dispersions. *Ergonomics* **1999**, *42*, 696–713. [CrossRef]
103. Killgore, W.D.; Kahn-Greene, E.T.; Lipizzi, E.L.; Newman, R.A.; Kamimori, G.H.; Balkin, T.J. Sleep deprivation reduces perceived emotional intelligence and constructive thinking skills. *Sleep Med.* **2008**, *9*, 517–526. [CrossRef]
104. Olsen, O.K.; Pallesen, S.; Eid, J. The impact of partial sleep deprivation on moral reasoning in military officers. *Sleep* **2010**, *33*, 1086–1090. [CrossRef]

105. Barnes, C.M.; Gunia, B.C.; Wagner, D.T. Sleep and moral awareness. *J. Sleep Res.* **2014**, *24*, 181–188. [CrossRef] [PubMed]

106. Vick, J.; Muchiri, E.; James, K. Insufficient Sleep and Depression in Adolescents. Family Nurse Practitioner Theses. 2015. 1. Available online: http://digitalcommons.northgeorgia.edu/fnp_etd/1 (accessed on 21 November 2018).

3

Mobile Phone Use and Mental Health: A Review of the Research that Takes a Psychological Perspective on Exposure

Sara Thomée

Department of Psychology, University of Gothenburg, 405 30 Gothenburg, Sweden;
sara.thomee@psy.gu.se;

Abstract: The purpose of this study was to carry out a review of observational studies that consider links between mobile phone use and mental health from a psychological or behavioral perspective. Systematic literature searches in PubMed and PsycINFO for articles published until 2017 were done. Exclusion criteria included: papers that considered radiofrequency fields, attention, safety, relational consequences, sexual behavior, cyberbullying, and reviews, qualitative, and case or experimental studies. A total of 4738 papers were screened by title and abstract, 404 were retrieved in full text, and 290 were included. Only 5% had any longitudinal design. Self-reporting was the dominating method of measurement. One third of the studies included children or youth. A majority of adult populations consisted of university students and/or self-selected participants. The main research results included associations between frequent mobile phone use and mental health outcomes, such as depressive symptoms and sleep problems. Mobile phone use at bedtime was associated with, e.g., shorter sleep duration and lower sleep quality. "Problematic use" (dependency) was associated with several negative outcomes. In conclusion, associations between mobile phone use and adverse mental health outcomes are found in studies that take a psychological or behavioral perspective on the exposure. However, more studies of high quality are needed in order to draw valid conclusions about the mechanisms and causal directions of associations.

Keywords: cell phone; epidemiology; psychology; behavioral addiction; depression; sleep

---

1. Introduction

Mobile phones have over only a few decades revolutionized how we communicate, interact, search for information, work, do chores, and pass time. The development of the smartphone with its multitude of functions, increased memory capacity and speed, and constant connectedness to the internet, has increased the time spent using the phone, implying a near ubiquitous usage. This fast development with changed exposure patterns has raised questions about potential health effects of the exposure [1,2]. The mobile phone communicates through emission of radio signals, and the exposure to radiofrequency electromagnetic fields has been proposed to be a health risk. There are today few indications that radiofrequency electromagnetic fields associated with mobile phones have any major health effects [3]. The World Health Organization (WHO) is currently undertaking a health risk assessment of radiofrequency electromagnetic fields, to be published as a monograph in the Environmental Health Criteria Series [4]. However, in addition to physiological aspects of the exposure, there is a growing research literature that takes a psychological or behavioral perspective on potential health effects of mobile phone use. The purpose of this literature review was to supplement the work of the WHO expert group by carrying out a literature review of quantitative observational studies that consider links between mobile phone use and mental health from a psychological or behavioral perspective. A formal systematic critical review with quality assessment of the papers was not done due to the large amount of included studies. The report presents an overview of the studies and examples of the main results. It does not include a comprehensive account of all included papers.

2. Materials and Methods

Two skilled university librarians performed systematic literature searches in PubMed and PsycINFO on 2 May 2016, with supplemental searches on 19 March 2018. The final search strategies (Table 1) aimed to identify scientific publications from 1993 to 31 December 2017 that included quantitative analyses of mobile phone use in relation to mental health outcomes and other psychological factors. Altogether, 4738 papers were identified, after automatic removal of duplicates. These were screened by title and abstract. Papers that considered radiofrequency electromagnetic fields (RF-EMF), attention or safety (while driving, working, or studying), consequences for relationships, sexual behavior (e.g., sexting), cyberbullying, as well as papers that were qualitative, case or experimental studies, literature reviews, or duplicates (not previously identified), were excluded. This left 404 articles to be retrieved in full text for evaluation. Another 114 papers were removed in accordance with the previously mentioned exclusion criteria, or if no mental health-related outcome could be distinguished, if mobile phone use could not be identified as a separate variable (e.g., was included in a composite variable such as "digital media" or "screen time"), if focused only on specific smartphone applications (e.g., Tinder, Facebook, camera) or phone loss scenarios, or were not in English. This left 290 studies [5–294] for closer scrutiny (Appendix A. PRISMA Flow Chart).

Table 1. Search strategies in PubMed and PsycINFO 2018-03-19.

Database	Search Strings
PubMed	"cell phones" [MeSH Terms] OR "mobile phone" [Text Word] OR "mobile telephone" [Text Word] OR "cell phone" [Text Word] OR "cellular phone" [Text Word] OR "cellular telephone" [Text Word] OR "mobile phones" [Text Word] OR "mobile telephones" [Text Word] OR "cellular phones" [Text Word] OR "cellular telephones" [Text Word] OR smartphone [MeSH Terms] OR smartphone [Text Word] AND Stress [Title/Abstract] OR Depress* [Title/Abstract] OR Sleep* [Title/Abstract] OR Addict* [Title/Abstract] OR problem* [Title/Abstract] OR Mental [Title/Abstract] OR psychol* [Title/Abstract] OR psychi* [Title/Abstract] OR insomnia [Title/Abstract] OR compuls* [Title/Abstract] OR patholog* [Title/Abstract] OR dependen* [Title/Abstract] OR anxi* [Title/Abstract] OR symptom* [Title/Abstract] AND ("1993/01/01" [PDat]: "2017/12/31" [PDat]) AND (English [lang] OR Norwegian [lang] OR Swedish [lang])
PsycINFO	ti ("cell phones" OR "mobile phone" OR "mobile telephone" OR "cell phone" OR "cellular phone" OR "cellular telephone" OR "mobile phones" OR "mobile telephones" OR "cellular phones" OR "cellular telephones" OR "smart phone" OR "smart phones" OR "smartphone" OR "smartphones") OR ab("cell phones" OR "mobile phone" OR "mobile telephone" OR "cell phone" OR "cellular phone" OR "cellular telephone" OR "mobile phones" OR "mobile telephones" OR "cellular phones" OR "cellular telephones" OR "smart phone" OR "smart phones" OR "smartphone" OR "smartphones") AND ti (Stress OR Depress* OR Sleep* OR Addict* OR problem* OR Mental OR psychol* OR psychi* OR insomnia OR compuls* OR patholog* OR dependen* OR anxi* OR symptom*) OR ab(Stress OR Depress* OR Sleep* OR Addict* OR problem* OR Mental OR psychol* OR psychi* OR insomnia OR compuls* OR patholog* OR dependen* OR anxi* OR symptom*) Filter Peer review, Eng, No 1993/01/01–2017/12/31

3. Results

The identified studies (n = 290) mainly dealt with frequency or duration of mobile phone use in relation to mental health symptoms (such as depression, anxiety, and insomnia), mobile phone use and sleep habits, and "problematic mobile phone use" (dependency/addiction). The number of published papers greatly increased during the time-period, especially the last five years (Table 2).

Table 2. Number of included papers (n = 290) by publication year.

2001	2002	2003	2004	2005	2006	2007	2008	2009	2010	2011	2012	2013	2014	2015	2016	2017 [1]
1	1	1	-	1	3	7	4	7	6	7	8	17	37	46	59	85

[1] Six papers were dated 2018 but had been published online previously and were categorized as 2017.

3.1. Study Designs and Populations

A massive majority of the retrieved studies had cross-sectional design. Only 14 studies, i.e., about 5% [26,65,95,123,132,144,148,156,184,249,268,269,274,286], were identified as having any form of longitudinal design, test-retest reliability studies excepted.

About one third of the studies were based on child or adolescent populations, mostly administered through schools. Of the more than 190 adult population studies, relatively few studies seemed to contain random or representative samples of adult populations. The majority were based on university or college student populations (>60%), or with students together with other groups (an additional 5%). Otherwise, participants were mainly recruited through advertisements, postings on websites (e.g., Mechanical Turk), mailing lists, or personal appeal, or were carried out in specific work places or health care units. Some papers lacked a description of the selection process of study participants altogether. The number of study participants varied from 40 to 120,115. Studies were performed on all continents.

3.2. Measurements

The vast majority of the studies were based on self-reported exposures and outcomes, mostly through pen-and-pencil or web questionnaires, but sometimes also through telephone or face-to-face interviews. For younger children, parental reports about the child's mobile phone use and health outcomes were used. The quantity of mobile phone use was mainly given in frequency and duration of calls and text messaging. However, with an increase of studies about smartphone usage, frequency and time spent on different apps and functions, including general screen time, were also examined. Many studies also included, for example, the type of phone, number of phones, from what age one had used a mobile phone, presence of a phone in the bedroom, what time the phone was used (e.g., time slots over the day, evening/nighttime use), and the size of the phone bill. A majority of the studies included scales or measurements of excessive or problematic mobile phone use (dependency/addiction), discussed further below.

Twelve studies could be identified as using objective measures for the quantity of mobile phone use. Three studies (conducted in the same population) used operator data for a subgroup of the participants [84,237,248]. The remaining studies used an app that was installed on the participants' phones to log usage [49,53,91,174–176,200,239,258]. Two studies included a procedure where participants responded to questions about activity, including mobile phone use, several times per day on a given signal [26,95].

Additional measurement methods for mental health variables included structured psychiatric interviews [49,126,177,196,197], actigraphy for sleep [83,205], and sleep diaries [5,83,144,205]. Two studies included magnetic resonance imaging of the participants' brains [110,283]. Further measurement methods occurred (e.g., body composition measurements, pedometers for physical activity, etc.), but did not pertain to mental health or psychological outcomes.

3.3. Main Research Findings

This section presents summaries and examples of the main findings in the included papers. The results have been clustered into three sections: (a) frequency/duration of mobile phone use and mental health outcomes, (b) bedtime mobile phone use, and (c) problematic mobile phone use. The main findings of each section are summarized in Tables 3–5. Table 6 summarizes the psychological factors that were most commonly associated with mobile phone use (all aspects).

3.3.1. Frequency/Duration of Mobile Phone Use and Mental Health Outcomes

Among the studies of children and adolescents, a longitudinal study with 126 US adolescents found that more time spent on mobile phone use at baseline was associated with increased depression, measured with Becks Depression Inventory for Primary care at the one-year follow-up, while controlling for baseline depression [26]. In another longitudinal study, adolescents who owned a smartphone compared to non-owners slept less and had more sleep problems at baseline. Following up after two years, there were no differences in sleep problems between smartphone owners, new owners, and non-owners, but those who had owned a smartphone since baseline, compared to those who still did not own a smartphone, had shorter sleep duration on weekdays [249]. Cross-sectional associations were seen between quantity of mobile phone use and depressive symptoms in a study with 2785 Japanese adolescents [113], a study with 1328 Spanish adolescents/young adults [244], and a study with 7292 Finnish adolescents [139]. Overall mobile phone use of more than 5 h per day among Japanese adolescents was not associated with depression after adjusting for confounders, while using the mobile phone for more than 2 h per day for social networking services or online chatting was [264]. In a large British study with 120,115 adolescents, smartphone use on the weekends was negatively associated with mental well-being, while the associations for weekday use was non-linear, in that only use above an extreme cut-off was negative for mental well-being [227]. In an Israeli study of 185 children, daily time spent on a smartphone was not associated with psychopathological outcomes [250]. Regarding sleep outcomes, a longitudinal study of Japanese adolescents found mobile phone use of 2 h per day to be associated with new insomnia onset at the two-year follow-up [274]. A cross-sectional German study with 7533 adolescents found associations between higher mobile phone use and sleep problems among the girls in the crude analysis, but these were not statistically significant when controlling for confounders [149]. In a study with 6247 Chinese schoolchildren, time spent on texting, playing games, or surfing the internet on the mobile phone was associated with later bedtimes, shorter sleep duration, difficulties initiating and maintaining sleep, and daytime tiredness [117]. Time spent on the mobile phone was associated with shorter sleep duration and tiredness also among Japanese adolescents [113], and with poor sleep quality and daytime sleepiness in adolescents in Hong Kong [187]. In a Finnish study, mobile phone use was associated with deteriorated sleep habits and daytime tiredness in 12–14 years old girls and boys, and in 16–18 years old girls [228].

Among the studies on adult populations, a prospective study with 1127 Swedish university students found frequent mobile phone use at baseline to be a risk factor for sleep problems and depressive symptoms at the one-year follow-up in the men, and prolonged stress in the women [268]. This study, however, did not account for any confounding factors. Another prospective cohort study with 4159 Swedish young adults which, besides sex, accounted for educational level, occupation, and relationship status, showed similar results: Frequent mobile phone use was a risk factor for new cases of sleep problems in men, and for depressive symptoms in both men and women at the one-year follow-up [269]. Among the cross-sectional studies, frequency and duration of mobile phone use, logged by an app on the participants' phones, was associated with depressed mood [239]. In another app log study, smartphone screen time was associated with depressed mood, but only before adjusting for confounders [53]. Cross-sectional associations were further seen between the frequency of calls and texts and perceived stress, sleep problems, and depressive symptoms among Swedish young adults [269]. A study that focused on work-related mobile phone use found that intensive mobile phone use among employees who had been provided by with a smartphone by the employer was associated with more work–home interference, less relaxation, less psychological detachment from work, and more exhaustion [65]. In other studies, time spent on the mobile phone was associated with anxiety [162], while the number of texts was associated with anxiety [29,162] and depressed mood [29]. A Finnish study with 6121 working-age participants, which examined mental symptoms in relation to the use of new technology, found associations between mobile phone use and depression in females 51–60 years, only [140]. Furthermore, in a US study with 308 adults, smartphone use frequency was negatively associated with depressive symptoms [74,75], and a Chinese study with 514 adults found that higher mobile use for calls was associated with higher mental well-being and positive affect [37].

Table 3. Frequency/duration of mobile phone use: summary of main results.

Outcomes	Study Designs and Citations
• Depression	L: [26,268,269] CS: [29,53,113,139,140,239,244,264,269] NA: [74,75]
• Sleep problems, lower sleep quality	L: [268,269,274] CS: [117,149,187,269]
• Later bedtimes, shorter sleep	CS: [103,113,117,228]
• Tiredness, reduced daytime function	CS: [65,113,117,187,228]
• Lower mental well-being	CS: [227] NA: [37]
• Stress	L: [268] CS: [269]
• Anxiety	CS: [29,162]

L = Longitudinal, CS = Cross-sectional, NA = Negative association. In crude, but not in adjusted, analyses: reference 53, 149. In subgroup of older women: reference 140.

Regarding personality, in one study, in which an app registered incoming and outgoing calls and text messages over five weeks among 49 German university students, associations between the number of calls and extraversion were seen, while no clear associations were found for the number of text messages and personality variables [200]. Another app log study found that smartphone use for calls was negatively associated with social anxiousness and loneliness [91]. One study concluded that lonely persons preferred to make voice calls rather than text messaging, while socially anxious persons preferred to text [231]. In a longitudinal study, increased mobile phone use over time was associated with decreased self-esteem and coping ability [286]. However, a one-week diary study that measured modes of social interaction found that meaningful text-based communication had a positive effect on self-esteem, compared to face-to-face communication and mobile phone voice communication [95]. Other studies found associations between time spent on mobile calls and extraversion [34] and low agreeableness [34,73], while text messaging was associated with neuroticism [34,73], extraversion [34], low self-esteem [73], low agreeableness [34], and low conscientiousness [34]. Time spent on mobile game playing was associated with low agreeableness [220,253].

3.3.2. Bedtime Mobile Phone Use

At least 35 studies addressed mobile phone use in the evening or at night: i.e., prior to bedtime, in bed, after "lights out", awakening at night because of the phone, or even just the presence of a phone in the bedroom. About two thirds of these studies were based on children or adolescent populations.

A longitudinal Australian study that included 1101 adolescents found cross-sectional associations between nighttime phone use, poor sleep behavior, and depressed mood [286], but in longitudinal analyses, changes in nighttime phone use was not directly associated with subsequent changes in depressed mood. However, changes in sleep behaviors acted as a mediator between night-time phone use and subsequent depressed mood [286]. Another longitudinal study found cross-sectional associations between nighttime awakenings by the phone and sleep problems, perceived stress, and depressive symptoms in young adults, but no statistically significant prospective associations were seen at the one-year follow-up [269]. A diary study of work-related smartphone use at night showed subsequent lower sleep quantity, which in turn was associated with greater fatigue the next morning and less engagement during the work day [148].

In cross-sectional studies with children, as well as with adults, bedtime mobile phone use (in the broad definition, above) was associated with later bedtimes [16,22,31,82,85,88,93,223,263], longer sleep onset latency [53,79,112,223,293], shorter sleep duration [14,15,22,36,71,82,86,148,161,202,210], insomnia or sleep problems [5,14,79,85,97,144,199,202,205,235,269,293], reduced sleep quality or sleep efficiency [5,32,53,71,79,82,83,167,202,205], and reduced daytime functioning or tiredness [79,86,93,112, 121,202,223,242,248,277,293]. In one study, keeping the phone close, rather than placing the phone at a distance from the bed, was associated with less sleep problems [235].

Almost all of the referred studies used self-reported sleep outcomes. However, two studies examined sleep by actigraphy in relation to self-reported mobile phone use [83,205]. Receiving night-time notifications on the phone predicted global sleep problems, subjective poor sleep quality, and sleep disruptions [205], and media use in bed or being awakened by the mobile phone at night negatively affected sleep efficiency [83].

Besides sleep outcomes, "bedtime" mobile phone use was associated with reduced mental health, suicidal feelings and self-injury [210], depressive symptoms [161,242,269,286], anxiety and stress [242], low self-esteem [286], and reduced cognitive performance in one study [235], but not in another [248].

Table 4. Bedtime mobile phone use: summary of main results.

Outcomes	Study Designs and Citations
• Sleep problems	CS: [5,14,79,85,97,144,199,202,205,235,269,293]
• Lower sleep quality/efficiency	CS: [5,32,53,71,79,82,83,167,202,205]
• Longer sleep onset latency	CS: [53,79,112,223,293]
• Poor sleep behavior	L: [286] CS: [286]
• Later bedtimes	CS: [16,22,31,82,85,88,93,223,263]
• Shorter sleep	CS: [14,15,22,36,71,82,86,148,161,202,210]
• Tiredness, reduced daytime function	L: [148] CS: [79,86,93,112,121,202,223,235,242,248,277,293]
• Depression	CS: [161,210,242,269,286]

L = Longitudinal, CS = Cross-sectional.

3.3.3. Problematic Mobile Phone Use

Approximately 70% of the papers in this literature review addressed what can be termed "excessive" or "problematic" mobile phone use. They explored health outcomes of excessive mobile phone use, predictors for excessive use, such as personality or other psychological factors, or were reliability and validity studies of scales. Research about overuse, excessive, dependent, addictive, problematic, or pathological mobile phone use has emerged in parallel with the increased mobile phone usage. The constructs are commonly referred to as behavioral addictions and are likened with other non-substance addictions such as gambling addiction. As such, it seems to be a case of impaired ability to regulate one's mobile phone use and can be associated with general symptoms of dependency, such as tolerance, withdrawal, escape, craving, using the mobile phone even when it is unsafe or prohibited, or functional consequences, such as financial or relational problems [295] (review, not included). A relationship can be seen with the concept of internet addiction, which was proposed as a specific psychiatric disorder in the 1990s by Young [296], who applied Diagnostic and Statistical Manual of Mental Disorders (DSM)-criteria for pathological gambling to internet use. Other constructs that have emerged include nomophobia and phubbing. Nomophobia is an abbreviation of "no mobile phone phobia" and refers to a phobia of not having access to a mobile phone [297]. It includes four dimensions: not being able to communicate, losing connectedness, not being able to access information, and giving up convenience [298]. The term "phubbing" comes from merging the words "phone" and "snubbing" and refers to when an individual is looking at or attending to his or her phone while in a conversation with others [124]. Yet another construct is "ringxiety", or "phantom ringing", which refers to perceiving that the phone rings even when it does not [260].

Excessive or problematic mobile phone use is usually associated with a high quantity of mobile phone use, while a high quantity of use does not necessarily imply problematic use. One of the papers concluded that mobile dependency was better predicted by personality factors (such as low self-esteem and extraversion) than actual phone use [108]. In one-month log data from 79 engineering students in Taiwan, a logarithm that combined frequency, duration, and frequency trend over time successfully predicted "smartphone addiction" [174,175]. Non-use patterns also predicted smartphone addiction [176]. Among functions that have been associated with excessive or problematic use are playing games [21,39,49,59,110,116,178] and the use of social networking sites (SNS) [33,39,49,116,183, 209,224,285,288]. Another log data study showed that dependent participants, besides games and SNS, also used the phone more for web surfing, shopping, and entertainment, and less for talking and texting, than non-dependent participants [49].

A whole array of scales (>50) were used for examining problematic use in the papers. The great number is partly due to the fact that some scales existed in several versions, and that different names for what appear to be the same scales occurred, perhaps due to translations between languages. Several of the scales follow diagnosis criteria from the International Statistical Classification of Diseases and Related Health Problems (ICD) or DSM for pathological gambling or substance dependence, and some scales are direct adaptations of Young's Internet Addiction Test [296], applied to mobile phones. Two of the most commonly referred to scales were the Mobile Phone Problem Use Scale (MPPUS) [25] and the Smartphone Addiction Scale (SAS) [146]. The MMPUS contains 27 items inspired from the addiction literature and covers areas such as tolerance, withdrawal, escape, craving, and negative consequences, giving a global score of problem use [25]. The SAS contains 48 items in six subscales: daily-life disturbance, positive anticipation, withdrawal, cyberspace-oriented relationship, overuse, and tolerance [146]. Several shortened versions of the scales were also used.

The prevalence of problematic mobile phone use varied greatly in the studies, which can be expected because the measures, definitions, and study populations varied. Most of the studies were cross-sectional. Among the exceptions was a longitudinal study with 1877 Korean adolescents that used three yearly measurements [123]. The study found bidirectional relationships between mobile phone addiction and depressive symptoms over time [123]; i.e., mobile phone addiction had an influence on depressive symptoms, and depressive symptoms influenced mobile phone addiction, over time. Another study in the same population showed that high mobile phone addiction was associated with an increase in incidence of poor sleep quality over time [156]. In a Swedish study, subjective overuse of the mobile phone at baseline was a prospective risk factor for sleep disturbances at the one-year follow-up in female young adults [269].

In addition, cross-sectional associations were seen between excessive or problematic use and depression [7,18,39,42,62,80,89,90,94,98,100,105,123,130,131,168,180,184,185,189,214,244,251,256, 267,269,282,290]. Conversely, in four studies, depression was negatively associated with problematic use [50,57,74,75]. Furthermore, associations were seen with anxiety [7,39,42,50,62,67,68,74–76,80,89, 100,108,115,135,157,180,184,189,198,214,245,267] (but, a negative association between text message dependency and anxiety in Reference [185]), sleep problems or insomnia [7,32,115,269], reduced sleep quality [38,39,62,80,110,195,240], shorter sleep duration [110,130,179,289], eveningness [64,229,273], stress [18,46,89,105,106,116,131,143,180,243,269,280,285], lower general mental wellbeing [20,23,76,80, 127,237], PTSD [55,56], suicidal thoughts [131,282,289], impulsivity or less self-control [27–30,33,46,56, 67,68,102,110,116,119,120,130,137,166,233,234,256,283,288,292], attention deficit hyperactivity disorder (ADHD)-symptoms [252], productivity loss at work [72], and perceived phantom ringing [142,260]. Moreover, problematic use was associated with other behavioral addictions (e.g., internet addiction [12, 19,43,45,50,52,63,100,105,118,127,145,146,154,178,186,198,217,236,266], shopping addiction [12,118, 188], gambling addiction [78,245], and general addiction proneness [126,245]). Two studies examined participants with magnetic resonance imaging; when comparing mobile phone dependent subjects with non-dependent participants, differences in white matter integrity of the brain were seen [110,283].

Table 5. Problematic mobile phone use: summary of main results.

Outcomes	Study Designs and Citations
• Depression	L: [123] (bidirectional) CS: [7,18,39,42,62,80,89,90,94,98,100,105,123,130,131,168,180,184,185,189,214,244,251,256,267,269,282,290] NA: [50,57,74,75]
• Anxiety	CS: [7,39,42,50,62,67,68,74–76,80,89,100,108,115,135,157,180,184,189,198,214,245,267] NA: [185]
• Sleep problems	L: [269] CS: [7,32,115,269]
• Lower sleep quality	L: [156] CS: [38,39,62,80,110,195,240]
• Shorter sleep	CS: [110,130,179,289]
• Stress	CS: [18,46,89,105,106,116,131,143,180,243,269,280,285]
• Lower mental wellbeing	CS: [20,23,76,80,127,237]
• Other behavioral addictions	CS: [12,19,43,45,50,52,63,78,100,105,118,126,127,145,146,154,178,186,188,198,217,236,245,266]

L = Longitudinal, CS = Cross-sectional, NA = Negative association.

Regarding psychological factors, several cross-sectional studies found associations between problematic mobile phone use and loneliness [24,91,98,129,133,158,270,279]. A longitudinal study with 288 participants 13–40 years of age examined causal relations between problematic use, loneliness, face-to-face-interaction, and the need for social assurance [132]. It found that loneliness predicted problematic use, while problematic use did not predict loneliness at the follow-up after four months. However, the authors concluded that loneliness increases problematic use, which in turn reduces face-to-face interactions and thus does not gratify increased needs for social assurance, and consequently, this process eventually leads to increased loneliness [132]. Other studies found associations with, e.g., shyness or social anxiousness [24,58,91,102,159], extraversion [12,13,18,25,46,64,81,108,255,256,261], fear of missing out [52,74,153,209,287], neuroticism [13,46,73,81,90,111,142,147,198,218,261,294], less self-esteem [13,25,100,108,256,281,289,291], low agreeableness [12,147], less openness [12,111,147,218,261], less conscientiousness [13,34,92,111,142,147,169,170], alexithymia [89], and less self-efficacy [99].

Table 6. Summary of the psychological factors most commonly associated with mobile phone use (all aspects).

Psychological Factors	Citations
• Impulsivity/less self-control	[27–30,33,46,56,67,68,102,110,114,116,119,120,130,137,166,233,234,256,283,288,292]
• Extraversion	[12,13,18,25,34,46,64,81,108,200,255,256,261]
• Neuroticism	[13,34,46,73,81,90,111,142,147,198,218,261,294]
• Less self-esteem	[13,25,73,100,108,256,281,286,289,291] NA: [95]
• Loneliness	[24,91,98,129,132,133,158,231,270,279] NA: [91]
• Less conscientiousness	[13,34,92,111,142,147,169,170]
• Low agreeableness	[12,34,73,147,220,253]
• Social anxiety, shyness	[24,58,91,102,159,231] NA: [91]
• Less openness	[12,111,147,218,261]
• Fear of missing out	[52,74,153,209,287]

NA = Negative association.

4. Discussion

The literature search showed that there is a vast—and increasing—amount of studies that explore links between mobile phone usage and mental health from a psychological or behavioral point of view. A high quantity of mobile phone use was associated with a wide range of mental health outcomes, such as depressive symptoms and sleep problems, in both children and adults. A relatively large proportion of the studies examined mobile phone use in relation to sleep habits; mobile phone use at bedtime or at night was associated with, e.g., shorter sleep and reduced quality of sleep. A dominating research field was excessive or problematic use, i.e., where intense mobile phone use is described as a behavioral addiction and/or pathological. A large amount of instruments to measure excessive or problematic use occurred, and problematic use was associated with several adverse outcomes, such as depression, anxiety, and sleep problems.

Only a few percent of the included studies had any form of longitudinal design. Cross-sectional studies limit the possibilities to draw valid conclusions about causal directions of associations. The found associations may thus be due to reversed causality, i.e., the outcome is causing what seems to be the risk factor, or the associations may be bi-directional or caused by common confounding factors not accounted for. For example, most of the studies on bedtime phone use and sleep variables were cross-sectional. In a longitudinal study with Canadian students [299] (not in the review due to the fact that mobile phone use was not analyzed separately), it was sleep problems that predicted media use and not the opposite. The researchers concluded that young adults used digital media to deal with sleep problems. Moreover, a study with 844 Belgian adults [300] (also not in the review) concluded that media, including mobile phones, was commonly used as a sleep aid.

Further, a majority of the papers were based on self-reporting, which implies that both exposures and outcomes may be subject to misclassification, recall difficulty, recall bias, and response-style bias. It is previously known that there is rather low agreement between self-reported mobile phone use for calling or texting compared to logged data (e.g., [301]), and this applies also to smartphone usage [297]. However, it seems that applications that log smartphone usage are becoming more available, and thus are increasingly used in research.

Strikingly, many of the studies on adult populations were done on university students or self-selected participants. This compromises generalizability of the results. Another observation was that in many studies, the found associations, although statistically significant, were small.

The current literature review focused on studies with mobile phone use as a specific entity. Broadening the search to include more general terms such as "screen time", "media use", "technology use", or "social media", would lead to a higher quantity of studies with results that probably could apply also to mobile phone usage. Several different technologies (such as computers, tablets, or other hand-held devices) are used for the same activities and in the same contexts, and results from studies that include other technologies are seen to show similar results. However, a broader definition of the exposure was outside the scope of this review.

Intense or frequent mobile phone usage is seen to be associated with a broad array of mental health related symptoms, behaviors, and psychological factors. Plausible behavioral and/or psychological mechanisms for the associations can be found in the review, such as impact on sleep habits, dependency/addiction issues, and individual personality traits. The extent to which mobile phone use interferes with the restorative functions of sleep can, of course, contribute to deteriorated health. Besides sleep being postponed, replaced, or disturbed by messages or calls at night, it is also conceivable that quantity as well as content of use can generate higher levels of psychological stress and physiological arousal. Higher levels of arousal can have a negative impact on sleep and recovery [302] and in other ways contribute to stress and ill health. In addition, there are studies [303,304] (not in the review) pointing to the fact that blue light emitted from screens may have an impact on melatonin levels and thus affect sleep and wakefulness.

It is also conceivable that the time spent on devices takes time from other activities and health-related behaviors, such as physical activity, supportive social interactions, or staying on task at work or school. In the current review, several relevant aspects were excluded in the literature search, for example, the impact of mobile phone use on attention, consequences for relationships, cyberbullying, cyber sexual behaviors, and physical health outcomes, all aspects likely to potentially have an impact on mental health. Furthermore, this report does not account for all factors analyzed in the included papers.

This review was done to supplement a systematic review of the potential health effects of exposure to radiofrequency electromagnetic fields (RF-EMF) from mobile phones. In light of this, it can be noted that there are several psychological and behavioral aspects that should be taken into consideration when assessing studies that examine health effects with RF-EMF exposure as the hypothesis. This is especially true given that many of the studies with an RF-EMF-perspective measure the exposures in the same manner as studies taking a psychological or behavioral perspective, i.e., with self-report.

5. Conclusions

Associations between mobile phone use and adverse mental health outcomes are found in studies that take a psychological or behavioral perspective on the exposure. However, more studies of high quality are needed—with longitudinal design, objective measurements, and well-defined study populations—in order to draw valid conclusions about mechanisms and causal directions of associations.

Appendix A

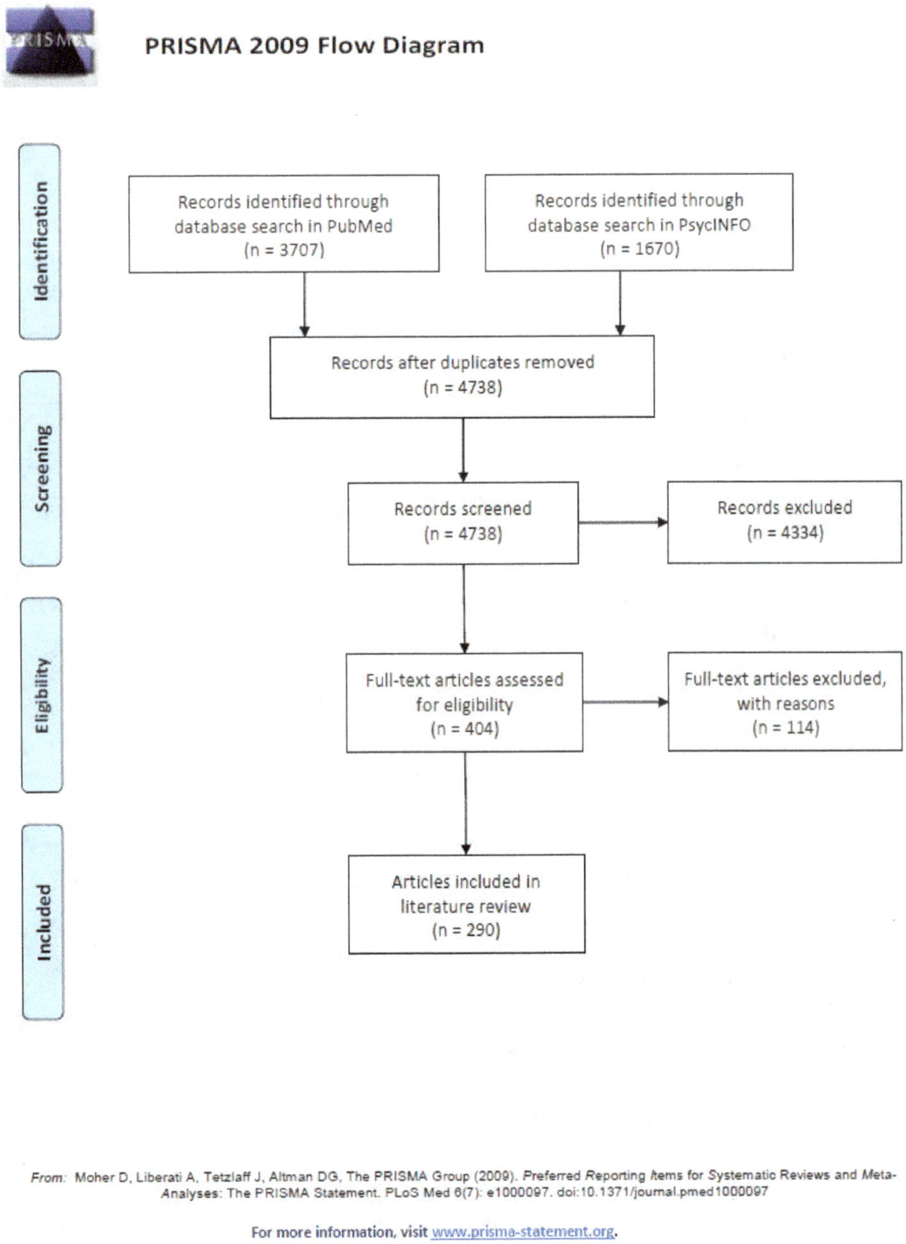

References

1. World Health Organization. Electromagnetic Fields and Public Health: Mobile Phones. Available online: http://www.who.int/en/news-room/fact-sheets/detail/electromagnetic-fields-and-public-health-mobile-phones (accessed on 12 November 2018).
2. US Food & Drug Administration (FDA). Health Issues: Do Cell Phones Pose a Health Hazard? Available online: https://www.fda.gov/Radiation-EmittingProducts/RadiationEmittingProductsandProcedures/HomeBusinessandEntertainment/CellPhones/ucm116282.htm (accessed on 12 November 2018).
3. Swedish Radiation Safety Authority. Recent Research on EMF and Health Risk. Twelfth Report from SSM's Scientific Council on Electromagnetic Fields. 2017. Available online: www.stralsakerhetsmyndigheten.se (accessed on 24 September 2018).
4. World Health Organization. Available online: http://www.who.int/peh-emf/research/rf_ehc_page/en/ (accessed on 24 September 2018).
5. Adams, S.K.; Kisler, T.S. Sleep quality as a mediator between technology-related sleep quality, depression, and anxiety. *Cyberpsychol. Behav. Soc. Netw.* **2013**, *16*, 25–30. [CrossRef] [PubMed]
6. Aggarwal, M.; Grover, S.; Basu, D. Mobile phone use by resident doctors: Tendency to addiction-like behaviour. *German J. Psychiatry* **2012**, *15*, 50–55.
7. Aker, S.; Sahin, M.K.; Sezgin, S.; Oguz, G. Psychosocial factors affecting Smartphone Addiction in university students. *J. Addict. Nurs.* **2017**, *28*, 215–219. [CrossRef] [PubMed]
8. Alavi, S.S.; Maracy, M.R.; Jannatifard, F.; Ojaghi, R.; Rezapour, H. The psychometric properties of cellular phone dependency questionnaire in students of Isfahan: A pilot study. *J. Educ. Health Promot.* **2014**, *3*, 71. [CrossRef] [PubMed]
9. Alavi, S.S.; Mohammadi, M.R.; Jannatifard, F.; Mohammadi Kalhori, S.; Sepahbodi, G.; BabaReisi, M.; Sajedi, S.; Farshchi, M.; KhodaKarami, R.; Hatami Kasvaee, V. Assessment of Semi-Structured Clinical Interview for Mobile Phone Addiction Disorder. *Iran. J. Psychiatry* **2016**, *11*, 115–119. [PubMed]
10. Aljomaa, S.S.; Al.Qudah, M.F.; Albursan, I.S.; Bakhiet, S.F.; Abduljabbar, A.S. Smartphone addiction among university students in the light of some variables. *Comput. Hum. Behav.* **2016**, *61*, 155–164. [CrossRef]
11. Alosaimi, F.D.; Alyahya, H.; Alshahwan, H.; Al Mahyijari, N.; Shaik, S.A. Smartphone addiction among university students in Riyadh, Saudi Arabia. *Saudi Med. J.* **2016**, *37*, 675–683. [CrossRef] [PubMed]
12. Andreassen, C.S.; Griffiths, M.D.; Gjertsen, S.R.; Krossbakken, E.; Kvam, S.; Pallesen, S. The relationships between behavioral addictions and the five-factor model of personality. *J. Behav. Addict.* **2013**, *2*, 90–99. [CrossRef] [PubMed]
13. Argumosa-Villar, L.; Boada-Grau, J.; Vigil-Colet, A. Exploratory investigation of theoretical predictors of nomophobia using the Mobile Phone Involvement Questionnaire (MPIQ). *J. Adolesc.* **2017**, *56*, 127–135. [CrossRef] [PubMed]
14. Arora, T.; Broglia, E.; Thomas, G.N.; Taheri, S. Associations between specific technologies and adolescent sleep quantity, sleep quality, and parasomnias. *Sleep Med.* **2014**, *15*, 240–247. [CrossRef] [PubMed]
15. Arora, T.; Hussain, S.; Hubert Lam, K.B.; Lily Yao, G.; Neil Thomas, G.; Taheri, S. Exploring the complex pathways among specific types of technology, self-reported sleep duration and body mass index in UK adolescents. *Int. J. Obes.* **2013**, *37*, 1254–1260. [CrossRef] [PubMed]
16. Arrona-Palacios, A. High and low use of electronic media during nighttime before going to sleep: A comparative study between adolescents attending a morning or afternoon school shift. *J. Adolesc.* **2017**, *61*, 152–163. [CrossRef] [PubMed]
17. Atwood, R.M.; Beckert, T.E.; Rhodes, M.R. Adolescent problematic digital behaviors associated with mobile devices. *N. Am. J. Psychol.* **2017**, *19*, 659–684.
18. Augner, C.; Hacker, G.W. Associations between problematic mobile phone use and psychological parameters in young adults. *Int. J. Public Health* **2012**, *57*, 437–441. [CrossRef] [PubMed]
19. Ayar, D.; Bektas, M.; Bektas, I.; Akdeniz Kudubes, A.; Selekoglu Ok, Y.; Sal Altan, S.; Celik, I. The Effect of Adolescents' Internet Addiction on Smartphone Addiction. *J. Addict. Nurs.* **2017**, *28*, 210–214. [CrossRef] [PubMed]
20. Babadi-Akashe, Z.; Zamani, B.E.; Abedini, Y.; Akbari, H.; Hedayati, N. The Relationship between Mental Health and Addiction to Mobile Phones among University Students of Shahrekord, Iran. *Addict. Health* **2014**, *6*, 93–99. [PubMed]

21. Bae, S.M. The relationship between the type of smartphone use and smartphone dependence of Korean adolescents: National survey study. *Child. Youth Serv. Rev.* **2017**, *81*, 207–211. [CrossRef]
22. Bartel, K.; Williamson, P.; van Maanen, A.; Cassoff, J.; Meijer, A.M.; Oort, F.; Knauper, B.; Gruber, R.; Gradisar, M. Protective and risk factors associated with adolescent sleep: Findings from Australia, Canada, and The Netherlands. *Sleep Med.* **2016**, *26*, 97–103. [CrossRef] [PubMed]
23. Beranuy, M.; Oberst, U.; Carbonell, X.; Chamarro, A. Problematic internet and mobile phone use and clinical symptoms in college students: The role of emotional intelligence. *Comput. Hum. Behav.* **2009**, *25*, 1182–1187. [CrossRef]
24. Bian, M.; Leung, L. Linking loneliness, shyness, smartphone addiction symptoms, and patterns of smartphone use to social capital. *Soc. Sci. Comput. Rev.* **2015**, *33*, 61–79. [CrossRef]
25. Bianchi, A.; Phillips, J.G. Psychological predictors of problem mobile phone use. *Cyberpsychol. Behav.* **2005**, *8*, 39–51. [CrossRef] [PubMed]
26. Bickham, D.S.; Hswen, Y.; Rich, M. Media use and depression: Exposure, household rules, and symptoms among young adolescents in the USA. *Int. J. Public Health* **2015**, *60*, 147–155. [CrossRef] [PubMed]
27. Billieux, J.; Gay, P.; Rochat, L.; Van der Linden, M. The role of urgency and its underlying psychological mechanisms in problematic behaviours. *Behav. Res. Ther.* **2010**, *48*, 1085–1096. [CrossRef] [PubMed]
28. Billieux, J.; van der Linden, M.; D'Acremont, M.; Ceschi, G.; Zermatten, A. Does impulsivity relate to perceived dependence on and actual use of the mobile phone? *Appl. Cogn. Psychol.* **2007**, *21*, 527–537. [CrossRef]
29. Billieux, J.; Van Der Linden, M.; Rochat, L. The role of impulsivity in actual and problematic use of the mobile phone. *Appl. Cogn. Psychol.* **2008**, *22*, 1195–1210. [CrossRef]
30. Bock, B.C.; Lantini, R.; Thind, H.; Walaska, K.; Rosen, R.K.; Fava, J.L.; Barnett, N.P.; Scott-Sheldon, L.A. The Mobile Phone Affinity Scale: Enhancement and Refinement. *JMIR mHealth uHealth* **2016**, *4*, e134. [CrossRef] [PubMed]
31. Brunborg, G.S.; Mentzoni, R.A.; Molde, H.; Myrseth, H.; Skouverøe, K.J.M.; Bjorvatn, B.; Pallesen, S. The relationship between media use in the bedroom, sleep habits and symptoms of insomnia. *J. Sleep Res.* **2011**, *20*, 569–575. [CrossRef] [PubMed]
32. Bruni, O.; Sette, S.; Fontanesi, L.; Baiocco, R.; Laghi, F.; Baumgartner, E. Technology Use and Sleep Quality in Preadolescence and Adolescence. *J. Clin. Sleep Med.* **2015**, *11*, 1433–1441. [CrossRef] [PubMed]
33. Burnell, K.; Kuther, T.L. Predictors of Mobile Phone and Social Networking Site Dependency in Adulthood. *Cyberpsychol. Behav. Soc. Netw.* **2016**, *19*, 621–627. [CrossRef] [PubMed]
34. Butt, S.; Phillips, J.G. Personality and self reported mobile phone use. *Comput. Hum. Behav.* **2008**, *24*, 346–360. [CrossRef]
35. Carbonell, X.; Chamarro, A.; Griffiths, M.; Oberst, U.; Cladellas, R.; Talarn, A. Problematic Internet and cell phone use in Spanish teenagers and young students. *Anales de Psicología* **2012**, *28*, 789–796.
36. Chahal, H.; Fung, C.; Kuhle, S.; Veugelers, P.J. Availability and night-time use of electronic entertainment and communication devices are associated with short sleep duration and obesity among Canadian children. *Pediatr. Obes.* **2013**, *8*, 42–51. [CrossRef] [PubMed]
37. Chan, M. Mobile phones and the good life: Examining the relationships among mobile use, social capital and subjective well-being. *New Media Soc.* **2015**, *17*, 96–113. [CrossRef]
38. Chang, A.K.; Choi, J. Predictors of sleep quality among young adults in Korea: Gender differences. *Issues Ment. Health Nurs.* **2016**, *37*, 918–928. [CrossRef] [PubMed]
39. Chen, B.; Liu, F.; Ding, S.; Ying, X.; Wang, L.; Wen, Y. Gender differences in factors associated with smartphone addiction: A cross-sectional study among medical college students. *BMC Psychiatry* **2017**, *17*, 341. [CrossRef] [PubMed]
40. Chen, C.; Zhang, K.Z.K.; Gong, X.; Zhao, S.J.; Lee, M.K.O.; Liang, L. Understanding compulsive smartphone use: An empirical test of a flow-based model. *Int. J. Inf. Manag.* **2017**, *37*, 438–454. [CrossRef]
41. Chen, C.; Zhang, K.Z.K.; Gong, X.; Zhao, S.J.; Lee, M.K.O.; Liang, L. Examining the effects of motives and gender differences on smartphone addiction. *Comput. Hum. Behav.* **2017**, *75*, 891–902. [CrossRef]
42. Chen, L.; Yan, Z.; Tang, W.; Yang, F.; Xie, X.; He, J. Mobile phone addiction levels and negative emotions among Chinese young adults: The mediating role of interpersonal problems. *Comput. Hum. Behav.* **2016**, *55*, 856–866. [CrossRef]

43. Ching, S.M.; Yee, A.; Ramachandran, V.; Sazlly Lim, S.M.; Wan Sulaiman, W.A.; Foo, Y.L.; Hoo, F.K. Validation of a Malay Version of the Smartphone Addiction Scale among Medical Students in Malaysia. *PLoS ONE* **2015**, *10*, e0139337. [CrossRef] [PubMed]
44. Chiu, S.I. The relationship between life stress and smartphone addiction on Taiwanese university student: A mediation model of learning self-Efficacy and social self-Efficacy. *Comput. Hum. Behav.* **2014**, *34*, 49–57. [CrossRef]
45. Chiu, S.I.; Hong, F.Y.; Chiu, S.L. An Analysis on the Correlation and Gender Difference between College Students' Internet Addiction and Mobile Phone Addiction in Taiwan. *ISRN Addict.* **2013**, *2013*, 360607. [CrossRef] [PubMed]
46. Cho, H.Y.; Kim, D.J.; Park, J.W. Stress and adult smartphone addiction: Mediation by self-control, neuroticism, and extraversion. *Stress Health* **2017**, *33*, 624–630. [CrossRef] [PubMed]
47. Cho, K.S.; Lee, J.M. Influence of smartphone addiction proneness of young children on problematic behaviors and emotional intelligence: Mediating self-assessment effects of parents using smartphones. *Comput. Hum. Behav.* **2017**, *66*, 303–311. [CrossRef]
48. Cho, S.; Lee, E. Development of a brief instrument to measure smartphone addiction among nursing students. *Comput. Inform. Nurs.* **2015**, *33*, 216–224. [CrossRef] [PubMed]
49. Choi, J.; Rho, M.J.; Kim, Y.; Yook, I.H.; Yu, H.; Kim, D.J.; Choi, I.Y. Smartphone dependence classification using tensor factorization. *PLoS ONE* **2017**, *12*, e0177629. [CrossRef] [PubMed]
50. Choi, S.W.; Kim, D.J.; Choi, J.S.; Ahn, H.; Choi, E.J.; Song, W.Y.; Kim, S.; Youn, H. Comparison of risk and protective factors associated with smartphone addiction and Internet addiction. *J. Behav. Addict.* **2015**, *4*, 308–314. [CrossRef] [PubMed]
51. Choliz, M.; Pinto, L.; Phansalkar, S.S.; Corr, E.; Mujjahid, A.; Flores, C.; Barrientos, P.E. Development of a Brief Multicultural Version of the Test of Mobile Phone Dependence (TMDbrief) Questionnaire. *Front. Psychol.* **2016**, *7*, 650. [CrossRef] [PubMed]
52. Chotpitayasunondh, V.; Douglas, K.M. How "phubbing" becomes the norm: The antecedents and consequences of snubbing via smartphone. *Comput. Hum. Behav.* **2016**, *63*, 9–18. [CrossRef]
53. Christensen, M.A.; Bettencourt, L.; Kaye, L.; Moturu, S.T.; Nguyen, K.T.; Olgin, J.E.; Pletcher, M.J.; Marcus, G.M. Direct Measurements of Smartphone Screen-Time: Relationships with Demographics and Sleep. *PLoS ONE* **2016**, *11*, e0165331. [CrossRef] [PubMed]
54. Chung, N. Korean adolescent girls' addictive use of mobile phones to maintain interpersonal solidarity. *Soc. Behav. Personal.* **2011**, *39*, 1349–1358. [CrossRef]
55. Contractor, A.A.; Frankfurt, S.B.; Weiss, N.H.; Elhai, J.D. Latent-level relations between DSM-5 PTSD symptom clusters and problematic smartphone use. *Comput. Hum. Behav.* **2017**, *72*, 170–177. [CrossRef] [PubMed]
56. Contractor, A.A.; Weiss, N.H.; Tull, M.T.; Elhai, J.D. PTSD's relation with problematic smartphone use: Mediating role of impulsivity. *Comput. Hum. Behav.* **2017**, *75*, 177–183. [CrossRef]
57. Csibi, S.; Griffiths, M.D.; Cook, B.; Demetrovics, Z.; Szabo, A. The psychometric properties of the Smartphone Application-Based Addiction Scale (SABAS). *Int. J. Ment. Health Addict.* **2018**, *16*, 393–403. [CrossRef] [PubMed]
58. Darcin, A.E.; Kose, S.; Noyan, C.O.; Nurmedov, S.; Yılmaz, O.; Dilbaz, N. Smartphone addiction and its relationship with social anxiety and loneliness. *Behav. Inf. Technol.* **2016**, *35*, 520–525. [CrossRef]
59. Das, A.; Sharma, M.K.; Thamilselvan, P.; Marimuthu, P. Technology Addiction among Treatment Seekers for Psychological Problems: Implication for Screening in Mental Health Setting. *Indian J. Psychol. Med.* **2017**, *39*, 21–27. [PubMed]
60. Dasgupta, P.; Bhattacherjee, S.; Dasgupta, S.; Roy, J.K.; Mukherjee, A.; Biswas, R. Nomophobic behaviors among smartphone using medical and engineering students in two colleges of West Bengal. *Indian J. Public Health* **2017**, *61*, 199–204. [PubMed]
61. Deleuze, J.; Rochat, L.; Romo, L.; Van der Linden, M.; Achab, S.; Thorens, G.; Khazaal, Y.; Zullino, D.; Maurage, P.; Rothen, S.; et al. Prevalence and characteristics of addictive behaviors in a community sample: A latent class analysis. *Addict. Behav. Rep.* **2015**, *1*, 49–56. [CrossRef] [PubMed]
62. Demirci, K.; Akgonul, M.; Akpinar, A. Relationship of smartphone use severity with sleep quality, depression, and anxiety in university students. *J. Behav. Addict.* **2015**, *4*, 85–92. [CrossRef] [PubMed]

63. Demirci, K.; Orhan, H.; Demirdas, A.; Akpinar, A.; Sert, H. Validity and reliability of the Turkish Version of the Smartphone Addiction Scale in a younger population. *Klinik Psikofarmakoloji Bülteni/Bull. Clin. Psychopharmacol.* **2014**, *24*, 226–234. [CrossRef]
64. Demirhan, E.; Randler, C.; Horzum, M.B. Is problematic mobile phone use explained by chronotype and personality? *Chronobiol. Int.* **2016**, *33*, 821–831. [CrossRef] [PubMed]
65. Derks, D.; Bakker, A.B. Smartphone use, work–home interference, and burnout: A diary study on the role of recovery. *Appl. Psychol. Int. Rev.* **2014**, *63*, 411–440. [CrossRef]
66. De-Sola, J.; Talledo, H.; Rodriguez de Fonseca, F.; Rubio, G. Prevalence of problematic cell phone use in an adult population in Spain as assessed by the Mobile Phone Problem Use Scale (MPPUS). *PLoS ONE* **2017**, *12*, e0181184. [CrossRef] [PubMed]
67. De-Sola, J.; Talledo, H.; Rubio, G.; de Fonseca, F.R. Development of a Mobile Phone Addiction Craving Scale and Its Validation in a Spanish Adult Population. *Front. Psychiatry* **2017**, *8*, 90. [CrossRef] [PubMed]
68. De-Sola, J.; Talledo, H.; Rubio, G.; de Fonseca, F.R. Psychological Factors and Alcohol Use in Problematic Mobile Phone Use in the Spanish Population. *Front. Psychiatry* **2017**, *8*, 11. [CrossRef] [PubMed]
69. Dixit, S.; Shukla, H.; Bhagwat, A.; Bindal, A.; Goyal, A.; Zaidi, A.K.; Shrivastava, A. A study to evaluate mobile phone dependence among students of a medical college and associated hospital of central India. *Indian J. Community Med.* **2010**, *35*, 339–341. [CrossRef] [PubMed]
70. Dlodlo, N. Salient indicators of mobile instant messaging addiction with selected socio-demographic attributes among tertiary students in South Africa. *S. Afr. J. Psychol.* **2015**, *45*, 207–222. [CrossRef]
71. Dube, N.; Khan, K.; Loehr, S.; Chu, Y.; Veugelers, P. The use of entertainment and communication technologies before sleep could affect sleep and weight status: A population-based study among children. *Int. J. Behav. Nutr. Phys. Act.* **2017**, *14*, 97. [CrossRef] [PubMed]
72. Duke, E.; Montag, C. Smartphone addiction, daily interruptions and self-reported productivity. *Addict. Behav. Rep.* **2017**, *6*, 90–95. [CrossRef] [PubMed]
73. Ehrenberg, A.; Juckes, S.; White, K.M.; Walsh, S.P. Personality and self-esteem as predictors of young people's technology use. *Cyberpsychol. Behav.* **2008**, *11*, 739–741. [CrossRef] [PubMed]
74. Elhai, J.D.; Levine, J.C.; Dvorak, R.D.; Hall, B.J. Fear of missing out, need for touch, anxiety and depression are related to problematic smartphone use. *Comput. Hum. Behav.* **2016**, *63*, 509–516. [CrossRef]
75. Elhai, J.D.; Levine, J.C.; Dvorak, R.D.; Hall, B.J. Non-social features of smartphone use are most related to depression, anxiety and problematic smartphone use. *Comput. Hum. Behav.* **2016**, *69*, 75–82. [CrossRef]
76. Emelin, V.A.; Rasskazova, E.I.; Tkhostov, A.S. Technology-related transformations of imaginary body boundaries: Psychopathology of the everyday excessive Internet and mobile phone use. *Psychol. Russ. State Art* **2017**, *10*, 177–189.
77. Emelin, V.A.; Tkhostov, A.S.; Rasskazova, E.I. Psychological adaptation in the info-communication society: The revised version of the Technology-Related Psychological Consequences Questionnaire. *Psychol. Russ. State Art* **2014**, *7*, 105–120. [CrossRef]
78. Enwereuzor, I.K.; Ugwu, L.I.; Ugwu, D.I. Role of smartphone addiction in gambling passion and schoolwork engagement: A Dualistic Model of Passion approach. *Asian J. Gambl. Issues Public Health* **2016**, *6*, 9. [CrossRef] [PubMed]
79. Exelmans, L.; Van den Bulck, J. Bedtime mobile phone use and sleep in adults. *Soc. Sci. Med.* **2016**, *148*, 93–101. [CrossRef] [PubMed]
80. Eyvazlou, M.; Zarei, E.; Rahimi, A.; Abazari, M. Association between overuse of mobile phones on quality of sleep and general health among occupational health and safety students. *Chronobiol. Int.* **2016**, *33*, 293–300. [CrossRef] [PubMed]
81. Ezoe, S.; Toda, M.; Yoshimura, K.; Naritomi, A.; Den, R.; Morimoto, K. Relationships of personality and lifestyle with mobile phone dependence among female nursing students. *Soc. Behav. Personal.* **2009**, *37*, 231–238. [CrossRef]
82. Falbe, J.; Davison, K.K.; Franckle, R.L.; Ganter, C.; Gortmaker, S.L.; Smith, L.; Land, T.; Taveras, E.M. Sleep duration, restfulness, and screens in the sleep environment. *Pediatrics* **2015**, *135*, e367–e375. [CrossRef] [PubMed]
83. Fobian, A.D.; Avis, K.; Schwebel, D.C. Impact of media use on adolescent sleep efficiency. *J. Dev. Behav. Pediatr.* **2016**, *37*, 9–14. [CrossRef] [PubMed]

84. Foerster, M.; Roser, K.; Schoeni, A.; Roosli, M. Problematic mobile phone use in adolescents: Derivation of a short scale MPPUS-10. *Int. J. Public Health* **2015**, *60*, 277–286. [CrossRef] [PubMed]
85. Fossum, I.N.; Nordnes, L.T.; Storemark, S.S.; Bjorvatn, B.; Pallesen, S. The association between use of electronic media in bed before going to sleep and insomnia symptoms, daytime sleepiness, morningness, and chronotype. *Behav. Sleep Med.* **2014**, *12*, 343–357. [CrossRef] [PubMed]
86. Fuller, C.; Lehman, E.; Hicks, S.; Novick, M.B. Bedtime Use of Technology and Associated Sleep Problems in Children. *Glob. Pediatr. Health* **2017**, *4*. [CrossRef] [PubMed]
87. Gallimberti, L.; Buja, A.; Chindamo, S.; Terraneo, A.; Marini, E.; Rabensteiner, A.; Vinelli, A.; Perez, L.J.; Baldo, V. Problematic cell phone use for text messaging and substance abuse in early adolescence (11- to 13-year-olds). *Eur. J. Pediatr.* **2016**, *175*, 355–364. [CrossRef] [PubMed]
88. Gamble, A.L.; D'Rozario, A.L.; Bartlett, D.J.; Williams, S.; Bin, Y.S.; Grunstein, R.R.; Marshall, N.S. Adolescent sleep patterns and night-time technology use: Results of the Australian Broadcasting Corporation's Big Sleep Survey. *PLoS ONE* **2014**, *9*, e111700. [CrossRef] [PubMed]
89. Gao, T.; Li, J.; Zhang, H.; Gao, J.; Kong, Y.; Hu, Y.; Mei, S. The influence of alexithymia on mobile phone addiction: The role of depression, anxiety and stress. *J. Affect. Disord.* **2018**, *225*, 761–766. [CrossRef] [PubMed]
90. Gao, T.; Xiang, Y.T.; Zhang, H.; Zhang, Z.; Mei, S. Neuroticism and quality of life: Multiple mediating effects of smartphone addiction and depression. *Psychiatry Res.* **2017**, *258*, 457–461. [CrossRef] [PubMed]
91. Gao, Y.; Li, A.; Zhu, T.; Liu, X.; Liu, X. How smartphone usage correlates with social anxiety and loneliness. *PeerJ* **2016**, *4*, e2197. [CrossRef] [PubMed]
92. Garcia-Oliva, C.; Piqueras, J.A. Experiential avoidance and technological addictions in adolescents. *J. Behav. Addict.* **2016**, *5*, 293–303. [CrossRef] [PubMed]
93. Garmy, P.; Ward, T.M. Sleep habits and nighttime texting among adolescents. *J. Sch. Nurs.* **2017**, *34*, 121–127. [CrossRef] [PubMed]
94. Ghasempour, A.; Mahmoodi-Aghdam, M. The Role of Depression and Attachment Styles in Predicting Students' Addiction to Cell Phones. *Addict. Health* **2015**, *7*, 192–197. [PubMed]
95. Gonzales, A.L. Text-based communication influences self-esteem more than face-to-face or cellphone communication. *Comput. Hum. Behav.* **2014**, *39*, 197–203. [CrossRef]
96. Gonzalez-Cabrera, J.; Leon-Mejia, A.; Perez-Sancho, C.; Calvete, E. Adaptation of the Nomophobia Questionnaire (NMP-Q) to Spanish in a sample of adolescents. *Actas Esp. Psiquiatr.* **2017**, *45*, 137–144. [PubMed]
97. Gradisar, M.; Wolfson, A.R.; Harvey, A.G.; Hale, L.; Rosenberg, R.; Czeisler, C.A. The sleep and technology use of Americans: Findings from the National Sleep Foundation's 2011 Sleep in America poll. *J. Clin. Sleep Med.* **2013**, *9*, 1291–1299. [CrossRef] [PubMed]
98. Güzeller, C.O.; Coşguner, T. Development of a Problematic Mobile Phone Use Scale for Turkish adolescents. *Cyberpsychol. Behav. Soc. Netw.* **2012**, *15*, 205–211. [CrossRef] [PubMed]
99. Gökçearslan, Ş.; Mumcu, F.K.; Haşlaman, T.; Çevik, Y.D. Modelling smartphone addiction: The role of smartphone usage, self-regulation, general self-efficacy and cyberloafing in university students. *Comput. Hum. Behav.* **2016**, *63*, 639–649. [CrossRef]
100. Ha, J.H.; Chin, B.; Park, D.-H.; Ryu, S.-H.; Yu, J. Characteristics of excessive cellular phone use in Korean adolescents. *Cyberpsychol. Behav.* **2008**, *11*, 783–784. [CrossRef] [PubMed]
101. Hadlington, L.J. Cognitive failures in daily life: Exploring the link with Internet addiction and problematic mobile phone use. *Comput. Hum. Behav.* **2015**, *51*, 75–81. [CrossRef]
102. Han, L.; Geng, J.; Jou, M.; Gao, F.; Yang, H. Relationship between shyness and mobile phone addiction in Chinese young adults: Mediating roles of self-control and attachment anxiety. *Comput. Hum. Behav.* **2017**, *76*, 363–371. [CrossRef]
103. Harada, T.; Morikuni, M.; Yoshii, S.; Yamashita, Y.; Takeuchi, H. Usage of mobile phone in the evening or at night makes Japanese students evening-typed and night sleep uncomfortable. *Sleep Hypn.* **2002**, *4*, 149–153.
104. Harada, T.; Tanoue, A.; Takeuchi, H. Epidemiological studies on dreams, sleep habits and mental symptoms in students aged 18–25 years and the 24 hour a day commercialization of Japanese society (1). *Sleep Biol. Rhythm.* **2006**, *4*, 274–281. [CrossRef]
105. Harwood, J.; Dooley, J.J.; Scott, A.J.; Joiner, R. Constantly connected—The effects of smart-devices on mental health. *Comput. Hum. Behav.* **2014**, *34*, 267–272. [CrossRef]

106. Haug, S.; Castro, R.P.; Kwon, M.; Filler, A.; Kowatsch, T.; Schaub, M.P. Smartphone use and smartphone addiction among young people in Switzerland. *J. Behav. Addict.* **2015**, *4*, 299–307. [CrossRef] [PubMed]
107. Hawi, N.S.; Samaha, M. To excel or not to excel: Strong evidence on the adverse effect of smartphone addiction on academic performance. *Comput. Educ.* **2016**, *98*, 81–89. [CrossRef]
108. Hong, F.-Y.; Chiu, S.-I.; Huang, D.-H. A model of the relationship between psychological characteristics, mobile phone addiction and use of mobile phones by Taiwanese university female students. *Comput. Hum. Behav.* **2012**, *28*, 2152–2159. [CrossRef]
109. Honkalampi, K.; Tanskanen, A.; Hintikka, J.; Haatainen, K.; Viinamäki, H. Does the cellular phone help to communicate when face-to-face contacts are difficult? *Can. J. Psychiatry* **2001**, *46*, 373. [CrossRef] [PubMed]
110. Hu, Y.; Long, X.; Lyu, H.; Zhou, Y.; Chen, J. Alterations in White Matter Integrity in Young Adults with Smartphone Dependence. *Front. Hum. Neurosci.* **2017**, *11*, 532. [CrossRef] [PubMed]
111. Hussain, Z.; Griffiths, M.D.; Sheffield, D. An investigation into problematic smartphone use: The role of narcissism, anxiety, and personality factors. *J. Behav. Addict.* **2017**, *6*, 378–386. [CrossRef] [PubMed]
112. Hysing, M.; Pallesen, S.; Stormark, K.M.; Jakobsen, R.; Lundervold, A.J.; Sivertsen, B. Sleep and use of electronic devices in adolescence: Results from a large population-based study. *BMJ Open* **2015**, *5*, e006748. [CrossRef] [PubMed]
113. Ikeda, K.; Nakamura, K. Association between mobile phone use and depressed mood in Japanese adolescents: A cross-sectional study. *Environ. Health Prev. Med.* **2014**, *19*, 187–193. [CrossRef] [PubMed]
114. Itani, O.; Kaneita, Y.; Munezawa, T.; Ikeda, M.; Osaki, Y.; Higuchi, S.; Kanda, H.; Nakagome, S.; Suzuki, K.; et al. Anger and Impulsivity Among Japanese Adolescents: A Nationwide Representative Survey. *J. Clin. Psychiatry* **2016**, *77*, e860–e866. [CrossRef] [PubMed]
115. Jenaro, C.; Flores, N.; Gómez-Vela, M.; González-Gil, F.; Caballo, C. Problematic internet and cell-phone use: Psychological behavioral, and health correlates. *Addict. Res. Theory* **2007**, *15*, 309–320. [CrossRef]
116. Jeong, S.H.; Kim, H.; Yum, J.Y.; Hwang, Y. What type of content are smartphone users addicted to? SNS vs. Games. *Comput. Hum. Behav.* **2016**, *54*, 10–17. [CrossRef]
117. Jiang, X.; Hardy, L.L.; Baur, L.A.; Ding, D.; Wang, L.; Shi, H. Sleep duration, schedule and quality among urban Chinese children and adolescents: Associations with routine after-school activities. *PLoS ONE* **2015**, *10*, e0115326. [CrossRef] [PubMed]
118. Jiang, Z.; Shi, M. Prevalence and co-occurrence of compulsive buying, problematic Internet and mobile phone use in college students in Yantai, China: Relevance of self-traits. *BMC Public Health* **2016**, *16*, 1211. [CrossRef] [PubMed]
119. Jiang, Z.; Zhao, X. Self-control and problematic mobile phone use in Chinese college students: The mediating role of mobile phone use patterns. *BMC Psychiatry* **2016**, *16*, 416. [CrossRef] [PubMed]
120. Jiang, Z.; Zhao, X. Brain behavioral systems, self-control and problematic mobile phone use: The moderating role of gender and history of use. *Personal. Individ. Differ.* **2017**, *106*, 111–116. [CrossRef]
121. Johansson, A.E.; Petrisko, M.A.; Chasens, E.R. Adolescent Sleep and the Impact of Technology Use Before Sleep on Daytime Function. *J. Pediatr. Nurs.* **2016**, *31*, 498–504. [CrossRef] [PubMed]
122. Jun, N.; Lee, A.; Baik, I. Associations of Caffeinated Beverage Consumption and Screen Time with Excessive Daytime Sleepiness in Korean High School Students. *Clin. Nutr. Res.* **2017**, *6*, 55–60. [CrossRef] [PubMed]
123. Jun, S. The reciprocal longitudinal relationships between mobile phone addiction and depressive symptoms among Korean adolescents. *Comput. Hum. Behav.* **2016**, *58*, 179–186. [CrossRef]
124. Karadağ, E.; Tosuntaş, Ş.B.; Erzen, E.; Duru, P.; Bostan, N.; Şahin, B.M.; Çulha, İ.; Babadağ, B. Determinants of phubbing, which is the sum of many virtual addictions: A structural equation model. *J. Behav. Addict.* **2015**, *4*, 60–74. [CrossRef] [PubMed]
125. Kawabe, K.; Horiuchi, F.; Ochi, M.; Oka, Y.; Ueno, S. Internet addiction: Prevalence and relation with mental states in adolescents. *Psychiatry Clin. Neurosci.* **2016**, *70*, 405–412. [CrossRef] [PubMed]
126. Khoury, J.M.; de Freitas, A.A.C.; Roque, M.A.V.; Albuquerque, M.R.; das Neves, M.C.L.; Garcia, F.D. Assessment of the accuracy of a new tool for the screening of smartphone addiction. *PLoS ONE* **2017**, *12*, e0176924. [CrossRef] [PubMed]
127. Kim, D.; Lee, Y.; Lee, J.; Nam, J.K.; Chung, Y. Development of Korean Smartphone Addiction Proneness Scale for youth. *PLoS ONE* **2014**, *9*, e97920. [CrossRef] [PubMed]
128. Kim, D.; Nam, J.K.; Oh, J.; Kang, M.C. A latent profile analysis of the interplay between PC and smartphone in problematic Internet use. *Comput. Hum. Behav.* **2016**, *56*, 360–368. [CrossRef]

129. Kim, E.; Cho, I.; Kim, E.J. Structural Equation Model of Smartphone Addiction Based on Adult Attachment Theory: Mediating Effects of Loneliness and Depression. *Asian Nurs. Res. (Korean Soc. Nurs. Sci.)* **2017**, *11*, 92–97. [CrossRef] [PubMed]
130. Kim, E.Y.; Joo, S.W.; Han, S.J.; Kim, M.J.; Choi, S.Y. Depression, Impulse Control Disorder, and Life Style According to Smartphone Addiction. *Stud. Health Technol. Inform.* **2017**, *245*, 1272. [PubMed]
131. Kim, H.J.; Min, J.Y.; Kim, H.J.; Min, K.B. Association between psychological and self-assessed health status and smartphone overuse among Korean college students. *J. Ment. Health* **2017**, 1–6. [CrossRef] [PubMed]
132. Kim, J.H. Longitudinal Associations among Psychological Issues and Problematic Use of Smartphones: A Two-Wave Cross-Lagged Study. *J. Media Psychol. Theor. Methods Appl.* **2017**. [CrossRef]
133. Kim, J.H. Smartphone-mediated communication vs. face-to-face interaction: Two routes to social support and problematic use of smartphone. *Comput. Hum. Behav.* **2017**, *67*, 282–291. [CrossRef]
134. Kim, J.-H.; Seo, M.; David, P. Alleviating depression only to become problematic mobile phone users: Can face-to-face communication be the antidote? *Comput. Hum. Behav.* **2015**, *51*, 440–447. [CrossRef]
135. Kim, R.; Lee, K.J.; Choi, Y.J. Mobile Phone Overuse among Elementary School Students in Korea: Factors Associated With Mobile Phone Use as a Behavior Addiction. *J. Addict. Nurs.* **2015**, *26*, 81–85. [CrossRef] [PubMed]
136. Kim, S.E.; Kim, J.W.; Jee, Y.S. Relationship between smartphone addiction and physical activity in Chinese international students in Korea. *J. Behav. Addict.* **2015**, *4*, 200–205. [CrossRef] [PubMed]
137. Kim, Y.; Jeong, J.E.; Cho, H.; Jung, D.J.; Kwak, M.; Rho, M.J.; Yu, H.; Kim, D.J.; Choi, I.Y. Personality Factors Predicting Smartphone Addiction Predisposition: Behavioral Inhibition and Activation Systems, Impulsivity, and Self-Control. *PLoS ONE* **2016**, *11*, e0159788. [CrossRef] [PubMed]
138. King, A.L.; Valenca, A.M.; Silva, A.C.; Sancassiani, F.; Machado, S.; Nardi, A.E. "Nomophobia": Impact of cell phone use interfering with symptoms and emotions of individuals with panic disorder compared with a control group. *Clin. Pract. Epidemiol. Ment. Health* **2014**, *10*, 28–35. [CrossRef] [PubMed]
139. Koivusilta, L.K.; Lintonen, T.P.; Rimpela, A.H. Orientations in adolescent use of information and communication technology: A digital divide by sociodemographic background, educational career, and health. *Scand. J. Public Health* **2007**, *35*, 95–103. [CrossRef] [PubMed]
140. Korpinen, L.; Paakkonen, R. Mental symptoms and the use of new technical equipment. *Int. J. Occup. Saf. Ergon.* **2009**, *15*, 385–400. [CrossRef] [PubMed]
141. Korpinen, L.; Paakkonen, R. Self-reported depression and anxiety symptoms and usage of computers and mobile phones among working-age Finns. *Int. J. Occup. Saf. Ergon.* **2015**, *21*, 221–228. [CrossRef] [PubMed]
142. Kruger, D.J.; Djerf, J.M. Bad vibrations? Cell phone dependency predicts phantom communication experiences. *Comput. Hum. Behav.* **2017**, *70*, 360–364. [CrossRef]
143. Kuang-Tsan, C.; Fu-Yuan, H. Study on relationship among university students' life stress, smart mobile phone addiction, and life satisfaction. *J. Adult Dev.* **2017**, *24*, 109–118. [CrossRef]
144. Kubiszewski, V.; Fontaine, R.; Rusch, E.; Hazouard, E. Association between electronic media use and sleep habits: An eight-day follow-up study. *Int. J. Adolesc. Youth* **2014**, *19*, 395–407. [CrossRef]
145. Kwon, M.; Kim, D.J.; Cho, H.; Yang, S. The smartphone addiction scale: Development and validation of a short version for adolescents. *PLoS ONE* **2013**, *8*, e83558. [CrossRef] [PubMed]
146. Kwon, M.; Lee, J.Y.; Won, W.Y.; Park, J.W.; Min, J.A.; Hahn, C.; Gu, X.; Choi, J.H.; Kim, D.J. Development and validation of a smartphone addiction scale (SAS). *PLoS ONE* **2013**, *8*, e56936. [CrossRef] [PubMed]
147. Lachmann, B.; Duke, É.; Sariyska, R.; Montag, C. Who's Addicted to the Smartphone and/or the Internet? *Psychol. Pop. Media Culture* **2017**. [CrossRef]
148. Lanaj, K.; Johnson, R.E.; Barnes, C.M. Beginning the workday yet already depleted? Consequences of late-night smartphone use and sleep. *Organ. Behav. Hum. Decis. Process.* **2014**, *124*, 11–23. [CrossRef]
149. Lange, K.; Cohrs, S.; Skarupke, C.; Gorke, M.; Szagun, B.; Schlack, R. Electronic media use and insomnia complaints in German adolescents: Gender differences in use patterns and sleep problems. *J. Neural Transm.* **2017**, *124*, 79–87. [CrossRef] [PubMed]
150. Lee, C.; Lee, S.J. Prevalence and predictors of smartphone addiction proneness among Korean adolescents. *Child. Youth Serv. Rev.* **2017**, *77*, 10–17. [CrossRef]
151. Lee, E.B. Facebook use and texting among African American and Hispanic teenagers: An implication for academic performance. *J. Black Stud.* **2014**, *45*, 83–101. [CrossRef]

152. Lee, E.B. Too much information: Heavy smartphone and Facebook utilization by African American young adults. *J. Black Stud.* **2015**, *46*, 44–61. [CrossRef]
153. Lee, H.; Kim, J.W.; Choi, T.Y. Risk Factors for Smartphone Addiction in Korean Adolescents: Smartphone Use Patterns. *J. Korean Med. Sci.* **2017**, *32*, 1674–1679. [CrossRef] [PubMed]
154. Lee, H.K.; Kim, J.H.; Fava, M.; Mischoulon, D.; Park, J.H.; Shim, E.J.; Lee, E.H.; Lee, J.H.; Jeon, H.J. Development and validation study of the Smartphone Overuse Screening Questionnaire. *Psychiatry Res.* **2017**, *257*, 352–357. [CrossRef] [PubMed]
155. Lee, J. Does stress from cell phone use increase negative emotions at work? *Soc. Behav. Personal.* **2016**, *44*, 705–716. [CrossRef]
156. Lee, J.E.; Jang, S.I.; Ju, Y.J.; Kim, W.; Lee, H.J.; Park, E.C. Relationship between Mobile Phone Addiction and the Incidence of Poor and Short Sleep among Korean Adolescents: A Longitudinal Study of the Korean Children & Youth Panel Survey. *J. Korean Med. Sci.* **2017**, *32*, 1166–1172. [PubMed]
157. Lee, K.E.; Kim, S.H.; Ha, T.Y.; Yoo, Y.M.; Han, J.J.; Jung, J.H.; Jang, J.Y. Dependency on Smartphone Use and Its Association with Anxiety in Korea. *Public Health Rep.* **2016**, *131*, 411–419. [CrossRef] [PubMed]
158. Lee, S.; Tam, C.L.; Chie, Q.T. Mobile phone usage preferences: The contributing factors of personality, social anxiety and loneliness. *Soc. Indic. Res.* **2014**, *118*, 1205–1228. [CrossRef]
159. Lee, Y.K.; Chang, C.T.; Lin, Y.; Cheng, Z.H. The dark side of smartphone usage: Psychological traits, compulsive behavior and technostress. *Comput. Hum. Behav.* **2014**, *31*, 373–383. [CrossRef]
160. Lee, Y.-K.; Chang, C.-T.; Cheng, Z.-H.; Lin, Y. Helpful-stressful cycle? Psychological links between type of mobile phone user and stress. *Behav. Inf. Technol.* **2016**, *35*, 75–86. [CrossRef]
161. Lemola, S.; Perkinson-Gloor, N.; Brand, S.; Dewald-Kaufmann, J.F.; Grob, A. Adolescents' electronic media use at night, sleep disturbance, and depressive symptoms in the smartphone age. *J. Youth Adolesc.* **2015**, *44*, 405–418. [CrossRef] [PubMed]
162. Lepp, A.; Barkley, J.E.; Karpinski, A.C. The relationship between cell phone use, academic performance, anxiety, and satisfaction with life in college students. *Comput. Hum. Behav.* **2014**, *31*, 343–350. [CrossRef]
163. Lepp, A.; Barkley, J.E.; Li, J. Motivations and experiential outcomes associated with leisure time cell phone use: Results from two independent studies. *Leis. Sci.* **2017**, *39*, 144–162. [CrossRef]
164. Lepp, A.; Li, J.; Barkley, J.E.; Salehi-Esfahani, S. Exploring the relationships between college students' cell phone use, personality and leisure. *Comput. Hum. Behav.* **2015**, *43*, 210–219. [CrossRef]
165. Leung, C. Assessing mobile phone dependency and teens' everyday life in Hong Kong. *Aust. J. Psychol.* **2017**, *69*, 29–38. [CrossRef]
166. Leung, L.; Liang, J. Psychological traits, addiction symptoms, and feature usage as predictors of problematic smartphone use among university students in China. *Int. J. Cyber Behav. Psychol. Learn.* **2016**, *6*, 57–74. [CrossRef]
167. Li, J.; Lepp, A.; Barkley, J.E. Locus of control and cell phone use: Implications for sleep quality, academic performance, and subjective well-being. *Comput. Hum. Behav.* **2015**, *52*, 450–457. [CrossRef]
168. Li, M.; Jiang, X.; Ren, Y. Mediator Effects of Positive Emotions on Social Support and Depression among Adolescents Suffering from Mobile Phone Addiction. *Psychiatr. Danub.* **2017**, *29*, 207–213. [CrossRef] [PubMed]
169. Lian, L. Alienation as mediator and moderator of the relationship between virtues and smartphone addiction among Chinese university students. *Int. J. Ment. Health Addict.* **2017**, *16*, 1208–1218. [CrossRef]
170. Lian, L.; You, X. Specific virtues as predictors of Smartphone addiction among Chinese undergraduates. *Curr. Psychol.* **2017**, *36*, 376–384. [CrossRef]
171. Lian, L.; You, X.; Huang, J.; Yang, R. Who overuses Smartphones? Roles of virtues and parenting style in smartphone addiction among Chinese college students. *Comput. Hum. Behav.* **2016**, *65*, 92–99. [CrossRef]
172. Lin, Y.H.; Chang, L.R.; Lee, Y.H.; Tseng, H.W.; Kuo, T.B.; Chen, S.H. Development and validation of the Smartphone Addiction Inventory (SPAI). *PLoS ONE* **2014**, *9*, e98312. [CrossRef] [PubMed]
173. Lin, Y.H.; Chiang, C.L.; Lin, P.H.; Chang, L.R.; Ko, C.H.; Lee, Y.H.; Lin, S.H. Proposed Diagnostic Criteria for Smartphone Addiction. *PLoS ONE* **2016**, *11*, e0163010. [CrossRef] [PubMed]
174. Lin, Y.H.; Lin, P.H.; Chiang, C.L.; Lee, Y.H.; Yang, C.C.H.; Kuo, T.B.J.; Lin, S.H. Incorporation of Mobile Application (App) Measures into the Diagnosis of Smartphone Addiction. *J. Clin. Psychiatry* **2017**, *78*, 866–872. [CrossRef] [PubMed]

175. Lin, Y.H.; Lin, Y.C.; Lee, Y.H.; Lin, P.H.; Lin, S.H.; Chang, L.R.; Tseng, H.W.; Yen, L.Y.; Yang, C.C.; Kuo, T.B. Time distortion associated with smartphone addiction: Identifying smartphone addiction via a mobile application (App). *J. Psychiatr. Res.* **2015**, *65*, 139–145. [CrossRef] [PubMed]
176. Lin, Y.H.; Lin, Y.C.; Lin, S.H.; Lee, Y.H.; Lin, P.H.; Chiang, C.L.; Chang, L.R.; Yang, C.C.; Kuo, T.B. To use or not to use? Compulsive behavior and its role in smartphone addiction. *Transl. Psychiatry* **2017**, *7*, e1030. [CrossRef] [PubMed]
177. Lin, Y.H.; Pan, Y.C.; Lin, S.H.; Chen, S.H. Development of short-form and screening cutoff point of the Smartphone Addiction Inventory (SPAI-SF). *Int. J. Methods Psychiatr. Res.* **2017**, *26*. [CrossRef] [PubMed]
178. Liu, C.H.; Lin, S.H.; Pan, Y.C.; Lin, Y.H. Smartphone gaming and frequent use pattern associated with smartphone addiction. *Medicine* **2016**, *95*, e4068. [CrossRef] [PubMed]
179. Liu, Q.Q.; Zhou, Z.K.; Yang, X.J.; Kong, F.C.; Niu, G.F.; Fan, C.Y. Mobile phone addiction and sleep quality among Chinese adolescents: A moderated mediation model. *Comput. Hum. Behav.* **2017**, *72*, 108–114. [CrossRef]
180. Long, J.; Liu, T.Q.; Liao, Y.H.; Qi, C.; He, H.Y.; Chen, S.B.; Billieux, J. Prevalence and correlates of problematic smartphone use in a large random sample of Chinese undergraduates. *BMC Psychiatry* **2016**, *16*, 408. [CrossRef] [PubMed]
181. Lopez-Fernandez, O. Short version of the Smartphone Addiction Scale adapted to Spanish and French: Towards a cross-cultural research in problematic mobile phone use. *Addict. Behav.* **2017**, *64*, 275–280. [CrossRef] [PubMed]
182. Lopez-Fernandez, O.; Honrubia-Serrano, L.; Freixa-Blanxart, M.; Gibson, W. Prevalence of problematic mobile phone use in British adolescents. *Cyberpsychol. Behav. Soc. Netw.* **2014**, *17*, 91–98. [CrossRef] [PubMed]
183. Lopez-Fernandez, O.; Kuss, D.J.; Romo, L.; Morvan, Y.; Kern, L.; Graziani, P.; Rousseau, A.; Rumpf, H.J.; Bischof, A.; Gassler, A.K.; et al. Self-reported dependence on mobile phones in young adults: A European cross-cultural empirical survey. *J. Behav. Addict.* **2017**, *6*, 168–177. [CrossRef] [PubMed]
184. Lu, X.; Katoh, T.; Chen, Z.; Nagata, T.; Kitamura, T. Text messaging: Are dependency and Excessive Use discretely different for Japanese university students? *Psychiatry Res.* **2014**, *216*, 255–262. [CrossRef] [PubMed]
185. Lu, X.; Watanabe, J.; Liu, Q.; Uji, M.; Shono, M.; Kitamura, T. Internet and mobile phone text-messaging dependency: Factor structure and correlation with dysphoric mood among Japanese adults. *Comput. Hum. Behav.* **2011**, *27*, 1702–1709. [CrossRef]
186. Mak, K.K.; Nam, J.K.; Kim, D.; Aum, N.; Choi, J.S.; Cheng, C.; Ko, H.C.; Watanabe, H. Cross-cultural adaptation and psychometric properties of the Korean Scale for Internet Addiction (K-Scale) in Japanese high school students. *Psychiatry Res.* **2017**, *249*, 343–348. [CrossRef] [PubMed]
187. Mak, Y.W.; Wu, C.S.; Hui, D.W.; Lam, S.P.; Tse, H.Y.; Yu, W.Y.; Wong, H.T. Association between screen viewing duration and sleep duration, sleep quality, and excessive daytime sleepiness among adolescents in Hong Kong. *Int. J. Environ. Res. Public Health* **2014**, *11*, 11201–11219. [CrossRef] [PubMed]
188. Martinotti, G.; Villella, C.; Di Thiene, D.; Di Nicola, M.; Bria, P.; Conte, G.; Cassano, M.; Petruccelli, F.; Corvasce, N.; Janiri, L.; et al. Problematic mobile phone use in adolescence: A cross-sectional study. *J. Public Health* **2011**, *19*, 545–551. [CrossRef]
189. Matar Boumosleh, J.; Jaalouk, D. Depression, anxiety, and smartphone addiction in university students—A cross sectional study. *PLoS ONE* **2017**, *12*, e0182239. [CrossRef] [PubMed]
190. Matsumoto, Y.; Uchimura, N.; Ishida, T.; Morimatsu, Y.; Mori, M.; Inoue, M.; Kushino, N.; Hoshiko, M.; Ishitake, T. The relationship of sleep complaints risk factors with sleep phase, quality, and quantity in Japanese workers. *Sleep Biol. Rhythm.* **2017**, *15*, 291–297. [CrossRef] [PubMed]
191. Mattila, A.K.; Luutonen, S.; Ylinen, M.; Salokangas, R.K.R.; Joukamaa, M. Alexithymia, human relationships, and mobile phone use. *J. Nerv. Ment. Dis.* **2010**, *198*, 722–727. [CrossRef] [PubMed]
192. Mazaheri, M.A.; Karbasi, M. Validity and reliability of the Persian version of mobile phone addiction scale. *J. Res. Med. Sci.* **2014**, *19*, 139–144. [PubMed]
193. McBride, J.; Derevensky, J. Internet gambling behavior in a sample of online gamblers. *Int. J. Ment. Health Addict.* **2009**, *7*, 149–167. [CrossRef]
194. Merlo, L.J.; Stone, A.M.; Bibbey, A. Measuring Problematic Mobile Phone Use: Development and Preliminary Psychometric Properties of the PUMP Scale. *J. Addict.* **2013**, *2013*, 912807. [CrossRef] [PubMed]

195. Mohammadbeigi, A.; Absari, R.; Valizadeh, F.; Saadati, M.; Sharifimoghadam, S.; Ahmadi, A.; Mokhtari, M.; Ansari, H. Sleep Quality in Medical Students; the Impact of Over-Use of Mobile Cell-Phone and Social Networks. *J. Res. Health Sci.* **2016**, *16*, 46–50. [PubMed]
196. Mohammadi Kalhori, S.; Mohammadi, M.R.; Alavi, S.S.; Jannatifard, F.; Sepahbodi, G.; Baba Reisi, M.; Sajedi, S.; Farshchi, M.; KhodaKarami, R.; Hatami Kasvaee, V. Validation and Psychometric Properties of Mobile Phone Problematic Use Scale (MPPUS) in University Students of Tehran. *Iran. J. Psychiatry* **2015**, *10*, 25–31. [PubMed]
197. Mohammadi, M.; Alavi, S.S.; Farokhzad, P.; Jannatifard, F.; Mohammadi Kalhori, S.; Sepahbodi, G.; Baba Reisi, M.; Sajedi, S.; Farshchi, M.; Khoda Karami, R.; et al. The Validity and Reliability of the Persian Version Test of Mobile Phone Dependency (TMD). *Iran. J. Psychiatry* **2015**, *10*, 265–272. [PubMed]
198. Mok, J.Y.; Choi, S.W.; Kim, D.J.; Choi, J.S.; Lee, J.; Ahn, H.; Choi, E.J.; Song, W.Y. Latent class analysis on internet and smartphone addiction in college students. *Neuropsychiatr. Dis. Treat.* **2014**, *10*, 817–828. [PubMed]
199. Monma, T.; Ando, A.; Asanuma, T.; Yoshitake, Y.; Yoshida, G.; Miyazawa, T.; Ebine, N.; Takeda, S.; Omi, N.; Satoh, M.; et al. Sleep disorder risk factors among student athletes. *Sleep Med.* **2018**, *44*, 76–81. [CrossRef] [PubMed]
200. Montag, C.; Błaszkiewicz, K.; Lachmann, B.; Andone, I.; Sariyska, R.; Trendafilov, B.; Reuter, M.; Markowetz, A. Correlating personality and actual phone usage: Evidence from psychoinformatics. *J. Individ. Differ.* **2014**, *35*, 158–165. [CrossRef]
201. Montag, C.; Sindermann, C.; Becker, B.; Panksepp, J. An affective neuroscience framework for the molecular study of Internet addiction. *Front. Psychol.* **2016**, *7*, 13. [CrossRef] [PubMed]
202. Munezawa, T.; Kaneita, Y.; Osaki, Y.; Kanda, H.; Minowa, M.; Suzuki, K.; Higuchi, S.; Mori, J.; Yamamoto, R.; Ohida, T. The association between use of mobile phones after lights out and sleep disturbances among Japanese adolescents: A nationwide cross-sectional survey. *Sleep* **2011**, *34*, 1013–1020. [CrossRef] [PubMed]
203. Munoz-Miralles, R.; Ortega-Gonzalez, R.; Lopez-Moron, M.R.; Batalla-Martinez, C.; Manresa, J.M.; Montella-Jordana, N.; Chamarro, A.; Carbonell, X.; Toran-Monserrat, P. The problematic use of Information and Communication Technologies (ICT) in adolescents by the cross sectional JOITIC study. *BMC Pediatr.* **2016**, *16*, 140. [CrossRef] [PubMed]
204. Murdock, K.K.; Gorman, S.; Robbins, M. Co-rumination via cellphone moderates the association of perceived interpersonal stress and psychosocial well-being in emerging adults. *J. Adolesc.* **2015**, *38*, 27–37. [CrossRef] [PubMed]
205. Murdock, K.K.; Horissian, M.; Crichlow-Ball, C. Emerging Adults' Text Message Use and Sleep Characteristics: A Multimethod, Naturalistic Study. *Behav. Sleep Med.* **2017**, *15*, 228–241. [CrossRef] [PubMed]
206. Nathan, N.; Zeitzer, J. A survey study of the association between mobile phone use and daytime sleepiness in California high school students. *BMC Public Health* **2013**, *13*, 840. [CrossRef] [PubMed]
207. Nathanson, A.I.; Beyens, I. The relation between use of mobile electronic devices and bedtime resistance, sleep duration, and daytime sleepiness among preschoolers. *Behav. Sleep Med.* **2018**, *16*, 202–219. [CrossRef] [PubMed]
208. Nikhita, C.S.; Jadhav, P.R.; Ajinkya, S.A. Prevalence of Mobile Phone Dependence in Secondary School Adolescents. *J. Clin. Diagn. Res.* **2015**, *9*, Vc06–Vc09. [CrossRef] [PubMed]
209. Oberst, U.; Wegmann, E.; Stodt, B.; Brand, M.; Chamarro, A. Negative consequences from heavy social networking in adolescents: The mediating role of fear of missing out. *J. Adolesc.* **2017**, *55*, 51–60. [CrossRef] [PubMed]
210. Oshima, N.; Nishida, A.; Shimodera, S.; Tochigi, M.; Ando, S.; Yamasaki, S.; Okazaki, Y.; Sasaki, T. The suicidal feelings, self-injury, and mobile phone use after lights out in adolescents. *J. Pediatr. Psychol.* **2012**, *37*, 1023–1030. [CrossRef] [PubMed]
211. Paik, S.H.; Cho, H.; Chun, J.W.; Jeong, J.E.; Kim, D.J. Gaming Device Usage Patterns Predict Internet Gaming Disorder: Comparison across Different Gaming Device Usage Patterns. *Int. J. Environ. Res. Public Health* **2017**, *14*, 1512. [CrossRef] [PubMed]
212. Paiva, T.; Gaspar, T.; Matos, M.G. Mutual relations between sleep deprivation, sleep stealers and risk behaviours in adolescents. *Sleep Sci.* **2016**, *9*, 7–13. [CrossRef] [PubMed]

213. Pamuk, M.; Atli, A. Development of a Problematic Mobile Phone Use Scale for university students: Validity and reliability study. *Düşünen Adam J. Psychiatry Neurol. Sci.* **2016**, *29*, 49–59. [CrossRef]
214. Panova, T.; Lleras, A. Avoidance or boredom: Negative mental health outcomes associated with use of Information and Communication Technologies depend on users' motivations. *Comput. Hum. Behav.* **2016**, *58*, 249–258. [CrossRef]
215. Park, N.; Kim, Y.C.; Shon, H.Y.; Shim, H. Factors influencing smartphone use and dependency in South Korea. *Comput. Hum. Behav.* **2013**, *29*, 1763–1770. [CrossRef]
216. Park, N.; Lee, H. Social implications of smartphone use: Korean college students' smartphone use and psychological well-being. *Cyberpsychol. Behav. Soc. Netw.* **2012**, *15*, 491–497. [CrossRef] [PubMed]
217. Pavia, L.; Cavani, P.; Di Blasi, M.; Giordano, C. Smartphone Addiction Inventory (SPAI): Psychometric properties and confirmatory factor analysis. *Comput. Hum. Behav.* **2016**, *63*, 170–178. [CrossRef]
218. Pearson, C.; Hussain, Z. Smartphone use, addiction, narcissism, and personality: A mixed methods investigation. *Int. J. Cyber Behav. Psychol. Learn.* **2015**, *5*, 17–32. [CrossRef]
219. Peiro-Velert, C.; Valencia-Peris, A.; Gonzalez, L.M.; Garcia-Masso, X.; Serra-Ano, P.; Devis-Devis, J. Screen media usage, sleep time and academic performance in adolescents: Clustering a self-organizing maps analysis. *PLoS ONE* **2014**, *9*, e99478. [CrossRef] [PubMed]
220. Phillips, J.G.; Butt, S.; Blaszczynski, A. Personality and self-reported use of mobile phones for games. *Cyberpsychol. Behav.* **2006**, *9*, 753–758. [CrossRef] [PubMed]
221. Phillips, J.G.; Ogeil, R.P.; Blaszczynski, A. Electronic interests and behaviours associated with gambling problems. *Int. J. Ment. Health Addict.* **2012**, *10*, 585–596. [CrossRef]
222. Phillips, J.G.; Sargeant, J.; Ogeil, R.P.; Chow, Y.-W.; Blaszczynski, A. Self-reported gambling problems and digital traces. *Cyberpsychol. Behav. Soc. Netw.* **2014**, *17*, 742–748. [CrossRef] [PubMed]
223. Pieters, D.; De Valck, E.; Vandekerckhove, M.; Pirrera, S.; Wuyts, J.; Exadaktylos, V.; Haex, B.; Michiels, N.; Verbraecken, J.; Cluydts, R. Effects of pre-sleep media use on sleep/wake patterns and daytime functioning among adolescents: The moderating role of parental control. *Behav. Sleep Med.* **2014**, *12*, 427–443. [CrossRef] [PubMed]
224. Piguet, C.; Berchtold, A.; Akre, C.; Suris, J.C. What keeps female problematic Internet users busy online? *Eur. J. Pediatr.* **2015**, *174*, 1053–1059. [CrossRef] [PubMed]
225. Pourrazavi, S.; Allahverdipour, H.; Jafarabadi, M.A.; Matlabi, H. A socio-cognitive inquiry of excessive mobile phone use. *Asian J. Psychiatry* **2014**, *10*, 84–89. [CrossRef] [PubMed]
226. Prasad, M.; Patthi, B.; Singla, A.; Gupta, R.; Saha, S.; Kumar, J.K.; Malhi, R.; Pandita, V. Nomophobia: A Cross-sectional Study to Assess Mobile Phone Usage Among Dental Students. *J. Clin. Diagn. Res.* **2017**, *11*, ZC34–ZC39. [CrossRef] [PubMed]
227. Przybylski, A.K.; Weinstein, N. A Large-Scale Test of the Goldilocks Hypothesis. *Psychol. Sci.* **2017**, *28*, 204–215. [CrossRef] [PubMed]
228. Punamaki, R.L.; Wallenius, M.; Nygard, C.H.; Saarni, L.; Rimpela, A. Use of information and communication technology (ICT) and perceived health in adolescence: The role of sleeping habits and waking-time tiredness. *J. Adolesc.* **2007**, *30*, 569–585. [CrossRef] [PubMed]
229. Randler, C.; Wolfgang, L.; Matt, K.; Demirhan, E.; Horzum, M.B.; Besoluk, S. Smartphone addiction proneness in relation to sleep and morningness-eveningness in German adolescents. *J. Behav. Addict.* **2016**, *5*, 465–473. [CrossRef] [PubMed]
230. Reed, D.D.; Becirevic, A.; Atchley, P.; Kaplan, B.A.; Liese, B.S. Validation of a novel delay discounting of text messaging questionnaire. *Psychol. Rec.* **2016**, *66*, 253–261. [CrossRef]
231. Reid, D.J.; Reid, F.J. Text or talk? Social anxiety, loneliness, and divergent preferences for cell phone use. *Cyberpsychol. Behav.* **2007**, *10*, 424–435. [CrossRef] [PubMed]
232. Roberts, J.A.; Petnji Yaya, L.H.; Manolis, C. The invisible addiction: Cell-phone activities and addiction among male and female college students. *J. Behav. Addict.* **2014**, *3*, 254–265. [CrossRef] [PubMed]
233. Roberts, J.A.; Pirog, S.F., 3rd. A preliminary investigation of materialism and impulsiveness as predictors of technological addictions among young adults. *J. Behav. Addict.* **2013**, *2*, 56–62. [CrossRef] [PubMed]
234. Roberts, J.A.; Pullig, C.; Manolis, C. I need my smartphone: A hierarchical model of personality and cell-phone addiction. *Personal. Individ. Differ.* **2015**, *79*, 13–19. [CrossRef]

235. Rosen, L.; Carrier, L.M.; Miller, A.; Rokkum, J.; Ruiz, A. Sleeping with technology: Cognitive, affective, and technology usage predictors of sleep problems among college students. *Sleep Health* **2016**, *2*, 49–56. [CrossRef] [PubMed]
236. Rosen, L.D.; Whaling, K.; Carrier, L.M.; Cheever, N.A.; Rokkum, J. The Media and Technology Usage and Attitudes Scale: An empirical investigation. *Comput. Hum. Behav.* **2013**, *29*, 2501–2511. [CrossRef]
237. Roser, K.; Schoeni, A.; Foerster, M.; Roosli, M. Problematic mobile phone use of Swiss adolescents: Is it linked with mental health or behaviour? *Int. J. Public Health* **2016**, *61*, 307–315. [CrossRef] [PubMed]
238. Rutland, J.B.; Sheets, T.; Young, T. Development of a scale to measure problem use of short message service: The SMS Problem Use Diagnostic Questionnaire. *Cyberpsychol. Behav.* **2007**, *10*, 841–843. [CrossRef] [PubMed]
239. Saeb, S.; Zhang, M.; Karr, C.J.; Schueller, S.M.; Corden, M.E.; Kording, K.P.; Mohr, D.C. Mobile Phone Sensor Correlates of Depressive Symptom Severity in Daily-Life Behavior: An Exploratory Study. *J. Med. Internet Res.* **2015**, *17*, e175. [CrossRef] [PubMed]
240. Sahin, S.; Ozdemir, K.; Unsal, A.; Temiz, N. Evaluation of mobile phone addiction level and sleep quality in university students. *Pak. J. Med. Sci.* **2013**, *29*, 913–918. [CrossRef] [PubMed]
241. Salehan, M.; Negahban, A. Social networking on smartphones: When mobile phones become addictive. *Comput. Hum. Behav.* **2013**, *29*, 2632–2639. [CrossRef]
242. Saling, L.L.; Haire, M. Are you awake? Mobile phone use after lights out. *Comput. Hum. Behav.* **2016**, *64*, 932–937. [CrossRef]
243. Samaha, M.; Hawi, N.S. Relationships among smartphone addiction, stress, academic performance, and satisfaction with life. *Comput. Hum. Behav.* **2016**, *57*, 321–325. [CrossRef]
244. Sanchez-Martinez, M.; Otero, A. Factors associated with cell phone use in adolescents in the community of Madrid (Spain). *Cyberpsychol. Behav.* **2009**, *12*, 131–137. [CrossRef] [PubMed]
245. Sapacz, M.; Rockman, G.; Clark, J. Are we addicted to our cell phones? *Comput. Hum. Behav.* **2016**, *57*, 153–159. [CrossRef]
246. Sato, M.; Sekine, T. The usage of cell phones and the feeling to them in modern Japanese college students. *J. Hum. Ergol.* **2010**, *39*, 23–33.
247. Savci, M.; Aysan, F. Technological addictions and social connectedness: Predictor effect of Internet addiction, social media addiction, digital game addiction and smartphone addiction on social connectedness. *Düşünen Adam J. Psychiatry Neurol. Sci.* **2017**, *30*, 202–216. [CrossRef]
248. Schoeni, A.; Roser, K.; Roosli, M. Symptoms and Cognitive Functions in Adolescents in Relation to Mobile Phone Use during Night. *PLoS ONE* **2015**, *10*, e0133528. [CrossRef] [PubMed]
249. Schweizer, A.; Berchtold, A.; Barrense-Dias, Y.; Akre, C.; Suris, J.C. Adolescents with a smartphone sleep less than their peers. *Eur. J. Pediatr.* **2017**, *176*, 131–136. [CrossRef] [PubMed]
250. Segev, A.; Mimouni-Bloch, A.; Ross, S.; Silman, Z.; Maoz, H.; Bloch, Y. Evaluating computer screen time and its possible link to psychopathology in the context of age: A cross-sectional study of parents and children. *PLoS ONE* **2015**, *10*, e0140542. [CrossRef] [PubMed]
251. Seo, D.G.; Park, Y.; Kim, M.K.; Park, J. Mobile phone dependency and its impacts on adolescents' social and academic behaviors. *Comput. Hum. Behav.* **2016**, *63*, 282–292. [CrossRef]
252. Seo, M.; Kim, J.H.; David, P. Always connected or always distracted? Adhd symptoms and social assurance explain problematic use of mobile phone and multicommunicating. *J. Comput. Mediat. Commun.* **2015**. [CrossRef]
253. Seok, S.; DaCosta, B. Predicting video game behavior: An investigation of the relationship between personality and mobile game play. *Games Culture* **2015**, *10*, 481–501. [CrossRef]
254. Sharma, M.K.; Rao, G.N.; Benegal, V.; Thennarasu, K.; Thomas, D. Technology Addiction Survey: An Emerging Concern for Raising Awareness and Promotion of Healthy Use of Technology. *Indian J. Psychol. Med.* **2017**, *39*, 495–499. [CrossRef] [PubMed]
255. Siddiqui, K. Personality influences mobile phone usage. *Interdiscip. J. Contemp. Res. Bus.* **2011**, *3*, 554–563.
256. Smetaniuk, P. A preliminary investigation into the prevalence and prediction of problematic cell phone use. *J. Behav. Addict.* **2014**, *3*, 41–53. [CrossRef] [PubMed]
257. Sohn, M.; Oh, H.; Lee, S.K.; Potenza, M.N. Suicidal Ideation and Related Factors among Korean High School Students: A Focus on Cyber Addiction and School Bullying. *J. Sch. Nurs.* **2017**, *34*, 310–318. [CrossRef] [PubMed]

258. Stachl, C.; Hilbert, S.; Au, J.Q.; Buschek, D.; De Luca, A.; Bischl, B.; Hussmann, H.; Bühner, M. Personality traits predict smartphone usage. *Eur. J. Personal.* **2017**, *31*, 701–722. [CrossRef]

259. Steelman, Z.R.; Soror, A.A. Why do you keep doing that? The biasing effects of mental states on IT continued usage intentions. *Comput. Hum. Behav.* **2017**, *73*, 209–223. [CrossRef]

260. Subba, S.H.; Mandelia, C.; Pathak, V.; Reddy, D.; Goel, A.; Tayal, A.; Nair, S.; Nagaraj, K. Ringxiety and the Mobile Phone Usage Pattern among the Students of a Medical College in South India. *J. Clin. Diagn. Res.* **2013**, *7*, 205–209. [CrossRef] [PubMed]

261. Takao, M. Problematic mobile phone use and big-five personality domains. *Indian J. Community Med.* **2014**, *39*, 111–113. [CrossRef] [PubMed]

262. Takao, M.; Takahashi, S.; Kitamura, M. Addictive personality and problematic mobile phone use. *Cyberpsychol. Behav.* **2009**, *12*, 501–507. [CrossRef] [PubMed]

263. Takeuchi, H.; Yamazaki, Y.; Oki, K.; Wada, K.; Noji, T.; Kawada, T.; Nakade, M.; Krejci, M.; Harada, T. Effects of chronotype and environmental factors upon sleep and mental health in Japanese students aged 18–40 yrs. *Biol. Rhythm. Res.* **2015**, *46*, 771–784. [CrossRef]

264. Tamura, H.; Nishida, T.; Tsuji, A.; Sakakibara, H. Association between Excessive Use of Mobile Phone and Insomnia and Depression among Japanese Adolescents. *Int. J. Environ. Res. Public Health* **2017**, *14*, 701. [CrossRef] [PubMed]

265. Tanis, M.; Beukeboom, C.J.; Hartmann, T.; Vermeulen, I.E. Phantom phone signals: An investigation into the prevalence and predictors of imagined cell phone signals. *Comput. Hum. Behav.* **2015**, *51*, 356–362. [CrossRef]

266. Tao, S.; Wu, X.; Zhang, S.; Tong, S.; Hao, J.; Tao, F. Association of alcohol use with problematic mobile phone use and depressive symptoms among college students in Anhui, China. *J. Public Health* **2017**, *25*, 103–112. [CrossRef]

267. Tao, S.; Wu, X.; Zhang, Y.; Zhang, S.; Tong, S.; Tao, F. Effects of Sleep Quality on the Association between Problematic Mobile Phone Use and Mental Health Symptoms in Chinese College Students. *Int. J. Environ. Res. Public Health* **2017**, *14*, 185. [CrossRef] [PubMed]

268. Thomée, S.; Eklöf, M.; Gustafsson, E.; Nilsson, R.; Hagberg, M. Prevalence of perceived stress, symptoms of depression and sleep disturbances in relation to information and communication technology (ICT) use among young adults—An explorative prospective study. *Comput. Hum. Behav.* **2007**, *23*, 1300–1321. [CrossRef]

269. Thomée, S.; Härenstam, A.; Hagberg, M. Mobile phone use and stress, sleep disturbances, and symptoms of depression among young adults—A prospective cohort study. *BMC Public Health* **2011**, *11*, 66. [CrossRef] [PubMed]

270. Titilope, A.O. Socio-psychological dimensions of mobile phone addiction and usage patterns amongst teenagers in higher institutions of learning in Kwara State. *Int. J. Inf. Commun. Technol. Educ.* **2014**, *10*, 1–3. [CrossRef]

271. Toda, M.; Ezoe, S.; Takeshita, T. Mobile phone use and stress-coping strategies of medical students. *Int. J. Cyber Behav. Psychol. Learn.* **2014**, *4*, 41–46. [CrossRef]

272. Toda, M.; Monden, K.; Kubo, K.; Morimoto, K. Mobile phone dependence and health-related lifestyle of university students. *Soc. Behav. Personal.* **2006**, *34*, 1277–1284. [CrossRef]

273. Toda, M.; Nishio, N.; Ezoe, S.; Takeshita, T. Chronotype and smartphone use among Japanese medical students. *Int. J. Cyber Behav. Psychol. Learn.* **2015**, *5*, 75–80. [CrossRef]

274. Tokiya, M.; Kaneita, Y.; Itani, O.; Jike, M.; Ohida, T. Predictors of insomnia onset in adolescents in Japan. *Sleep Med.* **2017**, *38*, 37–43. [CrossRef] [PubMed]

275. Tsimtsiou, Z.; Haidich, A.B.; Drontsos, A.; Dantsi, F.; Sekeri, Z.; Drosos, E.; Trikilis, N.; Dardavesis, T.; Nanos, P.; Arvanitidou, M. Pathological Internet use, cyberbullying and mobile phone use in adolescence: A school-based study in Greece. *Int. J. Adolesc. Med. Health* **2017**. [CrossRef] [PubMed]

276. Walsh, S.P.; White, K.M.; McD Young, R. Needing to connect: The effect of self and others on young people's involvement with their mobile phones. *Aust. J. Psychol.* **2010**, *62*, 194–203. [CrossRef]

277. Van den Bulck, J. Text messaging as a cause of sleep interruption in adolescents, evidence from a cross-sectional study. *J. Sleep Res.* **2003**, *12*, 263. [CrossRef] [PubMed]

278. Van Deursen, A.J.A.M.; Bolle, C.L.; Hegner, S.M.; Kommers, P.A.M. Modeling habitual and addictive smartphone behavior: The role of smartphone usage types, emotional intelligence, social stress, self-regulation, age, and gender. *Comput. Hum. Behav.* **2015**, *45*, 411–420. [CrossRef]

279. Wang, H.-H.; Wang, M.-C.; Wu, S.-Q. Mobile phone addiction symptom profiles related to interpersonal relationship and loneliness for college students: A latent profile analysis. *Chin. J. Clin. Psychol.* **2015**, *23*, 881–885.
280. Wang, J.L.; Wang, H.Z.; Gaskin, J.; Wang, L.H. The role of stress and motivation in problematic smartphone use among college students. *Comput. Hum. Behav.* **2015**, *53*, 181–188. [CrossRef]
281. Wang, P.; Zhao, M.; Wang, X.; Xie, X.; Wang, Y.; Lei, L. Peer relationship and adolescent smartphone addiction: The mediating role of self-esteem and the moderating role of the need to belong. *J. Behav. Addict.* **2017**, *6*, 708–717. [CrossRef] [PubMed]
282. Wang, P.W.; Liu, T.L.; Ko, C.H.; Lin, H.C.; Huang, M.F.; Yeh, Y.C.; Yen, C.F. Association between problematic cellular phone use and suicide: The moderating effect of family function and depression. *Compr. Psychiatry* **2014**, *55*, 342–348. [CrossRef] [PubMed]
283. Wang, Y.; Zou, Z.; Song, H.; Xu, X.; Wang, H.; d'Oleire Uquillas, F.; Huang, X. Altered Gray Matter Volume and White Matter Integrity in College Students with Mobile Phone Dependence. *Front. Psychol.* **2016**, *7*, 597. [CrossRef] [PubMed]
284. Warzecha, K.; Pawlak, A. Pathological use of mobile phones by secondary school students. *Arch. Psychiatry Psychother.* **2017**, *19*, 27–36. [CrossRef]
285. Venkatesh, E.; Jemal, M.Y.; Samani, A.S. Smart phone usage and addiction among dental students in Saudi Arabia: A cross sectional study. *Int. J. Adolesc. Med. Health* **2017**. [CrossRef] [PubMed]
286. Vernon, L.; Modecki, K.L.; Barber, B.L. Mobile Phones in the Bedroom: Trajectories of Sleep Habits and Subsequent Adolescent Psychosocial Development. *Child Dev.* **2018**, *89*, 66–77. [CrossRef] [PubMed]
287. Wolniewicz, C.A.; Tiamiyu, M.F.; Weeks, J.W.; Elhai, J.D. Problematic smartphone use and relations with negative affect, fear of missing out, and fear of negative and positive evaluation. *Psychiatry Res.* **2018**, *262*, 618–623. [CrossRef] [PubMed]
288. Wu, A.M.; Cheung, V.I.; Ku, L.; Hung, E.P. Psychological risk factors of addiction to social networking sites among Chinese smartphone users. *J. Behav. Addict.* **2013**, 2, 160–166. [CrossRef] [PubMed]
289. Yang, Y.S.; Yen, J.Y.; Ko, C.H.; Cheng, C.P.; Yen, C.F. The association between problematic cellular phone use and risky behaviors and low self-esteem among Taiwanese adolescents. *BMC Public Health* **2010**, *10*, 217. [CrossRef] [PubMed]
290. Yen, C.-F.; Tang, T.-C.; Yen, J.-Y.; Lin, H.-C.; Huang, C.-F.; Liu, S.-C.; Ko, C.-H. Symptoms of problematic cellular phone use, functional impairment and its association with depression among adolescents in Southern Taiwan. *J. Adolesc.* **2009**, *32*, 863–873. [CrossRef] [PubMed]
291. Yuchang, J.; Cuicui, S.; Junxiu, A.; Junyi, L. Attachment styles and smartphone addiction in Chinese college students: The mediating roles of dysfunctional attitudes and self-esteem. *Int. J. Ment. Health Addict.* **2017**, *15*, 1122–1134. [CrossRef]
292. Yun, I.; Kim, S.G.; Kwon, S. Low self-control among South Korean adolescents: A test of Gottfredson and Hirschi's Generality Hypothesis. *Int. J. Offender Ther. Comp. Criminol.* **2016**, *60*, 1185–1208. [CrossRef] [PubMed]
293. Zarghami, M.; Khalilian, A.; Setareh, J.; Salehpour, G. The Impact of Using Cell Phones After Light-Out on Sleep Quality, Headache, Tiredness, and Distractibility Among Students of a University in North of Iran. *Iran. J. Psychiatry Behav. Sci.* **2015**, *9*, e2010. [CrossRef] [PubMed]
294. Zhitomirsky-Geffet, M.; Blau, M. Cross-generational analysis of predictive factors of addictive behavior in smartphone usage. *Comput. Hum. Behav.* **2016**, *64*, 682–693. [CrossRef]
295. Billieux, J. Problematic use of the mobile phone: A literature review and a pathways model. *Curr. Psychiatry Rev.* **2012**, *8*, 299–307. [CrossRef]
296. Young, K.S. Internet addiction: The emergence of a new clinical disorder. *Cyberpsychol. Behav.* **1998**, *1*, 237–244. [CrossRef]
297. Andrews, S.; Ellis, D.A.; Shaw, H.; Piwek, L. Beyond self-report: Tools to compare estimated and real-world smartphone use. *PLoS ONE* **2015**, *10*, e0139004. [CrossRef] [PubMed]
298. Yildirim, C.; Correia, A.P. Exploring the dimensions of nomophobia: Development and validation of a self-reported questionnaire. *Comput. Hum. Behav.* **2015**, *49*, 130–137. [CrossRef]
299. Tavernier, R.; Willoughby, T. Sleep problems: Predictor or outcome of media use among emerging adults at university? *J. Sleep Res.* **2014**, *23*, 389–396. [CrossRef] [PubMed]

300. Exelmans, L.; Van den Bulck, J. The Use of Media as a Sleep Aid in Adults. *Behav. Sleep Med.* **2014**, *14*, 121–133. [CrossRef] [PubMed]
301. Boase, J.; Ling, R. Measuring Mobile Phone Use: Self-Report versus Log Data. *J. Comput. Mediat. Commun.* **2013**, *18*, 508–519. [CrossRef]
302. Riemann, D.; Spiegelhalder, K.; Feige, B.; Voderholzer, U.; Berger, M.; Perlis, M.; Nissen, C. The hyperarousal model of insomnia: A review of the concept and its evidence. *Sleep Med. Rev.* **2010**, *14*, 19–31. [CrossRef] [PubMed]
303. Chang, A.M.; Aeschbach, D.; Duffy, J.F.; Czeisler, C.A. Evening use of light-emitting eReaders negatively affects sleep, circadian timing, and next-morning alertness. *Proc. Natl. Acad. Sci. USA* **2015**, *112*, 1232–1237. [CrossRef] [PubMed]
304. Wood, B.; Rea, M.S.; Plitnick, B.; Figueiro, M.G. Light level and duration of exposure determine the impact of self-luminous tablets on melatonin suppression. *Appl. Ergon.* **2013**, *44*, 237–240. [CrossRef] [PubMed]

4

The Effect of Providing Free Eyeglasses on Children's Mental Health Outcomes in China: A Cluster-Randomized Controlled Trial

Hongyu Guan [1], Huan Wang [2,*], Kang Du [1], Jin Zhao [1], Matthew Boswell [2], Yaojiang Shi [1] and Yiwei Qian [3,*]

1 Center for Experimental Economics in Education, Shaanxi Normal University, Xi'an 710127, China; hongyuguan0621@gmail.com (H.G.); dukangceee@163.com (K.D.); zhaojinceee@163.com (J.Z.); shiyaojiang7@gmail.com (Y.S.)
2 Freeman Spogli Institute for International Studies, Stanford University, Stanford, CA 94305, USA; kefka@stanford.edu
3 Department of Economics, University of Southern California, Los Angeles, CA 90089, USA
* Correspondence: huanw@stanford.edu (H.W.); yiweiqia@usc.edu (Y.Q.)

Abstract: If children with common vision problems receive and use eyeglasses, their educational performance rises. Without proper treatment, visually impaired children may not achieve educational gains and could suffer from poor mental health. We use a randomized controlled trial to study the impact of an eyeglasses promotion program in rural China on the mental health of myopic primary school students. Three measures of mental health are used: learning anxiety, physical anxiety, and scores on the Mental Health Test (MHT). Our empirical analysis showed that on average, the treatment has small and insignificant for learning anxiety and MHT, and a small but significant reduction in physical anxiety. However, subgroup analysis reveals that myopic students who study more intensively see their learning anxiety and physical anxiety reduced after being provided with eyeglasses. In contrast, students with the lower study intensity suffer a rise in learning anxiety after receiving eyeglasses. A potential mechanism for the differing impacts is the increase in teasing reported among low study-intensity students that does not occur for high study-intensity students. Care should be taken to maximize the benefits and minimize the costs of in-school vision programs.

Keywords: myopia; eyeglasses; randomized controlled trial; health technology adoption; mental health

1. Introduction

Nearly half of the disabilities that affect children in developing countries are due to visual impairment [1]. The most common and easily treated cause of visual impairment is uncorrected refractive error. Among all children in the world who are visually impaired by refractive error, approximately half live in China [2]. Although eyeglasses offer a safe, effective, and inexpensive solution to visual impairment caused by refractive error, recent studies have shown that as few as one in six children in lower- and middle-income areas of the developing world who need eyeglasses actually own them [1].

In view of the large global burden of uncorrected pediatric refractive error, there is interest in addressing this condition and the subsequent impact on children's lives. A recent, large randomized controlled trial in rural western China demonstrated that providing eyeglasses could significantly improve children's educational outcomes [1,3]. The magnitude of the impact has been shown to be comparable to and potentially exceeding other in-school health care interventions, such as de-worming or nutritional supplements [4]. Providing eyeglasses also has been shown to reverse decrements in self-reported visual function in children with even modest abnormalities in visual acuity (<6/9) [5].

Although previous studies have focused mainly on the relationship between the correction of refractive error and educational outcomes, there is also concern that visual impairment and the absence of quality vision care for students may be a source of mental health problems [6]. In particular, the literature highlights competitive education systems as putting adolescents at risk of various mental health problems that may be exacerbated by anything that inhibits learning. For myopic students, the inability to see clearly could be a serious barrier to learning, especially in settings in which the blackboard, a common teaching tool, is positioned at the front of the classroom [1]. The inability to perform may itself be a source of anxiety, creating a cycle of poor achievement and worsening mental health [7].

There is a growing literature on the role of vision correction as an educational input [1,3,8]. A number of randomized studies have shown that correcting vision can improve scores on standardized tests. One study, for example, has shown that the provision of glasses in schools boosts standardized test scores among primary school students [1]. A similarly study found that the existence of systematic screening and referrals for free refraction and prescription eyeglasses at a local vision clinic raised test scores for children in surrounding schools [9]. Studies in other settings have shown similar positive results [1,3,4]

There is also a consensus on the link between poor vision and mental health. Studies among adults and the elderly have found that vision correction is associated with better mental health, less worry, reduced frustration, and a higher sense of well-being [10,11]. A smaller literature documents a correlation between uncorrected myopia and mental health among children [12].

However, comparatively little is known about how correcting vision may affect mental health in an educational context. The issue is especially important given the high degree of pressure to perform in many schooling environments, such as China, where only top-performing students in high-stake tests may enroll into high school and university, get recruited for satisfactory jobs, and enjoy opportunities that are off-limits to lower scoring students [13]. The literature shows that competitive education systems put adolescents at risk of various mental health problems that may be exacerbated by anything that inhibits learning. For myopic students, the inability to see clearly could be a serious barrier to learning, especially in settings in which the blackboard, a common teaching tool, is positioned at the front of the classroom [14]. The inability to perform in school might be a source of anxiety, creating a cycle of poor achievement and worsening mental health.

Despite the potential benefits of vision correction for mental health in these settings, there is also the possibility of negative impacts of wearing eyeglasses. Research suggests that a change in personal appearance due to eyeglasses wear can invite teasing from peers [15,16]. A recent study among students in the UK, for example, showed that students with glasses were far more likely to fall victim to bullying and name calling [15]. Additional research has reported the negative stereotypes associated with eyeglasses wear across a variety of contexts [17,18]. Children who wear eyeglasses can be accused of "putting on airs" or trying to appear overly intellectual. Such teasing may spur a decline in psychological well-being [15]. It is therefore possible that such negative impacts may obscure or even completely outweigh mental health gains accrued by being able to see clearly and improve in school.

For this reason, we are interested in particular about how study intensity serves to mediate the impact of vision correction on mental health. Study intensity, as reflected in the number of hours spent studying outside of class, has been shown to predict perseverance and passion for long-term goals [19–21]. Studies have found that students who spend more time studying outside of class tend to be more disciplined and capable of self-control [19], and have better academic performance and higher attendance in class [14,22]. Such students may be more likely to ignore teasing or concerns of personal appearance because the benefit gained in learning is perceived to be more important. Conversely, students that study less intensively, who often have lower levels of academic performance, may be relatively more concerned with appearance and peer interactions, and thus be more vulnerable to teasing or other "side effects" of glasses wear. In this way, study intensity may moderate the impact of glasses on mental health as much as, or more than, other student characteristics such as family background or household wealth.

The overall goal of this study is to evaluate the effect of correcting refractive error on the mental health of students in schools in rural China. In particular, given China's highly competitive schooling system, we are interested in exploring the differential impacts of vision correction on students with varying degrees of study intensity. To meet this goal, we have three specific objectives. First, we want to examine the average effect of correcting refractive error on the mental health condition of myopic students. Second, we seek to identify important heterogeneous effects of providing eyeglasses on mental health to determine whether vision correction affects the mental health of different types of children differently. Finally, we explore the mechanisms that might help to explain why correcting refractive error may have different effects on the mental health of students of different study intensity.

2. Sampling, Data Collection, and Analytical Approach

The setting for the study is the public school system in two of China's predominantly rural northwestern provinces, Shaanxi and Gansu. Success in China's competitive public school system is overwhelmingly dependent on performance on high-stakes tests [13], and only a fraction of students are able to move up through the school system and attend academic high school and college. Unfortunately, rural students often face a number of constraints, including poor access to quality health care, nutrition, and vision care. Further, rates of myopia are high among students in rural areas, approximately 20 to 30% in primary school, more than 50% in junior high, and as high as 90% upon completion of high school. As noted earlier, however, rates of eyeglasses wear remain very low among students.

We conducted a cluster-randomized controlled trial (hereafter, cluster-RCT) across 252 primary rural schools in China to study the impact of providing eyeglasses on the mental health of myopic students. In the trial, schools were randomly selected into the treatment group and the control group. Among 19,934 students in the 252 primary schools, 2851 myopic students who could potentially benefit from having eyeglasses were involved in the experiment. In the treatment group, fully subsidized eyeglasses were provided to eligible myopic students. In the control group, myopic students were given only eyeglasses prescriptions. Each myopic student was given a letter for their parents informing them of their child's myopia status and prescription. No other action was taken. If the students in the control group opted to purchases glasses, they would also have to travel to the county seat and select an optical shop and purchase the eyeglasses.

2.1. Sampling

Sampling was conducted immediately prior to the implementation of the study during the 2012–2013 school year in one prefecture in Gansu Province and one prefecture in Shaanxi Province. By choosing two provinces that differ in terms of wealth and development, as measured by GDP per capita (Gansu is relatively poor, and Shaanxi is close to China's overall average), we are able to increase the generalizability of our findings [23]. Gansu's GDP per capita, 3919 USD, was ranked the second poorest among China's 31 provincial administrative regions in 2013. Shaanxi's GDP per capita, 6883 USD, was ranked 12th [24]. One prefecture in each province was selected, Tianshui in Gansu Province and Yulin in Shaanxi Province. In total, we collected data in 18 of the 19 counties in the two prefectures. One county was not included due to the small size of its population, the surveying of which would have substantially raised the cost of the survey.

To choose the sample schools and students in these two prefectures, we followed a three-step protocol. First, we obtained a list of all rural primary schools in the two prefectures from local county education bureaus. Second, to eliminate the potential spillovers, we randomly selected only one school from each school district (or town) in the sample frame. Finally, within each school, we randomly selected one class in each of the fourth and fifth grades (likely age range was 9–12 years old). In total, 19,934 students from 252 rural primary schools were selected.

2.2. Experimental Design

To ensure a balanced sample and to improve the power of the experimental design, an intervention assignment was stratified by location (county), school size, and eye examination results (i.e., the proportion of myopic students in each school) collected in the baseline survey. In total, this yielded a total of 45 strata, and our analysis takes this stratified randomization procedure into account [25]. Two-thirds of the schools were randomly assigned to one of two treatment groups and the other one-third to a control group. Among the two treatment groups, half of the schools were assigned to a free eyeglasses treatment group and the other half to a voucher treatment group. Because the intervention in both treatment groups was almost the same (at least in the context of this study, as both sets of students received the same vision care and were given access to the kind of eyeglasses), we combined the two treatment groups into one.

Once the randomized assignment was completed, the implementation team launched the intervention. In the treatment group, every student was screened. Students with poor vision were identified through a two-step eye examination protocol (described in detail in Section 2.3). A prescription for eyeglasses for each student with poor vision was produced by a professional optometrist. A letter that described this vision care program and a prescription for the student was sent to parents. In addition, information about vision care and the importance of wearing eyeglasses was given to students in the form of an in-class training program. Based on the prescription, a pair of free eyeglasses was produced for each myopic student. About four weeks after the baseline (October 2012) program optometrists dispensed free eyeglasses at schools for the free treatment group, and free eyeglasses were ready for pickup at a shop of a local optometrist for the voucher treatment group. There were not large differences in acceptance or the wearing of eyeglasses or in the impact on academic outcomes between the two treatment groups, which further supports the decision to combine the two treatment groups in this study.

In the control group, only the letter and a prescription for the student were given to the parents. No additional training was provided to the students. The students and their families were blind to the cluster-RCT.

2.3. Data Collection

We conducted a total of two waves of surveys: one at baseline and one at post-treatment. Each survey was administrated to all sample students in the 252 schools. The baseline survey was conducted in September 2012 at the beginning of fall semester. The post-treatment survey was conducted in June 2013 at the end of the spring semester.

2.3.1. Baseline Survey

Baseline surveys were administered to all students in a classroom in two blocks. In the first block, examiners administered questionnaires to students in regard to age, gender, eyeglasses wear, awareness of refractive status, knowledge of vision care, and boarding status at school. The questionnaires also contained a place for an estimate of the number of hours that each student studied after class per day. In this study, we use this measure as a proxy for each student's study intensity. Each student was asked to record how much time he or she spends studying outside of school, drawing from a list of options that included "0–0.5 h," "0.5–2 h", or "more than 2 h." Students who recorded studying more than 2 h were considered to maintain high study intensity, whereas those who indicated studying for less than half an hour per day were considered students of low study intensity.

The first block of the survey also included a parent survey form in which parents reported their migration status, family asses, and education. We collected detailed information on the migration status of each student's parents. Specifically, the questions asked whether each parent had been migrated out of the area for work during the past six months. Field observations and interviews with key informants suggest that for most rural laborers in the study area, if they are working and living away from home for at least six months, it is almost certain that they were actually away from home for most or all of the entire year [26,27]. As a way of cross checking, we asked the homeroom teacher to verify the information on the parental migration status of each student. In our overall sample, around 12.5% of children are left behind children (that is, both parents have out-migrated), just a bit lower than estimates of the average of representative rural areas in China (15.7%) [28].

The household survey also collected information on value of family assets that students would likely have difficulty answering. Caregivers were asked to fill out a checklist of thirteen household consumption assets: automobile, truck, motor bike, tractor, farming equipment, computer, internet, television, camera, washing machine, air conditioner, water heater, gas stove, refrigerator, kitchen ventilator, and flushable toilet. A value was attached to each asset (based on the National Household Income and Expenditure Survey, which is organized and published by the China National Bureau of Statistics) to produce a single metric of household asset holdings. Summing the value of all household consumption assets then produced our proxy variable for family wealth value [29]. We did so because recent studies suggest using household asset indicators for household wealth is more reliable than self-reported income [30].

In the second block, examiners administered a test that we used to assess the mental health condition of each student. In our study, we measured mental health with an instrument that researchers in China term the Mental Health Test (MHT). The MHT was developed by Prof. Bucheng Zhou of East China Normal University, who adapted it from the General Anxiety Test developed by Kiyoshi Suzuki in Japan [31]. The MHT is a variation of the Children's Manifest Anxiety Scale, which is an internationally standardized test for the anxiety of children that has been widely used in the United States and other developed countries [32]. The MHT also has been widely applied in China [7,30]. The test has a reliability of 0.84–0.88 and a retest reliability of 0.78–0.86. Among the subcategories of the scale, we pay special attention to learning anxiety and physical anxiety, which are the two most common anxieties among rural students in China [30]. The use of eyeglasses would give myopic students a clear view of the blackboard and learning materials, thus potentially reducing their anxiety towards learning and physical health.

According to the MHT scale, learning anxiety refers to a student's fear of examinations or excessive concerns about test scores. Such as, worried about passing exams successfully, feel unhappy when the test scores are not good, feel anxious when student cannot remember what he/she has learned during an examination, and worry about getting a poor score when taking an exam. Physical anxiety refers to a student's excessive concerns about his/her body, such as: always worried about there is something wrong in his/her body, often think that other students are prettier or more handsome than him/her, find it difficult to sleep at night, and unwilling to take medicine.

During the analysis, we normalized the anxiety scores against the control group's baseline distribution. Higher scores represent higher levels of anxiety.

At the same time as the baseline survey, a two-step eye examination was administered to all students in the randomly selected classes in all sample schools. In the first step, a team of two trained staff administered visual acuity (VA) screenings, using Early Treatment Diabetic Retinopathy Study eye charts. Students who failed the VA screening test (the cutoff is a VA of either eye of less than or equal to 6/12, or 20/40) were enrolled in a second vision test that was conducted at each school one to two days after the first test. The second vision test was conducted by a team of one optometrist, one nurse, and one assistant. It involved cycloplegic automated refraction with subjective refinement to determine prescriptions for children's eligibility for eyeglasses (the cutoff for myopia is ≤ -0.5 diopters [D]). The eye examination team was trained by Zhongshan Ophthalmic Center (ZOC) at Sun Yat-sen University.

2.3.2. Post-Treatment Survey

In May 2013, approximately seven months after the eyeglasses were dispensed, a post-treatment survey was conducted. The post-treatment survey followed the same protocol as the baseline survey. As in the baseline survey, the examiners collected post-treatment MHT scores. As in the case of the baseline survey, we normalized scores, using the control group's baseline distribution.

As we were conducting the post-treatment survey, we also conducted an unannounced spot check to collect information on the eyeglasses wear of myopic students. We also conducted an unannounced spot check to collect information on the eyeglasses wear of myopic students. A team of two examiners was sent to schools in advance of the rest of the survey team. Examiners were given a list of the students diagnosed with myopia in the baseline and recorded individual-level information on whether each student wears eyeglasses regularly when studying and outside of class. Eyeglasses wear is a binary variable based on whether students wear eyeglasses regularly.

Right after the spot check, a survey that is similar to the baseline one was administered to all students in a classroom. In addition, being aware that misperceptions about wearing eyeglasses might lead myopic students to be teased by their classmates, we asked each student whether myopic students were being teased in his or her class. Being teased is a binary variable. We also collect data on whether students consider wearing eyeglasses to be good looking. Specifically, we define eyeglasses are good looking as a binary variable taking the value of one if a student thinks wearing eyeglasses is good looking.

2.4. Summary Statistics, Balance, and Attrition

Given our sampling strategy, the results of our baseline survey are representative of students in poor rural areas in China. As seen in Table 1, students in our sample are, on average, 10.51 years old (or 10 years, 6 months), which suggests that students started primary school (Grade 1), on average, at 7 years old. In our overall sample, 52% are male, which is similar to the sex ratio across poor areas of rural China [12]. In our sample, only 8.7% of mothers and 13.3% of fathers completed more than 12 years of education. For adults of this age, the levels of education are also typical as across China, where only 11.3% of individuals aged 25–64 from rural areas finished upper secondary education [30]. Finally, in our overall sample, 12.5% of children are left-behind children (that is, both parents have out-migrated). This level is similar to (or slightly lower than) estimates of the share of children who are left behind in China (15.7%) [18].

To identify students with vision problems, optometrists who worked with the survey team conducted eye examinations with all students in the 252 sample schools. Of the total number of students in the overall sample (19,934), 2851 (14.3%) were myopic to a degree that they could benefit from having eyeglasses; these students were included in our analysis (Table 1).

Random assignment successfully created a sample balanced between the treatment and control groups. Using student individual characteristics, family characteristics, and student mental health scores, Table 1 shows that the groups were similar in terms of the measured characteristics. A joint significance test across all baseline characteristics also confirms that the study arms are balanced. We test this by regressing treatment status on all baseline characteristics reported in Table 1 and test that the coefficients on all characteristics were jointly zero. The p-value of this test is 0.2344 (treatment group vs. control group). The attrition rate of the sample between baseline and post-treatment was 3.9%. In the RCT literature, this attrition rate is considered low [33].

Table A1 indicates that there are no statistically significant differences in the rates of attrition between the treatment group and control group. Further, as seen in Table A2, baseline characteristics are still well balanced between the control and treatment groups in terms of non-missing observations. In a later analysis, we control for these variables in the regression.

Table 1. Baseline Characteristics across Experimental Groups.

Variable	Entire Sample	Control Group	Treatment Group	Difference	p-Value
Student level					
Age (years)	10.507 (1.104)	10.547 (1.109)	10.487 (1.102)	−0.0597	0.4272
Male, 1 = yes	0.485 (0.5)	0.496 (0.5)	0.48 (0.5)	−0.0165	0.4097
Refractive error, D	−2.232 (1.245)	−2.277 (1.271)	−2.211 (1.232)	0.0659	0.2628
Wear eyeglasses at baseline, 1 = yes	0.154 (0.361)	0.145 (0.353)	0.159 (0.365)	0.0134	0.4808
Math score	0.239 (0.989)	0.244 (1.006)	0.236 (0.982)	−0.0079	0.9003
MHT score	−0.034 (1.042)	−0.037 (1.048)	−0.033 (1.04)	0.0041	0.4025
Learning anxiety score	−0.021 (1.014)	−0.052 (0.999)	−0.006 (1.022)	0.0461	0.948
Physical anxiety score	−0.045 (0.999)	−0.048 (1.028)	−0.043 (0.985)	0.0047	0.9365
Family level					
One or both parents with > 12 years education, 1 = yes	0.206 (0.404)	0.203 (0.403)	0.207 (0.405)	0.0039	0.8466
Family asset value, thousand RMB	32.06 (35.394)	30.763 (34.215)	32.679 (35.936)	1.9161	0.5567
Number of observations	2851	929	1922	2851	

Note: Standard deviations in parentheses.

2.5. Statistical Approach

We use ordinary least squares (OLS) regression analysis to estimate the treatment effect and heterogeneous impacts.

First, we compare the post-treatment standardized MHT scores and learning anxiety scores of students between the treatment and control schools, controlling for baseline standardized math test scores and a set of controls with strata effect and school effect.

The specification of the model is as follows:

$$Y_{1ijp} = \beta_0 + \beta_1 Z_{ijp} + \beta_2 Y_{0ijp} + X'_{ijp}\gamma + Strata_j + School_{jp} + \epsilon_{ijp} \quad (1)$$

where Y_{1ijp} is the post-treatment standardized MHT scores, learning anxiety scores, and physical anxiety scores for student i at school p in stratum j, treatment dummy Z_{ijp} takes the value of 1 if students were provided with free eyeglasses, and Y_{0ijp} is the standardized MHT, learning anxiety, and physical anxiety scores in the baseline. X_{ijp} is a vector of other baseline characteristics (described in Table 1).

Given that providing free eyeglasses might have a heterogeneous impact on students with different study intensity at baseline, we use the following model to estimate the heterogeneous treatment effect:

$$\begin{aligned} Y_{1ijp} = \beta_0 + \beta_1 Z_{ijp} + \beta_2 Z_{ijp} \times \mathbf{1}\{D_{0ijp} = 2\} + \beta_3 Z_{ijp} \times \mathbf{1}\{D_{0ijp} = 3\} + \\ \theta Y_{0ijp} + X'_{ijp}\gamma + Strata_j + School_{jp} + \epsilon_{ijp} \end{aligned} \quad (2)$$

where we add interaction terms of the treatment dummy and the indicator functions of the subgroup of study intensity at baseline D_{0ijp}, which takes three values: 1, 2 and 3. The parameter β_1 is a measure of the impact of providing free eyeglasses on the subgroup of students who study at a low level of intensity (0 to 0.5 h of studying per day after class); $\beta_1 + \beta_2$ measures the impact on the subgroup of students who study at a medium level of intensity (0.5 to 2 h of studying per day after class); and $\beta_1 + \beta_3$ measures the impact on the subgroup of students who study at a high level of intensity (greater than 2 h of studying per day after class).

3. Results

3.1. Impact of Providing Free Eyeglasses/Wearing Eyeglasses on Mental Health

The impact of the eyeglasses promotion program on mental health is presented in Table 2. Estimation from ordinary least squares regression analysis using model (1) show that the treatment has small and insignificant for Learning Anxiety and MHT. There is, however, a significant reduction in Physical Anxiety (Table 2, column 2).

Table 2. Impact of Providing Fully Subsidized Eyeglasses on Mental Health.

Dependent Variable	Post-Treatment		
	Learning Anxiety	Physical Anxiety	MHT
Treatment, 1 = yes	−0.0308 (0.0528)	−0.0763 † (0.0449)	−0.0781 (0.0492)
Variable controlled			
Baseline learning anxiety	Yes	No	No
Baseline physical anxiety	No	Yes	No
Baseline MHT	No	Yes	Yes
Student, family characteristics	Yes	Yes	Yes
Control mean	−0.1170	-0.1310	−0.1840
Number of observations	2557	2557	2557

Note: Standard deviations in parentheses. All coefficients are estimated with mixed-effect linear regression clustering at strata and school levels. † $p < 0.10$. MHT: Mental Health Test.

Although there is no impact of either providing free eyeglasses or wearing eyeglasses on mental health on average, it is worth considering whether there might be a heterogeneous treatment effect between different subgroups. It could be the case that there are heterogeneous treatment effects in subgroups with opposite signs that offset each other.

The results indicate that the treatment affects students of varying degrees of study intensity differently (Table 3). Treatment students who study at a low intensity level experience a 0.17 SD rise in Learning Anxiety, significant at the 5% level. Conversely, treatment students who study at a high intensity level experience a 0.25 SD decline in Learning Anxiety, significant at the 10% level; a 0.22 SD decline in Physical Anxiety, significant at the 10% level; and a 0.26 SD improvement in MHT score, significant at the 5% level. Echoing this trend, treatment students who study at a moderate degree of intensity experience a 0.13 decline in MHT score, significant at the 5% level.

In summary, the intervention of providing free eyeglasses, on average, does not improve the mental health condition of students. Even when we consider the effect of wearing eyeglasses on mental health (average treatment effect on the students), the estimated coefficient is still statistically insignificant, except for a small decline in Physical Anxiety. When we estimate the heterogeneous impacts as varying by study intensity, interestingly, we find the treatment worsens learning anxiety for students with low study intensity, whereas it improves the mental health condition for students with higher study intensity.

Table 3. Impact of Subsidized Eyeglasses on Mental Health by After-class Study Time.

Dependent Variable	Post-Treatment		
	Learning Anxiety	**Physical Anxiety**	**MHT**
Treatment, 1 = yes	0.1740 * (0.0857)	−0.0379 (0.0740)	0.0940 (0.0815)
Baseline study hours 0–0.5 h (as comparison)			
Baseline study hours 0.5–2 h, 1 = yes	0.1603 † (0.0829)	0.0245 (0.0722)	0.1314 (0.0799)
Baseline study hours >2 h, 1 = yes	0.3558 ** (0.1265)	0.1656 (0.1102)	0.2324 † (0.1219)
Treatment x (Baseline study hours 0.5–2 h)	−0.2696 ** (0.1001)	−0.0292 (0.0870)	−0.2258 * (0.0963)
Treatment x (Baseline study hours >2 h)	−0.4192 ** (0.1524)	−0.1789 (0.1325)	−0.3511 * (0.1466)
Variable controlled			
Baseline learning anxiety	Yes	No	No
Baseline physical anxiety	No	Yes	No
Baseline MHT	No	No	Yes
Student, family characteristics	Yes	Yes	Yes
Treatment effect for 0–0.5 h	0.1740 *	−0.0379	0.0940
p-value for 0–0.5 h	0.0420	0.6080	0.2490
Treatment effect for 0.5–2 h	−0.0960	−0.0670	−0.1320 *
p-value for 0.5–2 h	0.1440	0.2310	0.0320
Treatment effect for >2 h	−0.2450 †	−0.2170 †	−0.2570 *
p-value for >2 h	0.0620	0.0570	0.0410
N	2557	2557	2557
Control mean	−0.1170	−0.1310	−0.1840

Note: Cluster-robust standard errors in parentheses. All coefficients are estimated with mixed-effect linear regression clustering at strata and school levels. † $p < 0.10$, * $p < 0.05$, ** $p < 0.01$.

3.2. Mechanisms that Drive the Impact of Heterogeneity

The results presented in Table 4 concerns possible mechanisms for the heterogeneous impacts presented above. The results from regressions without controlling for baseline characteristics show a similar finding, see Tables A4 and A5. The analysis concerns secondary outcomes—Eyeglasses Wear, Change in Study Hours, Math Score, Being Teased, and Finding Eyeglasses Good Looking—among students of varying degrees of study intensity.

All students, regardless of their level of study intensity, experience a rise in wear of eyeglasses due to the intervention. Students who study at a high level of intensity experience an 18 percent rise in eyeglasses wear, significant at the 1% level, while moderate- and low-intensity students experience somewhat lower rate of wearing eyeglasses compare to their high study intensity peers (Table 4, column 1).

The analysis of the Being Teased outcome may shed light on why low intensity students experience a rise in Learning Anxiety, while their high intensity peers enjoy a decline in Learning Anxiety (as reported in Table 3). Students who study at a low intensity level experience a 13 percent rise in being teased from their peers due to the intervention, significant at the 1% level (Table 4, column 4). Moderate-intensity students see a similar, if more moderate, 11 percent rise in being teased, significant at the 1% level. High-intensity students experience no change in the amount that they are teased. A possible mechanism for this finding is that increasingly teased children internalize the notion that they are being perceived as more studious on account of wearing glasses, and therefore feel slightly more pressure to perform in school. No similar scenario unfolds for high intensity students, perhaps because they are already used to performing well in school. We examined the difference in baseline math test scores between different study intensity groups. Students who spend less time studying (low study intensity) at baseline were indeed the students who had worst test scores, they were 0.34 standard deviation behind the moderate study intensity students and 0.27 standard behind the high study intensity students, see Table A3. This interpretation is buttressed by the fact that high intensity students report a rise in believing that eyeglasses are good looking (Table 4, column 5)—after all, they are not being teased for wearing them.

Table 4. Impact of Providing Fully Subsidized Eyeglasses on Secondary Outcomes by Daily After-class Study Time.

Dependent Variables	Post-Treatment				
	(1) Wear Eyeglasses	(2) Change Study Hours	(3) Math Score	(4) Being Teased	(5) Eyeglasses Good-Looking
Treatment, 1 = yes	0.1073 ** (0.0378)	0.0006 (0.0368)	0.1248 † (0.0652)	0.1261 ** (0.0335)	0.0022 (0.0290)
Baseline Study hours 0–0.5 h	(as comparison)				
Baseline Study hours 0.5–2 h, 1 = yes	0.0265 (0.0324)	−0.2431 ** (0.0363)	0.1505 ** (0.0584)	0.0021 (0.0312)	0.0004 (0.0254)
Baseline Study hours >2 h, 1 = yes	0.0380 (0.0499)	0.2257 ** (0.0554)	0.1823 * (0.0899)	0.0422 (0.0479)	−0.0118 (0.0392)
Treatment * (Study hours 0.5–2 h)	0.0069 (0.0393)	0.0062 (0.0439)	−0.0419 (0.0709)	−0.0168 (0.0379)	0.0068 (0.0309)
Treatment * (Study hours >2 h)	0.0690 (0.0603)	−0.0057 (0.0667)	−0.0976 (0.1085)	−0.0545 (0.0578)	0.0707 (0.0473)
Variable Controlled:					
Baseline MHT, Learning Anxiety & Physical Anxiety	Yes	Yes	Yes	Yes	Yes
Student, Family Characteristics	Yes	Yes	Yes	Yes	Yes
Treatment effect for 0–0.5 h	0.1070 *	0.0010	0.1250 †	0.1260 **	0.0020
p-value for 0–0.5 h	0.0050	0.9870	0.0560	0.0000	0.9400
Treatment effect for 0.5–2 h	0.1140 **	0.0070	0.0830	0.1090 **	0.0090
p-value for 0.5–2 h	0.0000	0.8060	0.1140	0.0000	0.7040
Treatment effect for >2 h	0.1760 **	−0.0050	0.0270	0.0720	0.0730 †
p-value for >2 h	0.0010	0.9280	0.7770	0.1570	0.0860
N	2538	2631	2537	2536	2534
Control Mean	0.2690	0.4750	0.3280	0.1390	0.1150

Note: Cluster-robust standard errors in parentheses. All coefficients are estimated with mixed-effect linear regression clustering at strata and school levels. † $p < 0.10$, * $p < 0.05$, ** $p < 0.01$.

One seemingly contradictory finding from Table 4 is that students who get teased more as a consequence of wearing glasses still wear the eyeglasses. However, we see from the analysis that the vision correction intervention raised test scores by 0.13 SD among low study intensity myopic students, significant at the 1% level (Table 4, column 3). This reveals a possible explanatory factor for the apparently contradictory finding. The gains achieved in test score outcomes may be perceived as more important than the costs associated with increased teasing. Therefore, the children persist in wearing their glasses.

Finally, no students see any change in their hours of study due to the intervention. This appears to suggest that changes in the mental health outcomes among students in all three study intensity groups were not caused by any change in study time.

4. Conclusions

In this study, we use a cluster-RCT to measure the effect of an eyeglasses promotion program in 252 Chinese rural primary schools on the mental health condition of myopic students. On average, the treatment has small and insignificant for Learning Anxiety and MHT, and a small but significant reduction in Physical Anxiety.

These average treatment effects mask important heterogenous effects, however. Heterogeneous analysis on the amount of time that students spend in studying after school reveals that the program reduces both Learning Anxiety and Physical Anxiety among students who study with a high degree of intensity. Children who study less intensively are shown to experience an increase in Learning Anxiety. Increased teasing of less studious students following their acceptance of eyeglasses may explain their rise in anxiety.

The strengths of the current study include its large sample size and randomized design. The study of the mental health impacts of myopia correction also fills a gap in the literature concerning refractive error care among children, particularly as it relates to their study intensity. Although the sample area was large, caution must be used in extrapolating the results across all rural areas of China or beyond.

The study can inform policy on the provision of vision care in schools in important ways. It is clear from earlier analyses that the timely correction of myopia boosts academic outcomes for students [1]. In-school screenings and the subsidization of eyeglasses are also important drivers of eyeglasses acceptance and wear. Wear rates among students who need eyeglasses remain well below 100% in most contexts. To boost wear rates and minimize negative spillovers on mental health for some students, care should be taken in the classroom to eliminate teasing of students who are newly wearing eyeglasses, and encouragement should be offered to students of all types to recognize their eyeglasses as the valuable learning asset that they are.

Author Contributions: H.G., H.W., M.B. and Y.S. devised the research questions and analytical strategy. Y.Q. conducted the statistical analysis. All authors collaborated on the interpretation of the results and on writing and revising the paper.

Appendix A

Table A1. Attrition check.

Dependent Variable	Attrition, 1 = Yes
Treatment, 1 = yes	0.014 (0.009)
Control mean	2851
Number of observations	0.030
Overall attrition rate	0.039

Note. All coefficients are estimated with mixed-effect linear regression clustering at strata and school levels.

Table A2. Balance check of baseline characteristics of the remaining sample across experimental groups.

Variable	Control Group	Treatment Group	Difference	*p*-Value
Student level				
Age (years)	10.549 (1.1)	10.481 (1.084)	−0.0676	0.3673
Male, 1 = yes	0.502 (0.5)	0.481 (0.5)	−0.0207	0.3107
Refractive error, D	−2.285 (1.274)	−2.215 (1.236)	0.0699	0.2459
Wear eyeglasses at baseline, 1 = yes	0.142 (0.349)	0.16 (0.367)	0.0183	0.3356
Baseline math score	0.25 (1.002)	0.235 (0.981)	−0.0155	0.806

Table A2. *Cont.*

Variable	Control Group	Treatment Group	Difference	p-Value
Baseline MHT score	−0.057 (1.044)	−0.03 (1.038)	0.0274	0.6688
Baseline learning anxiety score	−0.068 (0.999)	−0.004 (1.022)	0.0645	0.2529
Baseline physical anxiety score	−0.061 (1.026)	−0.04 (0.981)	0.0208	0.7293
Family level				
One or both parents with > 12 years education, 1 = yes	0.202 (0.402)	0.203 (0.402)	0.0009	0.9662
Family asset value	30.422 (33.728)	32.884 (36.082)	2.4622	0.4482
Number of observations	901	1840	2741	

Note. Standard deviation in parentheses.

Table A3. Summary of student baseline math scores, by after-class study hours.

	Low Intensity (0–0.5 h)	Moderate Intensity (0.5–2 h)	High Intensity (>2 h)	Mild vs. Low	High vs. Low	High vs. Moderate
	(1)	(2)	(3)	(2)–(1)	(3)–(1)	(3)–(2)
Math Score	0.01 (0.974)	0.35 (0.969)	0.28 (1.028)	0.34 ** (0.042)	0.27 ** 0.0732	−0.071 (0.0639)

Note. Means with standard deviations reported in brackets; Cluster-robust standard errors adjusted for clustering at the school level in parentheses. ** $p < 0.01$.

Table A4. Impact of Providing Fully Subsidized Eyeglasses on Mental Health by Daily After-class Study Time (without controls).

Dependent Variable	Post-Treatment		
	Learning Anxiety	Physical Anxiety	MHT
Treatment, 1 = yes	0.1606 † (0.0923)	0.0100 (0.0813)	0.1279 (0.0937)
Baseline study hours 0–0.5 h		(as comparison)	
Baseline study hours 0.5–2 h, 1 = yes	0.1342 (0.0874)	0.0458 (0.0784)	0.1591 † (0.0897)
Baseline study hours >2 h, 1 = yes	0.3186 * (0.1327)	0.2482 * (0.1189)	0.3274 * (0.1362)
Treatment x (Baseline study hours 0.5–2 h)	−0.2066 † (0.1062)	−0.0334 (0.0953)	−0.2087 † (0.1091)
Treatment x (Baseline study hours >2 h)	−0.3058 † (0.1608)	−0.1802 (0.1440)	−0.3472 * (0.1649)
Variable controlled			
Baseline learning anxiety	No	No	No
Baseline physical anxiety	No	No	No
Baseline MHT	No	No	No
Student, family characteristics	No	No	No
Treatment effect for 0–0.5 h	0.1610 †	0.0100	0.1280
p-value for 0–0.5 h	0.0820	0.9020	0.1720
Treatment effect for 0.5–2 hrs	−0.0460	−0.0230	−0.0810

Table A4. *Cont.*

Dependent Variable	Post-Treatment		
	Learning Anxiety	Physical Anxiety	MHT
p-value for 0.5–2 h	0.5170	0.7040	0.2580
Treatment effect for >2 h	−0.1450	−0.1700	−0.2190
p-value for >2 h	0.2970	0.1690	0.1230
N	2765	2765	2765
Control mean	−0.1310	−0.1440	−0.1990

Note: Cluster-robust standard errors in parentheses. All coefficients are estimated with mixed-effect linear regression clustering at strata and school levels. † $p < 0.10$, * $p < 0.05$.

Table A5. Impact of Providing Fully Subsidized Eyeglasses on Secondary Outcomes by Daily After-class Study Time (without controls).

Dependent Variables	Post-Treatment				
	(1) Wear Eyeglasses	(2) Change Study Hours	(3) Math Score	(5) Being Teased	(6) Eyeglasses Good-Looking
Treatment, 1 = yes	0.1105 ** (0.0400)	−0.0060 (0.0359)	0.1110 (0.0802)	0.1173 ** (0.0329)	0.0173 (0.0280)
Baseline Study hours 0–0.5 h	(as comparison)				
Baseline Study hours 0.5–2 h, 1 = yes	0.0361 (0.0335)	−0.2529 ** (0.0347)	0.3745 ** (0.0702)	−0.0122 (0.0301)	0.0182 (0.0246)
Baseline Study hours >2 h, 1 = yes	0.0315 (0.0513)	0.2150 ** (0.0525)	0.2306 * (0.1074)	0.0534 (0.0459)	−0.0024 (0.0377)
Treatment * (Baseline Study hours 0.5−2 h)	−0.0050 (0.0410)	0.0099 (0.0423)	−0.0936 (0.0859)	−0.0077 (0.0368)	−0.0108 (0.0301)
Treatment * (Baseline Study hours >2 h)	0.0807 (0.0624)	−0.0052 (0.0636)	0.0222 (0.1305)	−0.0530 (0.0557)	0.0465 (0.0457)
Variable Controlled: Student, Family Characteristics	No	No	No	No	No
Treatment effect for 0−0.5 h	0.1110 **	−0.0060	0.1110	0.1170 **	0.0170
p-value for 0−0.5 h	0.006	0.8670	0.1670	0.0000	0.5350
Treatment effect for 0.5−2 h	0.1060 **	0.0040	0.0170	0.1100 **	0.0070
p-value for 0.5−2 h	0.001	0.8870	0.7880	0.0000	0.7700
Treatment effect for >2 h	0.1910 **	−0.0110	0.1330	0.0640	0.0640
p-value for >2 h	0.001	0.8370	0.2530	0.1880	0.1170
N	2740	2850	2739	2738	2739
Control Mean	0.2640	0.4840	0.3200	0.1400	0.1170

Note: Cluster-robust standard errors in parentheses. All coefficients are estimated with mixed-effect linear regression clustering at strata and school levels. * $p < 0.05$, ** $p < 0.01$.

References

1. Ma, X.; Zhou, Z.; Yi, H.; Pang, X.; Shi, Y.; Chen, Q.; Meltzer, M.E.; Le Cessie, S.; He, M.; Rozelle, S. Effect of providing free glasses on children's educational outcomes in China: Cluster randomized controlled trial. *BMJ* **2014**, *349*, g5740. [CrossRef] [PubMed]
2. Resnikoff, S.; Pascolini, D.; Mariotti, S.P.; Pokharel, G.P. Global magnitude of visual impairment caused by uncorrected refractive errors in 2004. *Bull. World Health Organ.* **2008**, *86*, 63–70. [CrossRef] [PubMed]
3. Glewwe, P.; Park, A.; Zhao, M. A better vision for development: Eyeglasses and academic performance in rural primary schools in China. *J. Dev. Econ.* **2016**, *122*, 170–182. [CrossRef]
4. McEwan, P.J. Improving learning in primary schools of developing countries: A meta-analysis of randomized experiments. *Rev. Educ. Res.* **2015**, *85*, 353–394. [CrossRef]
5. Esteso, P.; Castanon, A.; Toledo, S.; Rito, M.A.P.; Ervin, A.; Wojciechowski, R.; Congdon, N.G. Correction of moderate myopia is associated with improvement in self-reported visual functioning among Mexican school-aged children. *Investig. Ophthalmol. Vis. Sci.* **2007**, *48*, 4949–4954. [CrossRef] [PubMed]
6. Hesketh, T.; Ding, Q.J.; Jenkins, R. Suicide ideation in Chinese adolescents. *Soc. Psychiatr. Psychiatr. Epidemiol.* **2002**, *37*, 230–235. [CrossRef] [PubMed]

7. Zhang, L.; Kleiman-Weiner, M.; Luo, R.; Shi, Y.; Martorell, R.; Medina, A.; Rozelle, S. Multiple micronutrient supplementation reduces anemia and anxiety in rural China's elementary school children–4. *J. Nutr.* **2013**, *143*, 640–647. [CrossRef]
8. Congdon, N.; Zheng, M.; Sharma, A.; Choi, K.; Song, Y.; Zhang, M.; Wang, M.; Zhou, Z.; Li, L.; Liu, X.; et al. Prevalence and determinants of spectacle nonwear among rural Chinese secondary schoolchildren: The Xichang Pediatric Refractive Error Study Report 3. *Arch Ophthalmol.* **2008**, *126*, 1717–1723. [CrossRef]
9. Ma, Y.; Congdon, N.; Shi, Y.; Hogg, R.; Medina, A.; Boswell, M.; Rozelle, S.; Iyer, M. Effect of a local vision care center on eyeglasses use and school performance in rural china: A cluster randomized clinical trial. *JAMA Ophthalmol.* **2018**, *136*, 731–737. [CrossRef]
10. Broman, A.T.; Munoz, B.; Rodriguez, J.; Sanchez, R.; Quigley, H.A.; Klein, R.; Snyder, R.; West, S.K. The impact of visual impairment and eye disease on vision-related quality of life in a Mexican-American Population: Proyecto ver. *Investig. Ophthalmol. Vis. Sci.* **2002**, *43*, 3393–3398.
11. Coleman, A.L.; Yu, F.; Keeler, E.; Mangione, C.M. Treatment of uncorrected refractive error improves vision-specific quality of life. *J. Am. Geriatr. Soc.* **2006**, *54*, 883–890. [CrossRef] [PubMed]
12. Yi, H.; Zhang, L.; Ma, X.; Congdon, N.; Shi, Y.; Pang, X.; Zeng, J.; Wang, L.; Boswell, M.; Rozelle, S. Poor vision among China's rural primary school students: Prevalence, correlates and consequences. *China Econ. Rev.* **2015**, *33*, 247–262. [CrossRef]
13. Kirkpatrick, R.; Zang, Y. The negative influences of exam-oriented education on chinese high school students: Backwash from classroom to child. *Lang. Test. Asia* **2011**, *1*, 36. [CrossRef]
14. Stinebrickner, R.; Stinebrickner, T.R. Time-use and college outcomes. *J. Econ.* **2004**, *121*, 243–269. [CrossRef]
15. Horwood, J.; Waylen, A.; Herrick, D.; Williams, C.; Wolke, D. Common visual defects and peer victimization in children. *Investig. Ophthalmol. Vis. Sci.* **2005**, *46*, 1177–1181. [CrossRef] [PubMed]
16. Messer, D.H.; Mitchell, G.L.; Twelker, J.D.; Crescioni, M. Spectacle wear in children given spectacles through a school-based program. *Optom Vis Sci* **2012**, *89*, 19–26. [CrossRef]
17. Yabumoto, C.; Hopker, L.M.; Daguano, C.R.; Basilio, F.M.A.; Robl, R.; Rodrigues, D.B.; Jimenez, A.; Moreira, A.T.R.; Sakata, L.M.; Sakata, K. Factors associated with spectacles-use compliance in a visual screening program for children from Southern Brazil. *Investig. Ophthalmol. Vis. Sci.* **2009**, *50*, 2439.
18. Castanon Holguin, A.M.; Congdon, N.; Patel, N.; Ratcliffe, A.; Esteso, P.; Toledo Flores, S.; Gilbert, D.; Pereyra Rito, M.A.; Munoz, B. Factors associated with spectacle-wear compliance in school-aged Mexican children. *Investig. Ophthalmol. Vis. Sci.* **2006**, *47*, 925–928. [CrossRef]
19. Duckworth, A.L.; Peterson, C.; Matthews, M.D.; Kelly, D.R. Grit: Perseverance and passion for long-term goals. *J. Pers. Soc. Psychol.* **2007**, *92*, 1087–1101. [CrossRef]
20. Kuh, G.D.; Pace, C.R.; Vesper, N. The development of process indicators to estimate student gains associated with good practices in undergraduate education. *Res. High. Educ.* **1997**, *38*, 435–454. [CrossRef]
21. Kuh, G.D. The national survey of student engagement: Conceptual and empirical foundations. *New Dir. Inst. Res.* **2009**, *2009*, 5–20. [CrossRef]
22. Kember, D.; Jamieson, Q.W.; Pomfret, M.; Wong, E.T.T. Learning approaches, study time and academic performance. *High Educ.* **1995**, *29*, 329–343. [CrossRef]
23. Li, F.; Loyalka, P.K.; Yi, H.; Shi, Y.; Johnson, N.; Rozelle, S. Ability Tracking and Social Capital in China's Rural Secondary School System. Available online: https://reap.fsi.stanford.edu/publication/ability-tracking-and-social-capital-chinas-rural-secondary-school-system (accessed on 4 December 2018).
24. National Burea of Statsitics of China. *China Statistical Yearbook 2014*; National Burea of Statsitics of China: Beijing, China, 2014.
25. Bruhn, M.; McKenzie, D. In pursuit of balance: Randomization in practice in development field experiments. *Am. Econ. J. Appl. Econ.* **2009**, *1*, 200–232. [CrossRef]
26. Bai, Y.; Yi, H.; Zhang, L.; Shi, Y.; Ma, X.; Congdon, N.; Zhou, Z.; Boswell, M.; Rozelle, S. An investigation of vision problems and the vision care system in rural China. *Southeast Asian J. Trop. Med. Public Health* **2014**, *45*, 1464–1473. [PubMed]
27. Guan, H.; Wang, H.; Huang, J.; Du, K.; Zhao, J.; Boswell, M.; Shi, Y.; Iyer, M.; Rozelle, S. Health seeking behavior among rural left-behind children: Evidence from Shaanxi and Gansu Provinces in China. *Int. J. Environ. Res Public Health* **2018**, *15*, 883. [CrossRef] [PubMed]

28. Zhou, C.; Sylvia, S.; Zhang, L.; Luo, R.; Yi, H.; Liu, C.; Shi, Y.; Loyalka, P.; Chu, J.; Medina, A.; et al. China's Left-Behind Children: Impact of Parental Migration On Health, Nutrition, And Educational Outcomes. *Health Affairs* **2015**, *34*, 1964–1971. [CrossRef] [PubMed]
29. National Burea of Statistics of China. *China Statisitical Yearbook 2008*; National Burea of Statistics of China: Beijing, China, 2008.
30. Wang, H.; Yang, C.; He, F.; Shi, Y.; Qu, Q.; Rozelle, S.; Chu, J. Mental health and dropout behavior: A cross-sectional study of junior high students in northwest rural China. *Int. J. Educ. Dev.* **2015**, *41*, 1–12. [CrossRef]
31. Zhou, B. *Mental Health Test (MHT)*; East China Normal University Press: Shanghai, China, 1991.
32. Reynolds, C.R.; Richmond, B.O. What I think and feel: A revised measure of children's manifest anxiety. *J. Abnormal Child Psychol.* **1978**, *6*, 271–280. [CrossRef]
33. Duflo, E.; Glennerster, R.; Kremer, M. Using randomization in development economics research: A toolkit. *Handb. Dev. Econ.* **2007**, *4*, 3895–3962.

5

Impact of the Family Environment on Juvenile Mental Health: eSports Online Game Addiction and Delinquency

Chulhwan Choi [1], Mary A. Hums [2] and Chul-Ho Bum [3,*]

[1] Department of Golf Industry, College of Physical Education, Kyung Hee University, Seocheon-dong 1, Giheung-gu, Yongin-si, Gyeonggi-do 17104, Korea; chulhwanchoi@yahoo.com

[2] Department of Health and Sport Science, University of Louisville, SAC East 104Q, University of Louisville, Louisville, KY 40292, USA; mhums@louisville.edu

[3] Department of Sports Taekwondo, Graduate School of Physical Education, Kyung Hee University, Seocheon-dong 1, Giheung-gu, Yongin-si, Gyeonggi-do 17104, Korea

* Correspondence: bch2180@khu.ac.kr;

Abstract: Family types in Asian countries are rapidly changing as the society is changing. Thus, in this study, we analyzed and compared how the newly evolving family types (multicultural/dual-income) affect adolescents' online game addiction, delinquency, and online gaming (eSports) participation motivation. Multiple regression analysis was performed to examine the causal relationships between the variables, and multivariate analysis of variance and analysis of variance were performed for comparative analyses. The results indicate that adolescents from dual-income families scored significantly higher on all factors related to juvenile delinquency and addiction factors ("salience", "tolerance" and "withdrawal"). Additionally, adolescents from multicultural families revealed significantly higher scores on an addiction factor, "mood modification". Lastly, adolescents in dual-income families were motivated to play online games to pass the time, and adolescents in multicultural families play online games to engage in social interaction. Results of this study may provide the answers required to help address societal issues related to adolescents in a changing society.

Keywords: eSports; family form; game addiction; juvenile delinquency; participation

---

1. Introduction

In Asian countries in this age, significant changes are occurring in the existing family system. For example, the entry of foreign migrant workers and an increase of international marriages have led to a shift from a traditional "single ethnic society" to a "multicultural society" [1]. According to the South Korean Ministry of the Interior and Safety [2], one out of 10 new marriages is international. This type of multicultural family is defined as a family composed of members belonging to different ethnicities or cultural backgrounds [3].

Moon et al. [4] have suggested that multicultural families are, unfortunately, experiencing financial difficulties, reaching only 59% of the income earned in other households. In particular, these authors found that the lower the economic level, the higher the probability that both husband and wife worked, with most couples working long hours for low wages.

Although such dual-income couples can be a positive factor in financial terms, considerable problems have been found to occur in the home [5]. In dual-income households, both husband and wife have jobs and must simultaneously perform the role of worker, spouse, and parent [6]. In this respect, Peterson and Hennon [7] pointed out the major challenges that dual-income couples experience include role overload from dealing with work and family at the same time and, at a deeper level, difficulties with parenting.

Previous research has found that children of dual-career parents who work long hours generally spend a great amount of time watching TV after school, using the internet, and playing online games [8]. Compared to adults, adolescents in particular are more likely to be addicted to online games as they consist of content that can stimulate curiosity and competition [9]. Ultimately, adolescents' addiction to online games has been shown to have a major impact on their lives [10–13]. In particular, adolescents addicted to online games tend to exhibit behaviors related to juvenile delinquency, such as drinking and smoking, and tend to hang out with friends who are also addicted [14].

With the high penetration rate of PCs as well as the expansion of high-speed information/communication networks in recent years, modern humans in developed countries live in an environment where they can easily access the internet [15]. In particular, as cutting-edge technology began to influence the electronics industry, electronic sports, or eSports for short, which are video games played in a virtual space, have dramatically increased in popularity [16,17].

Therefore, the study examined which online game addiction factors drive juvenile delinquency. Additionally, the present study investigated the effects of the changed family form (e.g., single-income/dual-income households and multicultural/monocultural families) on eSports game addiction, delinquency, and eSports participation motivation.

2. Literature Review

2.1. Online Game Addiction

As the social issue of online game addiction emerged with the growing popularity of eSports [18], playing online games became negatively perceived, similar to gambling addiction or alcoholism [19]. The definition of game addiction refers to an "excessive and compulsive use of video games that results in social and/or emotional problems; despite these problems, the gamer is unable to control this excessive use" [20] (p. 78). In other words, online game addiction can be determined based on how much one depends psychologically or emotionally on online games. Most previous studies have claimed that mental illness [21–28] and inactive lifestyle [29] are the consequences of game addiction. The problems mentioned above are also found in adolescents, and their excessive online gaming has been discussed from a negative perspective [30].

2.2. Juvenile Delinquency

In general, the consistent opinions, attitudes, and behaviors that are expected by society are called social norms, and any behavior that deviates from these norms are considered deviant behaviors. In other words, when adolescents take part in delinquent behaviors that deviate from social norms, this is explained as juvenile delinquency [31]. Since there is no consistent definition of juvenile delinquency in previous studies, the majority of studies, including the present study, focus on the deviant behaviors themselves rather than the actual person. Drinking, smoking, and unauthorized absenteeism are the main types of delinquent behaviors among adolescents. While these behaviors are not considered problematic for adults, they are considered delinquent based on their status as adolescents [32]. Because drinking and smoking behaviors tend to decrease naturally over the course of adulthood, some studies see these behaviors as normal behaviors with transitional traits [33]. On the other hand, according to some studies, it is difficult to rule out the potential for these adolescents to become criminals as adults [34]. Lastly, unauthorized absenteeism often occurs due to stress from academics or family matters [35], and repeated unauthorized absenteeism may develop into more serious delinquency or crimes in the future [31].

"Adolescents are confronted with a variety of cumulated stressors such as physical and hormonal changes, as well as shifts in personal value and belief systems" ([36], p. 3–4). Research has shown that online games are used as a tool for coping with such stress, and that addiction to online games leads to behavioral issues in adolescents, including displays of aggressive tendencies and a decrease in self-control [37]. While some researchers argue that excessive online gaming is strongly associated with adolescent misconduct [38], others maintain that the evidence of such relationship is not only weak, but almost nonexistent [39,40].

2.3. Participation Motivation in eSports

Motivation plays a critical role in understanding consumer behavior. It is defined as the factor that influences people's unconscious determination of behavior in a given situation [41]. Research on sport participation motivation explores why consumers participate in sports and what benefits they gain from participation [42]. The reasons why people participate in sports are determined by the active choice to satisfy their needs, and hence, uses and gratification theory has been utilized as a basic theoretical framework for explaining people's propensity to participate [43].

As the number of eSports fans has now exceeded 205 million worldwide [44], it is interesting to track participation in eSports as well. However, as motivation to participate in eSports tends to be different from participation in general sports activities, it is not appropriate to apply participation motivation in traditional sports to the understanding of eSports [45]. In this context, Lee and Schoenstedt [45] developed 14 eSports participation motives from modifying and supplementing participation motivation factors of existing general sports, such as baseball, that are relevant to eSports (Social Interaction, Fantasy, Identification with Sport, Diversion, Competition, Entertainment, Sport Knowledge Application, Arousal, Design/Graphics, Pass Time, Control, Skill Building for Playing Actual Sport, Permanence, and Peer Pressure). Comparative analysis with traditional sport consumption motives revealed the significant influence of three factors (i.e., competition, peer pressure, and skill building for playing actual sport).

2.4. Significance of the Study and Research Questions

Family types are changing in Asian countries to accommodate diverse cultures and evolving environments. The purpose of this study was to examine how new family types in our Korean society (multicultural families and dual-income families) affect adolescent behavior. Specifically, this research focused on: (a) online game addiction (b) juvenile delinquency, (c) influence of online game addiction on juvenile delinquency, and (d) eSports participation motivation. Participants consisted of four groups: (a) monocultural, single-income families, (b) monocultural, dual-income families, (c) multicultural, single-income families, and (d) multicultural, dual-income families. Through this study, we will be able to interpret adolescents' online game addiction and delinquency from the perspective of changing family types, while presenting solutions to the problem. This study will be guided by the following research questions:

RQ1. What online game addiction factors drive juvenile delinquency?

RQ2. What are the differences in online game addiction, juvenile delinquency, and eSports participation motivation among the forms of families?

3. Materials and Methods

3.1. Participants

Much like in Western countries, multicultural families have become more common in Asian countries due to the increased inflow of foreigners following changes in the social flow [1]. Unfortunately, most of these families experience financial difficulties, and both men and women work full time [3]. This has been reported to potentially have a considerable impact on how children are raised [5]. Hence, in order to analyze these social phenomena, adolescents were selected as the subject of this study. Adolescence in this study refers, as is typical, to the ages of 13 to 18 [46,47]. Although there are cultural differences [47], people in this age group mostly include students in middle and high school. Thus, in light of Korean culture, this study limited the age of participants to 12–18, to coincide with middle and high school in Korea.

The participants selected for this study were 12 to 18-year-old adolescents from either monocultural or multicultural families. A pilot test was conducted to modify sentences and word choice that might have been somewhat difficult for adolescents to understand. Following the research aim, a purposive sampling method was employed at two middle/high schools in southern Gyeonggi Province during five multicultural family day events, from the second half of 2017 to the first half of 2018, with the help of multicultural support centers operated by the city or county. Participation in the survey was voluntary, and each questionnaire was completed using the self-administered method. Through these procedures, a total of 300 questionnaires were distributed, of which 268 were returned (response rate approximately 89%). After excluding 22 unfinished questionnaires, the final 246 surveys were used for analysis.

3.2. *Measures*

3.2.1. Online Game Addiction

This measure consisted of factors identified by Lemmens et al. [20] to assess game addiction in adolescents, including salience (e.g., "Have you felt addicted to eSports?"), tolerance (e.g., "Did you play longer than intended?"), mood modification (e.g., "Did you play eSports to forget about real life?"), relapse (e.g., "Were you unable to reduce time to play eSports?"), withdrawal (e.g., "Have you felt bad when you were unable to play?"), conflict (e.g., "Did you have fights with others over your time spent on eSports?"), and problem (e.g., "Did you feel bad after playing for a long time?"). There are 21 items, showing acceptable Cronbach's alphas ranging from 0.84 to 0.90 in the previous study, in total with three items per factor utilizing 5-point Likert scale with 1 point for "Strongly disagree", 2 for "Disagree", 3 for "Neither agree nor disagree", 4 for "Agree", and 5 for "Strongly agree".

3.2.2. Juvenile Delinquents

Three items used by Lee [31] were modified and utilized in this measure asking if one has engaged in delinquent behaviors (smoking, $\alpha = 0.82$; drinking, $\alpha = 0.89$; school absence, $\alpha = 0.87$ in the previous study) during the past year. This study employed a 5-point Likert scale with 1 point for "Never", 2 for "Rarely", 3 for "Sometimes", 4 for "Often", and 5 for "Very often".

3.2.3. eSports Participation Motivation

Based on various previous studies [48,49], the present study used eight factors regarding motivation to participate in eSports, which were used by Lee and Schoenstedt showing acceptable Cronbach alphas ranging from 0.71 to 0.86 [45]. These factors include entertainment (e.g., "I play eSport because it is enjoyable"), competition (e.g., "I like to play to prove to others that I am the best"), permanence (e.g., "I tend to play eSport because they are readily available"), pass time (e.g., "I often play eSport because there is nothing else to do"), social interaction (e.g., "I use eSport as a reason to get together with others"), diversion (e.g., "Playing eSport gives me a break from my regular routine"), arousal (e.g., "I play eSport because they excite me"), and peer pressure (e.g., "My friends force me to play eSport"). Social interaction and arousal each consisted of four items, while the other factors consisted of three items each, for a total of 26 items applying 7-point Likert scale with 1 point for "Strongly disagree", 2 for "Disagree", 3 for "Somewhat disagree", 4 for "Neutral", 5 for "Somewhat agree", 6 for "Agree", and 7 for "Strongly agree".

3.3. *Data Analysis*

In a confirmatory factor analysis (CFA), Comparative fit index (CFI), Tucker-Lewis index (TLI), root mean square residual (RMR), and root mean square error of approximation (RMSEA) were used to test model fitness. In addition, reliability analysis was conducted using Cronbach's alpha to test the internal consistency of the items. Multivariate analysis of variance (MANOVA) including post-hoc analyses were performed to compare and analyze the differences in online game addiction, juvenile delinquency, and participation motivation among adolescents across the four groups. Additionally, multiple regression analysis was conducted to examine the causal relationships between variables.

4. Results

4.1. Socio-Demographic Statistics

A total of 246 questionnaires were utilized, consisting of responses from 202 boys (82%) and 44 girls (18%). Participation was limited to adolescents of ages 12 to 18 ($M = 14.40$, $SD = 1.924$), fitting the goal of the research study. Family types could be divided into monocultural ($n = 131$, 53%) and multicultural ($n = 115$, 47%) families, as well as single-income ($n = 133$, 54%) and dual-income ($n = 113$, 46%) families. Finally, the four family-type groups that participated in the study were (a) monocultural/single-income ($n = 70$, 28%), (b) monocultural/dual-income ($n = 61$, 25%), (c) multicultural/single-income ($n = 63$, 26%), and multicultural/dual-income ($n = 52$, 21%) (Table 1).

Table 1. Frequency of distributions for socio-demographic variables.

Variables	Categories	Frequency (n = 246)	Percentage (100%)
Gender	Male	202	82
	Female	44	18
Culture	Single	131	53
	Multiple	115	47
Income	Single	133	54
	Double	113	46

4.2. Scale Validity and Reliability

From the results of the confirmatory factor analysis, all critical ratios in the regression weights were found to be greater than ±1.96. In addition, the values of squared multiple correlations (SMC) for all items were found to be greater than 0.4. In general, a SMC value closer to 1 explains the variance of the measured variables Tests of model fit were: Chi-square = 1145.097, DF = 1055, $p = 0.027$, Chi-square/DF = 1.095, CFI = 0.988, TLI = 0.986, RMR = 0.064, and RMSEA = 0.019. The model is considered to be a good fit if CFI and TLI values exceeded the criterion of 0.900, and RMR and RMSEA values are conservatively smaller than 0.05. As shown above, the results of this study mostly satisfy these figures, and thus this model is a fit.

Lastly, all Cronbach's alpha showed good internal consistency for reliability based on the 0.70 cutoff [50]: (a) online game addiction (Salience, $\alpha = 0.923$; Tolerance, $\alpha = 0.891$; Mood Modification, $\alpha = 0.873$; Relapse, $\alpha = 0.888$; Withdrawal, $\alpha = 0.848$; Conflict, $\alpha = 0.858$; Problem, $\alpha = 0.823$), (b) juvenile delinquency ($\alpha = 0.901$), and (c) participation motivation (Entertainment, $\alpha = 0.854$; Competition, $\alpha = 0.840$; Permanence, $\alpha = 0.894$; To pass time, $\alpha = 0.919$; Social interaction, $\alpha = 0.848$; Diversion, $\alpha = 0.887$; Arousal, $\alpha = 0.902$; Peer pressure, $\alpha = 0.900$).

4.3. Multiple Regression Analysis

Multiple regression analysis resulted in a regression model where $F = 8.559$, $p = 0.000$, and $R^2 = 0.201$, explaining 20.1% of the variance. More specifically, in adolescent online game addiction, salience ($t = 5.24$, $p = 0.000$), withdrawal ($t = 3.02$, $p = 0.003$), and tolerance ($t = 2.01$, $p = 0.045$) were found to increase delinquent behavior, while the other subfactors were not statistically significant (Table 2).

Table 2. Results of multiple regression: effects of online game addiction on juvenile delinquency.

DV	IV	B	β	t	p	R^2	F	p
Juvenile Delinquency						0.20	8.559	0.000 ***
	Salience	0.30	0.32	5.24	0.000 ***			
	Withdrawal	0.19	0.18	3.02	0.003 **			
	Tolerance	0.12	0.12	2.01	0.045 *			

Note. * $p < 0.05$, ** $p < 0.01$, *** $p < 0.001$.

4.4. *Multivariate Analysis of Variance (MANOVA) for Online Game Addiction*

The multivariate test indicated statistically significant differences based on the forms of family on the eSports addiction [Wilks' lambda = 0.460, $F(21, 678.215) = 10.044$, $p = 0.00$, partial $\eta^2 = 0.228$]. Based on adjusted alpha level using Bonferroni correction ($p = 0.05/7 = 0.007$), univariate tests for (a) Salience, (b) Tolerance, (c) Mood Modification, (d) Withdrawal, and (e) Problem were statistically significant. However, the rest of the tests were not statistically significant: (a) Relapse and (b) Conflict. Results are shown in Table 3.

Table 3. Results of MANOVA: Differences in addiction in esports between four groups based on the forms of families.

Source	DV	df	F	p	η^2
Addiction	Salience	3	24.394	0.000 ***	0.232
	Tolerance	3	15.265	0.000 ***	0.159
	Mood modification	3	9.126	0.000 ***	0.102
	Relapse	3	1.333	0.264	0.016
	Withdrawal	3	17.171	0.000 ***	0.176
	Conflict	3	1.213	0.306	0.015
	Problem	3	8.052	0.000 ***	0.091

Note. *** $p < 0.001$.

Follow-up Tukey post hoc analyses revealed that salience, tolerance, and withdrawal scores were higher in the two dual-income family groups than in the two single-income family groups. The mood modification score was higher in the two multi-cultural family groups than in the two monocultural family groups. Lastly, the problem score was significantly lower in the monocultural/single-income family group compared to the rest of the groups (Table 4).

Table 4. Mean scores for addiction in esports among groups and scale reliability.

	Salience	Tolerance	Mood Modification	Relapse	Withdrawal	Conflict	Problem
Group1	1.83	1.82	1.85	2.91	1.69	1.80	1.69
Group2	**2.96**	**2.69**	1.85	2.97	**2.40**	1.79	**2.32**
Group3	1.82	1.77	**2.46**	2.83	1.71	1.90	**2.41**
Group4	**2.69**	**2.52**	**2.47**	3.15	**2.56**	1.62	**2.22**

Note. Group1 = Single cultural/Single income, Group2 = Single cultural/Double income, Group3 = Multi cultural/Single income, Group4 = Multi cultural/Double income. Statistically significant higher mean scores between groups in bold.

4.5. *Analysis of Variance (ANOVA) for Juvenile Delinquency*

There was a statistically significant difference among the four groups on juvenile delinquency [$F(3,242) = 48.100$, $p = 0.000$]. A Tukey post hoc test found that the two dual-income family groups scored higher on measures of juvenile delinquency than the two single-income family groups. There was no statistically significant difference between monocultural and multicultural families ($p > 0.05$). More detailed information is shown in Table 5.

Table 5. Result of ANOVA, mean scores, and scale reliability: Differences in juvenile delinquency in esports between four groups based on the forms of families.

	SS	*Df*	*MS*	*F*	*p*
Between Groups	89.280	3	29.760	48.100	0.000 ***
Within Groups	149.728	242	0.619		
Total	239.008	245			

	Group1	Group2	Group3	Group4
Juvenile Delinquency	1.62	**2.97**	1.70	**2.73**

Note. *** $p < 0.001$. Group1 = Single cultural/Single income, Group2 = Single cultural/Double income, Group3 = Multi cultural/Single income, Group4 = Multi cultural/Double income. Statistically significant higher mean scores between groups in bold.

4.6. Multivariate Analysis of Variance (MANOVA) for Participation Motivation

The multivariate test revealed statistically significant differences based on the forms of family on eSports participation motivation [Wilks' lambda = 0.445, $F(24, 682.173) = 9.154$, $p = 0.00$, partial $\eta^2 = 0.237$]. Based on adjusted alpha level using Bonferroni correction ($P = 0.05/8 = 0.006$), univariate tests for (a) To pass time and (b) Social interaction were statistically significant. However, the rest of the tests were not statistically significant: (a) Entertainment, (b) Competition, (c) Permanence, (d) Diversion, (e) Arousal, and (f) Peer pressure as shown in Table 6.

Table 6. Results of MANOVA: Differences in participation motivations in esports between four groups based on the forms of families.

Source	DV	*df*	F	*p*	η^2
Participation Motivation	Entertainment	3	0.972	0.407	0.012
	Competition	3	1.952	0.122	0.024
	Permanence	3	2.608	0.052	0.031
	To pass time	3	40.703	0.000 ***	0.335
	Social interaction	3	28.530	0.000 ***	0.261
	Diversion	3	1.789	0.150	0.022
	Arousal	3	0.331	0.803	0.004
	Peer pressure	3	0.069	0.976	0.001

Note. ***$p < 0.001$.

Follow-up Tukey post hoc analyses revealed that the two dual-income family groups scored higher on "pass time" than the two single-income family groups, and the two multicultural family groups scored higher on "social interaction" than the two monocultural family groups (Table 7).

Table 7. Mean scores for participation motivations in esports among groups and scale reliability.

	1	2	3	4	5	6	7	8
Group1	4.91	4.79	3.67	3.21	3.16	3.98	4.48	3.92
Group2	4.63	4.82	3.47	**4.97**	3.07	3.88	4.32	3.92
Group3	4.77	4.40	3.15	3.34	**4.34**	3.96	4.29	3.95
Group4	4.54	4.45	3.12	**4.97**	**4.77**	4.44	4.46	3.84

Note. Group1 = Single cultural/Single income, Group2 = Single cultural/Double income, Group3 = Multi cultural/Single income, Group4 = Multi cultural/Double income. 1 = Entertainment, 2 = Competition, 3 = Permanence, 4 = To pass time, 5 = Social interaction, 6 = Diversion, 7 = Arousal, 8 = Peer pressure. Statistically significant higher mean scores between groups in bold.

5. Discussion

5.1. Online Game Addiction due to Differences in Family Environment

In this study, the family type was found to have a significant effect on online game addiction. More specifically, "salience", "tolerance", and "withdrawal" scores were higher among adolescents from dual-income families than those from single-income families. This shows that, for adolescents from dual-income families whose parents have relatively little control [14], engagement in online games lasts longer, due to being difficult to self-control, which can lead to an unstable psychological state when gaming ceased. In addition, aside from single-income and dual-income families, the "mood modification" score was higher for adolescents from multicultural families than those from monocultural families. This shows that adolescents from multicultural families experienced mood modifications like stress relief and a temporary escape through online games relatively more than adolescents from monocultural families.

In the case of the "problem" factor referred as problems caused by excessive game play (e.g., "Did you feel bad after playing for a long time"), only adolescents from monocultural/single-income families showed a significantly lower average value than the other groups. This means that adolescents from monocultural/single-income families, who were free from both the multicultural family and dual-income family factors (selected as the independent variables in this study), were less likely to experience the "problem" factor than other groups.

Previous studies have shown that children from multicultural families often experience group bullying because of their exotic appearance [51]. Continuation of such isolation can lead to a decrease in self-competence [52] and social avoidance tendencies [53]. Eventually, those with poor interpersonal relationships are more likely to escape reality and become addicted to the internet [54] and go on to become addicted to online games [55]. In addition to the factors mentioned above, previous studies have shown that children are more immersed in internet use and online games when their parents work long hours due to dual-careers [8].

The results of the present study are largely similar to previous research. This is because adolescents are not only more influenced by external contextual factors than adults but also, to some extent, lack the ability to control their own needs [56]. In this context, these results will contribute to the data for adolescent education, as they indicate that the most important factors in adolescent game addiction tendency, which has recently emerged as a social issue, are derived from society or their parents, rather than being their own fault.

5.2. Delinquency/Deviance due to Differences in Family Environment

In this study, being from a multicultural family was not a significant factor concerning juvenile delinquency. However, the dual-income family environment was found to be a critical factor in juvenile delinquency. Specifically, adolescents from dual-income families scored significantly higher on all factors including smoking, drinking, and school absence compared to those from single-income families. This result was consistent with the previous literature that dual-income families tend to have problems regarding child-rearing in spite of a better financial status [4].

Ashford and Lecroy [57] argued that the main characteristics of juvenile delinquents included more rebelliousness, more hostility, and poorer self-regulatory abilities compared with typical adolescents. Among the important factors of adolescent engagement in delinquent behaviors, the role of parents has been reported to be particularly important [58]. Therefore, parental interest toward children, and the total amount of time spent with them seem to be critical in reducing juvenile delinquency, rather than invisible social discrimination or prejudice toward children from multicultural families. In particular, considering that, the factors related to addiction, "salience", "tolerance" and "withdrawal" were found to be significant predictors of juvenile delinquency, it is apparent that the role of parents is very important in addition to adolescents' self-control.

5.3. Participation Motivation due to Differences in Family Environment

The MANOVA showed statistically significant differences between the groups in "pass time" and "social interaction". Follow-up analysis found that monoculturalism/multiculturalism had no effect on "pass time" but dual-income/single-income did, meaning that adolescents in dual-income families were motivated to play online games to pass the time. This suggests that adolescents in dual-income families whose parents are not at home after school tend to send more time to play online games, which is consistent with results of previous literature [14].

There was no effect of dual-/single-income on "social interaction" but there was an effect from multi/monoculturalism, suggesting that adolescents in multicultural families play online games to engage in social interaction. This result suggests that adolescents in multicultural families pursue social interaction in the online environment characterized by anonymity.

In conclusion, adolescents from dual-income families showed a tendency to rely on online games when alone [6], and those from multicultural families participated in online games for self-expression [59]. In addition, while there were no significant differences between groups, "entertainment", "competition" and "arousal" had higher mean scores than other factors, which suggests that, regardless of family types, adolescents generally enjoy online games with the motives of "entertainment", "competition" and "arousal" characteristics of such games.

6. Conclusions

This study focused on the family form (double-income and multicultural family) that is changing in Asian countries due to various reasons, just like in their Western counterparts. In other words, this study compared and analyzed how such changes in family form have an impact on online game addiction and delinquency in children who are going through their sensitive adolescent stage. Further, we conducted an empirical examination of the significant cause-and-effect relationship between online game addiction and delinquency in adolescents. As mentioned above, this study interestingly found that not only does this new family form have a considerable impact on adolescents, but also that online game addition increases delinquent behaviors. This is a significant finding that implies the need for more focus and training on adolescents, as they have not yet grown into adults. Specifically, it is necessary to provide programs for afterschool care and education by employing helpers for dual income families at the school level or establishing systems to prevent indiscreet game addiction among adolescents by limiting the hours of use and ensuring online activity occurs under their real names. Moreover, this study will serve useful for developing efficient social welfare plans by the Education Ministry and the government.

There are several limitations regarding external validity and research design. This study was conducted in South Korea, a country at a top global rank in terms of internet communication network supply rate and average speed. Therefore, while it is true that Korean adolescents play several online games, it is necessary to see the results for adolescents in other Asian countries where the internet is not yet widely commercialized. Since the preferences and characteristics of adolescents may differ according to their country, even if they are from the same continent, a more in-depth follow-up study must be conducted on these differences. Also, if an in-depth interview or other qualitative research method is implemented, it will be a good opportunity to solve the social and psychological issues of future adolescents on the basis of more diverse opinions. Moreover, this study has limitations that prevent generalizing the results to other Asian countries because the research was conducted exclusively in Korea. Accordingly, for follow-up research, an in-depth study must be conducted based on comparative analyses of Asian countries. Lastly, the cross-sectional data may not support cause and effect relationships in this study conducted for a relatively short period of time. Thus, a future research with longitudinal study design will be able to capture mentality and behaviors of adolescents.

Author Contributions: C.C. and C.-H.B. developed research questions. Also, C.C. was in charge of method and interpreted the results. M.A.H. covered literature review and edited the paper. All authors read and approved the final manuscript.

References

1. Jo, H.Y.; Seo, D.H.; Kwon, S.H. An ethnographic study on the academic performance of children of migrants. *Korean J. Soc. Educ.* **2008**, *18*, 105–134.
2. Ministry of the Interior and Safety. Employment Extension of Public Officer for Foreigners and North Korean Defectors. 2009. Available online: http://www.mois.go.kr/frt/bbs/type010/commonSelectBoardArticle.do?bbsId=BBSMSTR_000000000008&nttId=26822 (accessed on 25 August 2018).
3. Kim, B.S. An ethnographic study on the kindergarten life of the children of multicultural family. *Res. Cent. Korean Youth Cult.* **2008**, *18*, 98–138.
4. Moon, H.J.; Choi, Y.K.; Seo, S.J. Children in Korean multi-cultural families. *Korean Assoc. Child Stud.* **2009**, *30*, 85–97.
5. Choi, Y.J.; Choi, M.; Choi, S.B. The effect of dual earner couple's role assignment on work-family conflict, family life satisfaction, and depression. *J. Soc. Res.* **2018**, *19*, 47–93.
6. Lee, J.H.; Lee, E.H. The moderating effect of coping strategies upon multiple role conflicts and depression within dual employed couples. *Korean J. Health Psychol.* **2000**, *5*, 287–303.
7. Peterson, G.W.; Hennon, C.B. Conceptualizing parenting stress with family stress theory. In *Families and Change*, 3rd ed.; McKenry, P.C., Price, S.J., Eds.; Sage: Thousand Oaks, CA, USA, 2005; pp. 25–48.
8. Pǎǎkkőnen, H. Alone at home. *Int. J. Time Use Res.* **2008**, *5*, 43–64. [CrossRef]
9. King, S.A. Is the Internet Addictive, or Are Addicts Using the Internet? *1996.* Available online: http://www.concentric.net/~{}Astorm/iad.html (accessed on 13 May 2018).
10. Brenner, V. Psychology of computer use: XLVII. Parameters of Internet use, abuse and addiction: The first 90 days of the Internet Usage Survey. *Psychol. Rep.* **1997**, *80*, 879–882. [CrossRef]
11. Hauge, M.R.; Gentile, D.A. Video game addiction among adolescents: Associations with academic performance and aggression. In Proceedings of the Society for Research in Child Development Conference, Tampa, FL, USA, 24–27 April 2003.
12. Young, K.S. Internet addiction: The emergence of a new clinical disorder. *Cyberpsychol. Behav.* **1996**, *1*, 237–244. [CrossRef]
13. Kim, Y.E.; Park, S.H. A study on the online game use influences in game flow and addiction: Focusing on the uses and gratifications approach. *Korean J. Commun. Stud.* **2007**, *51*, 355–496.
14. Kim, D. An analysis on the difference of juvenile delinquency by online-game addiction. *Korean Crim. Psychol. Res.* **2012**, *8*, 5–33.
15. Noh, S.-J. Analyzing socio-psychological factors affecting internet addiction in university students. *J. Korean Educ.* **2010**, *37*, 235–261.
16. Bányai, F.; Griffiths, M.D.; Király, O.; Demetrovics, Z. The psychology of esports: A systematic literature review. *J. Gambl. Stud.* **2018**, 1–15. [CrossRef] [PubMed]
17. Taylor, T. *Raising the Stakes: E-Sports and the Professionalization of Computer Gaming*; The MIT Press: Cambridge, MA, USA, 2012.
18. Xu, Z.; Turel, O.; Yuan, Y. Online game addiction among adolescents: Motivation and prevention factors. *Eur. J. Inf. Syst.* **2012**, *21*, 321–340. [CrossRef]
19. Choi, S.W.; Kim, H.S.; Kim, G.Y.; Jeon, Y.; Park, S.M.; Lee, J.Y.; Jung, H.Y.; Sohn, B.K.; Choi, J.S.; Kim, D.J. Similarities and differences among Internet gaming disorder, gambling disorder and alcohol use disorder: A focus on impulsivity and compulsivity. *J. Behav. Addict.* **2014**, *3*, 246–253. [CrossRef] [PubMed]
20. Lemmens, J.S.; Valkenburg, P.M.; Peter, J. Development and validation of a game addiction scale for adolescents. *Media Psychol.* **2009**, *12*, 77–95. [CrossRef]
21. Wei, H.T.; Chen, M.H.; Huang, P.C.; Bai, Y.M. The association between online gaming, social phobia, and depression: An internet survey. *BMC Psychiatry* **2012**, *12*, 92–98. [CrossRef]
22. Loton, D.; Borkoles, E.; Lubman, D.; Polman, R.C.J. Video game addiction, engagement and symptoms of stress, depression and anxiety: The mediating role of coping. *Int. J. Ment. Health Addict.* **2016**, *14*, 565–578. [CrossRef]

23. Guo, J.; Chen, L.; Wang, X.; Liu, Y.; Kwan, C.H.; He, H.; Qu, Z.; Tian, D. The relationship between Internet addiction and depression among migrant children and left-behind children in China. *Cyberpsychol. Behav. Soc. Netw.* **2012**, *15*, 585–590. [CrossRef]
24. Young, K.; Pistner, M.; O'Mara, J.; Buchanan, J. Cyber-Disorders: The mental health concern for the new millennium. *Cyberpsychol. Behav.* **2000**, *3*, 475–479. [CrossRef]
25. Grüsser, S.M.; Tahlemann, R.; Griffiths, M.D. Excessive computer game playing: Evidence for addiction and aggression? *Cyberpsychol. Behav.* **2007**, *10*, 290–292. [CrossRef]
26. Lo, S.; Wang, C.; Fang, W. Physical interpersonal relationships and social anxiety among online game players. *Cyberpsychol. Behav.* **2005**, *8*, 15–20. [CrossRef] [PubMed]
27. Ko, C.N.; Liu, T.L.; Wang, P.W.; Chen, C.S.; Yen, C.F.; Yen, J.Y. The exacerbation of depression, hostility, and social anxiety in the course of internet addiction among adolescents: A prospective study. *Compr. Psychiatry* **2014**, *55*, 1377–1384. [CrossRef] [PubMed]
28. Beranuy, M.; Carbonell, X.; Griffiths, M. A qualitative analysis of online gaming addicts in treatment. *Int. J. Ment. Health Addict.* **2013**, *11*, 149–161. [CrossRef]
29. Henchoz, Y.; Studer, J.; Deline, S.; N'Goran, A.A.; Baggio, S.; Gmel, G. Video gaming disorder and sport and exercise in emerging adulthood: A longitudinal study. *Behav. Med.* **2016**, *42*, 105–111. [CrossRef] [PubMed]
30. Griffiths, M.D.; Davies, M.; Chappell, D. Online computer gaming: A comparison of adolescent and adult gamers. *J. Adolesc.* **2004**, *27*, 87–96. [CrossRef] [PubMed]
31. Lee, H.J. The effects of social supports and strains on adolescent delinquency. Master's Thesis, Myongji University, Seoul, South Korea, 2014.
32. Senna, J.; Siegel, L. *Juvenile Delinquency: Theory, Practice and Law*, 7th ed.; Wadsworth: Stamford, CT, USA, 2014.
33. Cho, Y.S.; Shin, Y.S. Causal pathway analysis of adolescence status delinquency. *J. Korean Acad. Soc. Nurs. Educ.* **2001**, *7*, 379–390.
34. Robert, A. Desisting from crime: Continuity and change in long-term crime patterns of serious chronic offenders. *Contemp. Crisis* **2005**, *44*, 205–209.
35. Moon, J.W. Factors affecting runaway impulse and experience of adolescents. *Korean Public Health Res.* **2012**, *38*, 19–34.
36. Kuss, D.J.; Griffiths, M.D. Online gaming addiction in children and adolescents: A review of empirical research. *J. Behav. Addict.* **2012**, *1*, 3–22. [CrossRef]
37. Kim, E.J.; Kee, N.; Ku, T.; Kim, S.J. The relationship between online game addiction and aggression, self-control and narcissistic personality traits. *Eur. Psychiatry* **2008**, *23*, 212–218. [CrossRef]
38. Anderson, C.; Sakamoto, A.; Gentile, D.; Ihori, N.; Shibuya, A.; Yukawa, S.; et al. Longitudinal effects of violent video games on aggression in Japan and the United States. *Pediatrics* **2008**, *122*, 1067–1072. [CrossRef] [PubMed]
39. Etchells, P.J.; Gage, S.H.; Rutherford, A.D.; Munafò, M.R. Prospective investigation of video game use in children and subsequent conduct disorder and depression using data from the Avon longitudinal study of parents and children. *PLoS ONE* **2016**, *11*, e0147732. [CrossRef] [PubMed]
40. Kutner, L.; Olson, C. *Grand Theft Childhood: The Surprising Truth About Violent Video Games and What Parents Can Do*; Simon & Schuster: New York, NY, USA, 2008.
41. Ko, Y.J.; Park, H.; Claussen, C.L. Action sports participation: Consumer motivation. *Int. J. Sports Mark. Spons.* **2008**, *9*, 111–124.
42. Shank, M.M. Fan or fanatic: Refining a measure of sports involvement. *J. Sport Manag.* **1998**, *21*, 435–443.
43. Rubin, A.M. Media uses and effects: A uses and gratifications perspective. In *Media Effects: Advances in Theory and Research*; Bryant, I.J., Zillmann, D., Eds.; Lawrence Erlbaum Associates: Hillsdale, NJ, USA, 1994; pp. 417–436.
44. Casselman, B. Resistance Is Futile: eSports Is Massive ... and Growing. 2015. Available online: http://www.espn.com/espn/story/_/id/13059210/esports-massive-industry-growing (accessed on 20 May 2018).
45. Lee, D.; Schoenstedt, L.J. Comparison of eSports and traditional sports consumption motives. *ICHPER-SD J. Res.* **2011**, *6*, 39–44.
46. Stanford Children's Care. Available online: https://www.stanfordchildrens.org/en/topic/default?id=the-growing-child-adolescent-13-to-18-years-90-P02175 (accessed on 3 December 2018).
47. WHO. Available online: http://www.who.int/maternal_child_adolescent/topics/adolescence/development/en/ (accessed on 3 December 2018).

48. Kim, Y.; Ross, S.D. An exploration of motives in sport video gaming. *Int. J. Sports Mark. Spons.* **2006**, *8*, 28–40. [CrossRef]
49. Sherry, J.L.; Lucas, K.; Greenberg, B.S.; Lachlan, K. Video game uses and gratifications as predictors of use and game preference. In *Playing Video Games: Motives, Responses, and Consequences*; Vorderer, P., Bryant, J., Eds.; Lawrence Erlbaum Associates, Inc.: Nahwah, NJ, USA, 2006.
50. Nunnally, J.C.; Bernstein, I.H. *Psychometric Theory*, 3rd ed.; McGraw-Hill: New York, NY, USA, 1994.
51. Seol, D.H. International marriage migration and national identity: Marriage-based immigrants' and their children's self-identification of Koreanness with regard to ethnic and civic nationhood in South Korea. *Econ. Soc.* **2006**, *103*, 278–312.
52. Kurdek, L.A.; Krile, D. A developmental analysis of the relation between peer acceptance and both interpersonal understanding and perceived social self-competence. *Child Dev.* **1982**, *53*, 1485–1591. [CrossRef]
53. Asher, S.R.; Parkhurst, J.T.; Hymel, S.; Williams, G.A. Peer rejection and loneliness in childhood. In *Peer Rejection in Childhood*; Asher, A.R., Coie, J.D., Eds.; Cambridge University Press: New York, NY, USA, 1990; pp. 253–273.
54. Young, K.S. Internet addiction: Symptoms, evaluation and treatment. In *Innovations in Clinical Practice: A Source Book*; Van de Creek, L., Jackson, X., Eds.; Professional Resource Press: Sarasota, FL, USA, 1997; Volume 17L, pp. 19–31.
55. Chak, K.; Leung, L. Shyness and locus of control as predictors of internet addiction and internet use. *CyberPsychol. Behav.* **2004**, *7*, 559–570. [CrossRef]
56. Gupta, R.; Derevensky, J.L. Adolescents with gambling problems: From research to treatment. *J. Gambl. Stud.* **2000**, *16*, 315–342. [CrossRef]
57. Ashford, J.B.; LeCroy, C.W. Juvenile recidivism: A comparison of three prediction instruments. *Adolescence* **1990**, *25*, 441–450. [PubMed]
58. Steinberg, L.; Silverberg, S.B. The vicissitudes of autonomy in early adolescence. *Child Dev.* **1986**, *57*, 841–851. [CrossRef] [PubMed]
59. Park, S.B.; Chung, N.H. A factor affecting self-presentation desire and participation intention in online game. *e-Bus. Stud.* **2010** *11*

6

What Predicts Stable Mental Health in the 18–29 Age Group Compared to Older Age Groups? Results from the Stockholm Public Health Cohort 2002–2014

Regina Winzer [1,2,*], Kimmo Sorjonen [3] and Lene Lindberg [1,4]

1 Department of Public Health Sciences, Karolinska Institutet, 17165 Stockholm, Sweden; lene.lindberg@ki.se
2 Department of Living Conditions and Lifestyles, Public Health Agency of Sweden, 17182 Solna, Sweden
3 Department of Clinical Neuroscience, Karolinska Institutet, 17165 Stockholm, Sweden; kimmo.sorjonen@ki.se
4 Center for Epidemiology and Community Medicine, Stockholm County Council, 10431 Stockholm, Sweden
* Correspondence: regina.winzer@folkhalsomyndigheten.se;

Abstract: Mental health has decreased in young people since the 1990s, and mental health promotion is an urgent matter. A first step is to identify which social determinants could be of importance for intervention. We used the Stockholm Public Health Cohort, a longitudinal population-based health survey, completed by 31,000 inhabitants in the Stockholm County. We focused on the 18–29 age group, n = 3373 (60% females, 40% males) and aimed at assessing which social determinants predict stable mental health, measured as scoring <3 points on the General Health Questionnaire 12 at all time points: 2002, 2007, 2010, and 2014. Forty-six percent of males and 36% of females reported stable mental health. Among the 17 predictors on sociodemographics, socioeconomics, social capital, health behavior, and victimization, six predicted stable mental health in the following order: occupation and especially employment, emotional support, male gender, being born in Sweden, absence of financial strain, and consumption of fruit and berries. In the 30–84 age group, 66% males and 55% females reported stable mental health. Nine determinants in the following rank predicted stable mental health: absence of financial strain, occupation and especially being self-employed, emotional support, male gender, physical activity, instrumental support, interpersonal trust, community trust, and absence of hazardous alcohol consumption. Interaction analysis showed significant difference between the younger and older group regarding physical activity and absence of financial strain with importance being higher for the older group. Our findings indicate that the determinants of health differ across the life-course with fewer predictors related to social capital and health behavior in the younger group compared to the older. We conclude that health-promoting interventions should be lifespan-sensitive.

Keywords: longitudinal study; young adults; stable mental health; social determinants

---

1. Introduction

Promoting mental health and preventing mental ill-health in populations has been a public-health issue for decades. Young people have been especially in focus since a decrease in their mental health in many Western societies has been observed since the 1990s [1–5], and internalizing problems in adolescents, especially in girls, seem to have increased during the 21th century [6]. For self-rated mental ill-health in adolescents, a global rise is evident between 1980 and 2000, with stabilization between 2000 and 2010. However, an exception is observed for Northern Europe, where a continuous increase in adolescents' mental and somatic complaints in 1982–2013 has been shown [7]. Compared to older age groups, young adults 16–29 years in Sweden report the highest levels of psychological distress, 54% in women and 33% in men, according to the National Public Health Survey 2016 [8]. This pattern is similar to other Nordic countries as Denmark [9] and Finland [10].

Less well-known, and in contrast to studies about social determinants of health [11], is the fact that symptoms of mental ill-health also highly affect students during their tertiary education. According to systematic reviews, the prevalence of depressive symptoms among students varies between 27.2% and 30.6% [12,13], with even higher rates for anxiety and distress [14,15]. Furthermore, students in higher education report up to 4.4 times higher distress than age-matched peers do [14,16], significantly higher rates compared to those actively working [17], and elevated levels compared to the general population [12,13].

To develop positive mental health during childhood, adolescence, and young adulthood is an important outcome in its own right, but it also constitutes a predictor for educational attainment and perceived competence [18], future income levels [19], personal finances [20], occupational attainment, life satisfaction, and quality of relationships [21] in later life.

When applying the biopsychosocial model [22], it becomes evident that it is possible to promote mental health by an array of actions, e.g., through the social determinants of health. Social determinants have considerable impact in peoples' lives [23,24] and are important predictors for general health [25] as well as for mental health [26]. A review by Allen et al. on the determinants for mental health indicates a social gradient, meaning that worldwide mental distress affects those with lower socioeconomic status proportionally worse compared with those with higher status. Furthermore, female gender and low educational attainment, low household income, financial debt, and unemployment also have an association with mental distress and disorder [11]. However, the social determinants of health also include features related to the concept of social capital, e.g., participation in organizations, emotional and social support, trust, and social harmony [27]. A large body of research indicates that health behavior factors—i.e., physical activity [28,29], tobacco and alcohol consumption [30,31], and nutrition [32–34]—are also associated with mental health. A problem in the study of social determinants of health is that those factors available to analyze account for risk factors for mental ill-health rather than promotive factors for mental health. Though they may be related, risk and promotive factors have diverse features, i.e., they do not represent different sides of the same coin [35,36].

Regarding factors related to social capital, previous studies have found associations with young people's positive development and mental health. Hawkins et al. found that social-capital constructs, such as civic action and engagement, trust and tolerance of others, and trust in authorities and organizations, were consistently related to positive development in 19–20-year-old young adults [37]. In the same cohort, precursors for positive development in emerging adulthood were investigated and identified as the following: stronger family and peer relationships, better adjustment to school settings, higher family socioeconomic status, and better emotional control [38]. Findings on the association between immigrant status and mental distress are inconclusive. Some studies indicate that immigrants perceive less distress compared to nonimmigrants [39,40], while a systematic review found higher levels of mental ill-health in immigrants in 13 of 21 included studies. The authors concluded that the differences in mental distress versus native populations could be related to stressful conditions during the migration process and in the host countries [41]. A longitudinal study found that ethnic minority status in adolescents, despite economic disadvantage and racism, predicted a better mental health outcome at 21–23 years of age compared to the British majority. A mediating factor for this association was family connectedness and support [42]. In contrast, poor family relationships in adolescence predicted mental ill-health later in life [43]. Social support together with internal resources were also positively correlated with mental health in a cross-sectional study among university students, while perceived stress showed a negative association with mental health [44]. According to an overview article, chronic arousal due to stress has been identified as a key factor for mental ill-health irrespective of age group [26]. Victimization in young people differs between males and females regarding their perpetrators and places of victimization, but their adverse mental-health associations are similar [45–47] and have longstanding consequences for adulthood [48].

As shown, many studies have focused on mental ill-health, whereas mental health has been examined to a lesser extent. However, with the exception of one study, which investigated the absence of a diagnosis as a measure for endurance in mental health [21], according to our knowledge, stability in mental health has not been investigated as an effect of former health determinants, though stability in mental health seems to be an important factor for future positive and negative life events. In a longitudinal study, Keyes et al. found that relatively small declines in mental health predicted future mental illness, and the researchers underscored the importance of investing in mental-health promotion and protection [49]. Another longitudinal study revealed that seven-year mortality was more strongly predicted by the absence of positive wellbeing than the presence of psychological symptoms [35]. With our study, we wanted to examine sociodemographic factors, social capital, and health behavior and exposure to violence, and their association with the stability of mental health.

The aim of this study was to assess which determinants of health contribute to a stable mental health in the 18–29 age group. More precisely, we wanted to investigate the determinants contributing to a state free from psychological distress. Furthermore, we investigated if these determinants differ from those observed in the older population, 30 years and older.

2. Methods

2.1. *Sampled Participants and Procedures*

The sample consisted of the Stockholm Public Health Cohort (SPHC), a population-based postal and/or web survey set up in 2002. The cohort profile, including the questionnaire, has been described in detail elsewhere [50]. In brief, the survey included an area-based random sample of 50,000 inhabitants in the Stockholm County aged 18–84 years in 2002, and was followed up in 2007, 2010, and 2014. The response rate was 62% in 2002 (n = 31,182), and the resurveyed rates for the follow-up years were 79, 77, and 71%, respectively. Data collection was conducted by Statistics Sweden in collaboration with the Department of Public Health Sciences at Karolinska Institutet. Survey data were supplemented by register data, and participants gave their informed consent to future contacts and record linkages. The study was approved by the Stockholm Regional Ethical Review Board (no. 2010/1879-31/5, no. 2007/545-31, no. 2018/1569-32).

We used data for the 12-year period, 2002–2014, and analyzed the 18–29 age group. In 2002, our age group comprised 3373 persons, 2012 women (59.7%) and 1361 men (40.3%), equaling a response rate of 53.9%. For the following surveys, see Figure 1. As a non-response analysis was not available we were able to comment on the attrition characteristics.

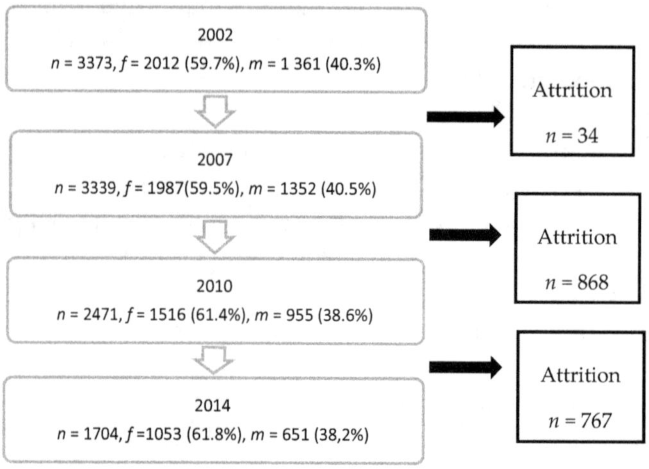

Figure 1. Flow-chart of respondents in the 18–29 age group of the Stockholm Public Health Cohort 2002, 2007, 2010, and 2014.

The 18–29 age group was compared with the rest of the population, 30 years and older, 7237 men (43.6%) and 9377 women (56.4%). (Supplementary Materials, Figure S1. Flow-chart of the respondents in the 30 years and older age group of the Stockholm Public Health Cohort 2002, 2007, 2010, and 2014).

In the following, we present our data using the STROBE Statement and provide the checklist of items that should be included in reports of cohort studies (Supplementary Materials, Table S1).

2.2. Study Variables

Our outcome variable, absence of psychological distress, was measured by the General Health Questionnaire (GHQ-12). This 12-item self-report questionnaire, which originated from earlier versions (60, 30, and 28 items), was created to assess psychiatric morbidity in clinical and community settings [51]. The instrument has been validated and applied in various international population surveys [52–56], as well as in Swedish contexts [57,58]. The included items of the instrument capture symptoms of anxiety, depression, social dysfunction, and stress-related problems, i.e., psychological distress. They have a severity range from 0 = better than usual, to 3 = much worse than usual. Following the results of a recent validation [58], we used the Standard GHQ-12 Scoring method, in the range of 0–12 points. Following earlier analyses of the same cohort, a cut-off of ≥3 points was chosen for symptoms of mental ill-health [59]. We defined 'absence of psychological distress' as a GHQ-12 score < 3 at all four measuring points, 2002, 2007, 2010, and 2014 referred as 'stable mental health' in the following.

A comparison was made with those reporting psychological distress at one to three time points during the four measuring points, referred as 'unstable mental health'. However, we excluded the respondents reporting psychological distress at all four measurement points (i.e., a constant stable negative mental health) as we considered the numbers being too small to be included in the statistical analyses. The stable mental health and unstable mental health groups were compared separately in the 18–29 and 30–84 age groups in order to assess if the determinants among the younger and older age groups differed from each other. The potential social determinants of health—i.e., the survey items, their response alternatives, and categorization measured in 2002—are described and commented in Supplementary Materials, Table S2.

2.3. Statistical Analysis

Logistic regression analysis predicting stable mental health was conducted separately for the 18–29 age group and the 30 years and older age group (Table 1). For missing data no imputations were carried out. Case-wise deletion, the default in SPSS, was employed, i.e., only respondents with complete data were included in the analyses. For 15 out the 17 variables, the attrition rate varied from 0.0–2.8%. Attrition was highest for community trust, with 7.5% in the younger group, and 8.4% in the older group, and further, hazardous alcohol consumption, with 9.7% and 10.2%, respectively.

Interaction analysis was performed for presumptive differences in health determinants between the two groups (Table 1). All analyses were performed on IBM/SPSS Statistics version 22.0 (IBM Corp., Armonk, NY, USA). We used the level of statistical significance at $p < 0.05$.

Table 1. Determinants for stable mental health in the 18–29 years and 30 years and older age groups.

Determinants	18–29 Years			≥30 Years			Interaction between the Determinant and the 18–29 Year and ≥30 Year Age Groups		
	OR	95% CI	Sig.	OR	95% CI	Sig.	OR	95% CI	Sig.
Gender									
Male (Reference: female)	1.91	1.54–2.36	0.000 ***	1.64	1.51–1.78	0.000 ***	1.00	0.81–1.24	0.975
Country of birth			0.111			0.474			0.266
Sweden	1.86	1.07–3.26	0.029 *	1.02	0.80–1.29	0.901	1.60	0.88–2.88	0.121
Other Nordic Countries	1.46	0.52–4.09	0.476	1.15	0.87–1.51	0.330	1.07	0.37–3.07	0.898
Other Europe	1.26	0.54–2.95	0.597	1.07	0.79–1.45	0.656	1.13	0.46–2.77	0.784
Outside Europe (Reference)	1			1			1		
Occupational status			0.005 **			0.000 ***			0.056
Employed	2.63	1.46–4.76	0.001 ***	1.70	1.29–2.24	0.000 ***	1.39	0.73–2.65	0.318
Own business	1.79	0.78–4.08	0.170	2.25	1.67–3.04	0.000 ***	0.78	0.33–1.85	0.570
Student/Trainee	1.93	1.06–3.53	0.033 *	0.97	0.64–1.46	0.877	1.89	0.92–3.90	0.085
Leave of absence/Parental leave	2.54	1.15–5.63	0.021 *	1.07	0.74–1.56	0.716	2.04	0.86–4.85	0.107
Outside labor market	2.22	0.97–5.12	0.060	2.21	1.66–2.93	0.000 ***	0.95	0.40–2.28	0.908
Unemployed (Reference)	1			1			1		
Financial strain			0.007 **			0.000 ***			0.003 **
No financial strain	1.56	1.07–2.28	0.021 *	2.79	2.25–3.47	0.000 ***	0.53	0.35–0.80	0.002 **
Some financial strain	1.16	0.79–1.71	0.448	1.66	1.32–2.10	0.000 ***	0.67	0.43–1.04	0.072
Major financial strain (Reference)	1			1			1		
Housing			0.983			0.429			0.443
Own	0.98	0.74–1.30	0.877	1.20	0.90–1.60	0.207	0.78	0.53–1.15	0.213
Rented	0.97	0.73–1.30	0.858	1.18	0.88–1.58	0.273	0.83	0.56–1.25	0.377
Lodger/Dormitory/Other (Reference)	1			1			1		
Emotional support			0.000 ***			0.000 ***			0.072
High emotional support	1.95	1.08–3.53	0.027 **	1.91	1.62–2.27	0.000 ***	0.93	0.55–1.57	0.779
Moderate emotional support	1.14	0.63–2.05	0.672	1.49	1.27–1.74	0.000 ***	0.70	0.40–1.22	0.204
Low emotional support (Reference)	1			1			1		
Instrumental support			0.373			0.001 **			0.206
High instrumental support	1.03	0.41–2.58	0.954	1.45	1.19–1.78	0.000 ***	0.66	0.29–1.52	0.329
Moderate instrumental support	0.84	0.34–2.09	0.711	1.29	1.06–1.57	0.009 *	0.55	0.23–1.29	0.167
Low instrumental support (Reference)	1			1			1		
Interpersonal trust			0.001 **			0.033 *			0.018 *
Strong interpersonal trust	1.33	0.96–1.83	0.084	1.23	1.04–1.44	0.014 *	1.02	0.73–1.43	0.909
Fair interpersonal trust	0.87	0.65–1.16	0.345	1.14	0.98–1.33	0.089	0.75	0.55–1.03	0.072
Weak interpersonal trust (Reference)	1			1			1		

Table 1. *Cont.*

Determinants	18–29 Years			≥30 Years			Interaction between the Determinant and the 18–29 Year and ≥30 Year Age Groups		
	OR	95% CI	Sig.	OR	95% CI	Sig.	OR	95% CI	Sig.
Community trust			0.864			0.044 *			0.699
Strong community trust	1.01	0.81–1.27	0.927	1.11	1.02–1.21	0.019 *	0.91	0.72–1.15	0.432
Fair community trust	1.07	0.83–1.38	0.598	1.08	0.98–1.19	0.112	1.00	0.76–1.31	0.996
Weak community trust (Reference)	1			1			1		
Societal participation									
Yes (Reference: did not participate)	0.94	0.75–1.19	0.611	0.97	0.90–1.05	0.496	0.93	0.74–1.16	0.505
Voting									
Yes (Reference: did not vote)	0.86	0.61–1.21	0.384	0.98	0.84–1.16	0.847	0.95	0.66–1.37	0.773
Nutrition—consumption of breakfast			0.548			0.829			0.994
Daily consumption of breakfast	1.26	0.81–1.96	0.303	1.06	0.87–1.31	0.561	1.03	0.64–1.64	0.912
Weekly consumption of breakfast	1.17	0.73–1.87	0.513	1.04	0.83–1.32	0.717	1.03	0.61–1.72	0.921
Seldom consumption of breakfast (Reference)	1			1			1		
Nutrition—consumption of fruit and berries			0.071			0.168			0.900
Daily consumption of fruit and berries	1.39	1.05–1.84	0.021 *	1.13	1.00–1.28	0.060	1.07	0.81–1.42	0.649
Weekly consumption of fruit and berries	1.25	0.94–1.67	0.127	1.09	0.95–1.25	0.207	1.04	0.77–1.42	0.784
Rare consumption of fruit and berries (Reference)	1			1			1		
Physical activity			0.438			0.000 ***			0.030 *
Regular physical activity	0.99	0.68–1.44	0.960	1.54	1.31–1.80	0.000 ***	0.65	0.44–0.94	0.023 *
Moderate physical activity	0.87	0.63–1.20	0.395	1.34	1.19–1.51	0.000 ***	0.65	0.47–0.90	0.010 *
Sedentary physical behavior (Reference)	1			1			1		
Tobacco smoking									
No (Reference: Daily smoking)	0.72	0.51–1.01	0.058	0.95	0.85–1.07	0.396	0.70	0.50–0.97	0.033 *
Hazardous alcohol consumption									
No (Reference: Hazardous alcohol consumption)	0.93	0.75–1.16	0.522	1.11	1.02–1.21	0.012 *	0.846	0.68–1.06	0.138
Victim of threat and violence			0.447			0.000 ***			0.736
Not victim of threat and violence	1.09	0.50–2.39	0.823	1.25	0.82–1.90	0.306	0.80	0.33–1.92	0.621
Victim of threat	0.80	0.33–1.92	0.611	0.74	0.46–1.21	0.229	1.04	0.39–2.83	0.934
Victim of violence	0.86	0.34–2.20	0.754	1.11	0.64–1.92	0.709	0.79	0.27–2.32	0.673
Victim of threat and violence (Reference)	1			1			1		

Data are presented as: OR, Odds Ratio; CI, Confidence Interval; reference value = 1. *p*-values indicate the following: $p > 0.05$ nonsignificant, * $p \leq 0.05$, ** $p \leq 0.01$, *** $p \leq 0.001$.

3. Results

Out of the 18–29-year-old study population, i.e., 3373 individuals (Figure 1), the GHQ-12 was completed by 2471 individuals. According to frequency analyses for the 18–29 age group, stable mental health was reported by 434, i.e., 46.2% out of a total of 939 men, and 524, i.e., 35.7% out of 1466 women. Sixty-six individuals reporting stable mental ill health were excluded from the analysis. In the 30–84 age group, i.e., 20,421 individuals (Supplementary Materials, Figure S1), the GHQ-12 was completed by 16,857 individuals. In our corresponding frequency analyses, stable mental health was reported by 4757, i.e., 65.7% out of a total of 7237 men, and 5140, i.e., 54.9% out of 9377 women for the 30–84 age group. In total, 243 individuals reporting stable mental ill health were excluded from the analysis. All 17 potential determinants were included in the regression analysis presented in Table 1.

The analysis showed that occupational status was the strongest predictor for stable mental health for 18–29 years. Different kinds of occupational status showed significant difference in odds for correlation with stable mental health compared to unemployment. The most robust associations were found for employment (OR = 2.63, 95% CI = 1.46–4.76), leave of absence/parental leave (OR = 2.54, 95% CI = 1.15–5.63), and being a student (OR = 1.93, 95% CI = 1.06–3.53). High emotional support, compared to low emotional support, appeared to be the second strongest predictor for stable mental health (OR = 1.95, 95% CI = 1.08–3.53). Furthermore, the male gender was a predictor for stable mental health compared to the female gender (OR = 1.91, 95% CI = 1.54–2.36), followed by being born in Sweden compared to born outside Europe (OR = 1.86, 95% CI = 1.07–3.26). Other determinants for stable mental health were experiencing no financial strain compared to the experience of major financial strain (OR = 1.56, 95% CI = 1.07–2.28), and, lastly, daily consumption of fruit and berries compared to seldom consumption of fruit and berries (OR = 1.39, 95% CI = 1.05–1.84). Physical activity, no daily tobacco smoking, and absence of hazardous alcohol consumption were not associated with stability in mental health.

In the regressed data, the findings in the older age group contrasted from the younger, revealing that experiencing no financial strain, compared to the experience of major financial strain was a principal predictor for stable mental health (OR = 2.79, 95% CI = 2.25–3.47), as shown in Table 1. Having some, rather than major financial strain, also yielded stable mental health in the older age group (OR = 1.66, 95% CI = 1.32–2.10). Secondly, occupational status predicted stable mental health, especially the status of running one's own business (OR = 2.25, 95% CI = 1.67–3.04), a position outside the labor market (OR = 2.21, 95% CI = 1.66–2.93), or being employed (OR = 1.70, 95% CI = 1.29–2.34) compared to unemployment. In third place, high and also moderate emotional support related to stable mental health (OR = 1.91, 95% CI = 1.62–2.27; and OR = 1.49, 95% CI = 1.27–1.74, respectively). The male gender, compared to female, ranked in fourth place (OR = 1.64, 95% CI = 1.51–1.78). Regular (OR = 1.54, 95% CI = 1.31–1.80) and moderate physical activity (OR = 1.34, 95% CI = 1.19–1.51) compared to sedentary physical behavior contributed to stable mental health. Further, high instrumental support (OR = 1.45, 95% CI = 1.19–1.78) and moderate instrumental support (OR = 1.29, 95% CI = 1.06–1.57) compared to weak instrumental support, as well as trust in terms of strong interpersonal trust (OR = 1.23, 95% CI = 1.04–1.44) compared to weak interpersonal trust, and strong community trust (OR = 1.11, 95% CI = 1.02–1.21) compared to weak community trust, were associated to stable mental health. Lastly, the absence of hazardous alcohol consumption (OR = 1.11, 95% CI = 1.02–1.21) produced stable mental health.

The interaction analyses displayed in Table 1 showed that significant differences between the younger and older groups were obvious only for three determinants of health. These were physical activity, where regular physical activity (OR = 0.65, 95% CI = 0.44–0.94) and moderate physical activity (OR = 0.65, 95% CI = 0.47–0.90) yielded a difference and were of importance for a stable mental health only in the older age group. The effect of absence of financial strain (OR = 0.53, 95% CI = 0.35–0.80) also differed between the younger and older groups, and was more important among the latter. Although to refrain from tobacco smoking was not a significant predictor for stable mental health in either age group, the effect differed significantly between the groups (OR = 0.70, 95% CI = 0.50–0.97), with smoking being a more important predictor in the younger group (OR = 0.72, 95% CI = 0.51–1.01).

4. Discussion

Our results show that every second male and every third female in the 18–29 age group reported stable mental health in the period of 2002–2014. Our findings may be compared with the Dunedin Cohort, where only 17% of the participants (57% males) at no time point did fulfill any criteria for a psychiatric diagnosis during the six waves of investigation, i.e., a period of nearly 30 years [21]. Six determinants were associated with this stability, namely, occupational status and especially employment, being absent or on parental leave, emotional support, the male gender, being of Swedish origin, experiencing no financial strain, and having healthy food intake, illustrated by a regular consumption of fruit and berries. It is noteworthy that only one of the determinants could be assigned to social capital and health behavior, emotional support and nutrition, respectively, whereas physical activity, the absence of daily tobacco smoking and of hazardous alcohol consumption, were not of importance for stability in mental health. These findings are comparable with those in an Australian cohort study, where positive development in young adulthood was to a very small extent associated with trust in authorities, civic action, and engagement in social groups [60]. Another study of the same cohort showed, in accordance with our study, that hazardous alcohol use had no relationship with positive development in young people [61]. The authors suggest that alcohol use among young people is rather normative and does not compromise positive functioning in other domains, an explanation shared by our findings. Regarding our results on the association between the regular consumption of fruit and berries and a stable mental health may be seen as a proxy for a healthy nutritional behavior on the whole. There is emerging evidence on healthy nutrition indicated by the consumption of fruit and vegetables as a factor associated with positive mental health and wellbeing [62–64]. Emerson and Carbert showed in their large sample of immigrants in Canada that a higher intake of vegetables and fruit was associated with lower odds of having psychiatric disorders, lower levels of distress, and higher levels of self-rated good mental health. Furthermore, these protective findings for nutrition and mental health were independent of sociodemographic, physical health, and health behavior such as physical activity and alcohol consumption [65].

Not surprisingly, occupational status in terms of employment is the main factor predicting future stability in mental health and unemployment may cause mental ill-health according to meta-analyses [66]. Employment entails a steady income and enables a young person to establish themselves in society. According to cross-sectional studies, employment has been associated with better mental health compared to being a student [14,16,17,67].

In line with many studies and a systematic review, emotional support is of profound importance for mental health and associated with protection from depression during one's lifespan [68,69]. Furthermore, in accordance with our findings, emotional support, but not practical support, had a stress-buffering effect in a longitudinal sample of young people [70]. The inequity in self-reported mental health between males and females, in favor of males, has been reported in research worldwide [71,72] and is also confirmed by us. Absence of financial strain also yielded stability in mental health, which could be seen as self-evident. However, the association between stability in mental health and healthy nutrition, illustrated by the consumption of fruit and berries, may not be well-known, though there is emerging evidence on this correlation [64]. Comparing our results of the younger group with the 30 years and older age group, stable mental health was experienced by a higher proportion in both males and females, which is in line with earlier findings, indicating less psychological distress in older age groups compared to the younger [73,74]. In contrast to the younger age group, more determinants related to social capital—beyond emotional support, instrumental support, interpersonal trust, and community trust—were also of importance for the older group. Furthermore, absence of financial strain was a more important determinant in the older age group compared to the younger, while country of birth had no significant association with stable mental health.

Running one's own business—i.e., being self-employed—seems to be of pronounced importance for the older group and their stability in mental health. Gevaert et al. investigated the phenomenon of self-employed people's wellbeing in 28 European countries [75]. Their findings highlight individual characteristics, such as motivation and the ability to identify opportunities, and, furthermore, that medium and large employers present high levels of wellbeing, but not self-employed in dependencies, such as farmers and freelancers. The fact that a position outside the labor market favored a stable mental health in the older group may be surprising. However, the 30 years and older age group, on the whole consisted of 26% outside the labor market; among those above 65 years of age, 91% were in that position, most likely pensioners. Health behavior, especially physical activity and absence of hazardous alcohol consumption, seems essential for stability in mental health at older age. Physical activity was critical for the older group and showed, together with financial strain, a significant difference between the younger and older groups. We hypothesize that a reason for the significance of physical activity in the older age group might be, that sedentary behavior often increases with age and has to be compensated by a choice for physical activity in order to achieve stable mental health. Regarding the importance of absence of financial strain in the older group, we refer to Wilkinson and Pickett, illustrating how people in equivalent groups compare one selves with each other and how relative inequalities get "under the skin" and are sentenced as stigma [76]. In younger ages financial difficulties are common and normalized among students and those not being established in working life. However, financial strain becomes more seldom with increasing age and therefore, might be sentenced as a shame for those experiencing the status.

It may be surprising that participation in social organizations and in elections produced no association with stable mental health in either group. Fiorillo et al. in a longitudinal study on participation in social groups, demonstrated that it was not sufficient to only be active in associations or a member in organizations to present good mental health [77]. Instead, both membership and active participation were required. As our survey did not include items concerning membership, we were not able to assess to what degree our responders were active participants.

The strengths of our study include the longitudinal study design upon which the results are based. Furthermore, the population sample entails a relatively large sample size, and the items measuring the determinants of health are well-established and cover different aspects of public health, e.g., sociodemographics, socioeconomics, social capital, and health behavior. Their frequent use of population surveys enables our results to be compared with other studies. Our study also has limitations. Firstly, this is a correlational study that does not give conclusive indications of causality. For example, the found association between unemployment and unstable mental health could be due to unemployment affecting mental health, mental health affecting the likelihood of unemployment, or both unemployment and mental health being affected by some confounding factor. It would, of course, be interesting to study if actively helping people out of unemployment affects their mental health. Secondly, the determinants of health are restricted to the items available from 2002. Important data related to socioeconomics—i.e., income and education—were also not relevant to use for our young study population, as these records do not tend to stabilize until later in life. Thirdly, our outcome variable 'stable mental health' is not optimal, as it just expresses freedom from mental distress, but not flourishing mental health. The lack of items on positive mental health restricted us from measuring wellbeing and flourishing in this population sample, and choosing 'stability in mental health' was our second-best choice. Lastly, our comparison age group, 30 years and older, may be too wide. We could have divided our comparison group into three or more subgroups, but to make assessments of determinants of health and stable mental health in all specific age groups was not the aim of our study. Our focus was the 18–29 age group, and future studies should make more specific comparisons among different age groups.

5. Conclusions

Our findings showed that, for young people, occupational status, especially being employed, is of major importance to developing stable mental health. Other factors are emotional support, male gender, being of Swedish origin, absence of financial strain, and nutrition. These determinants differ from the older age group, where absence of financial strain is the key determinant for stability in mental health. Furthermore, occupational status, particularly running one's own business and determinants related to social capital and physical activity were crucial for stability in mental health in the older age group. Our findings indicate that predictors for mental health differ over the life-course, and in order to address health-promoting interventions as efficiently as possible, policy-makers should be aware of which determinants to target in diverse age groups. Nevertheless, our study warrants replications.

Author Contributions: R.W. conceived and designed the study, performed the statistical analyses, and wrote the original article. K.S. supervised the methodology and statistical analyses. L.L. supervised the study. All authors read and approved the final manuscript.

Acknowledgments: We are especially grateful to Peeter Fredlund, who is in charge of the administration of the Stockholm Public Health Cohort and provided us with a dataset of the necessary variables for this study. Furthermore, we wish to thank The Public Health Agency for offering us the publication fee.

References

1. Eckersley, R. Troubled youth: An island of misery in an ocean of happiness, or the tip of an iceberg of suffering? *Early Interv. Psychiatry* **2011**, *5*, 6–11. [CrossRef] [PubMed]
2. Collishaw, S.; Maughan, B.; Natarajan, L.; Pickles, A. Trends in adolescent emotional problems in England: A comparison of two national cohorts twenty years apart. *J. Child Psychol. Psychiatry* **2010**, *51*, 885–894. [CrossRef] [PubMed]
3. Sweeting, H.; Young, R.; West, P. GHQ increases among Scottish 15 year olds 1987–2006. *Soc. Psychiatry Psychiatr. Epidemiol.* **2009**, *44*, 579–586. [CrossRef] [PubMed]
4. Soest, T.; Wichstrøm, L. Secular Trends in Depressive Symptoms Among Norwegian Adolescents from 1992 to 2010. *J. Abnorm. Child Psychol.* **2014**, *42*, 403–415. [CrossRef] [PubMed]
5. Friberg, P.; Hagquist, C.; Osika, W. Self-perceived psychosomatic health in Swedish children, adolescents and young adults: An internet-based survey over time. *BMJ Open* **2012**, *2*. [CrossRef] [PubMed]
6. Bor, W.; Dean, A.J.; Najman, J.; Hayatbakhsh, R. Are child and adolescent mental health problems increasing in the 21st century? A systematic review. *Aust. N. Z. J. Psychiatry* **2014**. [CrossRef] [PubMed]
7. Potrebny, T.; Wiium, N.; Lundegard, M.M. Temporal trends in adolescents' self-reported psychosomatic health complaints from 1980–2016: A systematic review and meta-analysis. *PLoS ONE* **2017**, *12*, e0188374. [CrossRef]
8. Public Health Agency of Sweden. Mental Health. Available online: https://www.folkhalsomyndigheten.se/the-public-health-agency-of-sweden/living-conditions-and-lifestyle/mental-health/ (accessed on 1 December 2018).
9. Danish Health Authority. Den Nationale Sundhetsprofil 2017. Available online: https://www.sst.dk/da/udgivelser/2018/~/media/73EADC242CDB46BD8ABF9DE895A6132C.ashx (accessed on 1 December 2018).
10. National Institute for Health and Welfare of Finland. Statistical Yearbook on Social Welfare and Health Care 2017. Available online: http://www.julkari.fi/bitstream/handle/10024/135959/URN_ISBN_978-952-302-970-5.pdf?sequence=1&isAllowed=y (accessed on 1 December 2018).
11. Allen, J.; Balfour, R.; Bell, R.; Marmot, M. Social determinants of mental health. *Int. Rev. Psychiatry* **2014**, *26*, 392–407. [CrossRef]
12. Rotenstein, L.S.; Ramos, M.A.; Torre, M.; Segal, J.B.; Peluso, M.J.; Guille, C.; Sen, S.; Mata, D.A. Prevalence of Depression, Depressive Symptoms, and Suicidal Ideation Among Medical Students: A Systematic Review and Meta-Analysis. *JAMA* **2016**, *316*, 2214–2236. [CrossRef]

13. Ibrahim, A.K.; Kelly, S.J.; Adams, C.E.; Glazebrook, C. A systematic review of studies of depression prevalence in university students. *J. Psychiatr. Res.* **2013**, *47*, 391–400. [CrossRef]
14. Dyrbye, L.N.; Thomas, M.R.; Shanafelt, T.D. Systematic review of depression, anxiety, and other indicators of psychological distress among U.S. and Canadian medical students. *Acad. Med.* **2006**, *81*, 354–373. [CrossRef] [PubMed]
15. Hope, V.; Henderson, M. Medical student depression, anxiety and distress outside North America: A systematic review. *Med. Educ.* **2014**, *48*, 963–979. [CrossRef] [PubMed]
16. Leahy, C.M.; Peterson, R.F.; Wilson, I.G.; Newbury, J.W.; Tonkin, A.L.; Turnbull, D. Distress levels and self-reported treatment rates for medicine, law, psychology and mechanical engineering tertiary students: Cross-sectional study. *Aust. N. Z. J. Psychiatry* **2010**, *44*, 608–615. [CrossRef] [PubMed]
17. Winzer, R.; Lindblad, F.; Sorjonen, K.; Lindberg, L. Positive versus negative mental health in emerging adulthood: A national cross-sectional survey. *BMC Public Health* **2014**, *14*, 1238. [CrossRef] [PubMed]
18. O'Connor, M.; Sanson, A.V.; Toumbourou, J.W.; Norrish, J.; Olsson, C.A. Does Positive Mental Health in Adolescence Longitudinally Predict Healthy Transitions in Young Adulthood? *J. Happiness Stud.* **2017**, *18*, 177–198. [CrossRef]
19. De Neve, J.E.; Oswald, A.J. Estimating the influence of life satisfaction and positive affect on later income using sibling fixed effects. *Proc. Natl. Acad. Sci. USA* **2012**, *109*. [CrossRef] [PubMed]
20. Moffitt, T.E.; Arseneault, L.; Belsky, D.; Dickson, N.; Hancox, R.J.; Harrington, H.; Houts, R.; Poulton, R.; Roberts, B.W.; Ross, S.; et al. A gradient of childhood self-control predicts health, wealth, and public safety. *Proc. Natl. Acad. Sci. USA* **2011**, *108*, 2693–2698. [CrossRef] [PubMed]
21. Schaefer, J.D.; Caspi, A.; Belsky, D.W.; Harrington, H.; Houts, R.; Horwood, L.J.; Hussong, A.; Ramrakha, S.; Poulton, R.; Moffitt, T.E. Enduring mental health: Prevalence and prediction. *J. Abnorm. Psychol.* **2017**, *126*, 212–224. [CrossRef] [PubMed]
22. Havelka, M.; Lucanin, J.D.; Lucanin, D. Biopsychosocial model—The integrated approach to health and disease. *Coll. Antropol.* **2009**, *33*, 303–310.
23. *Social Determinants of Health: The Solid Facts*, 2nd ed.; WHO Regional Office for Europe: Copenhagen, Denmark, 2003.
24. Viner, R.M.; Ozer, E.M.; Denny, S.; Marmot, M.; Resnick, M.; Fatusi, A.; Currie, C. Adolescence and the social determinants of health. *Lancet* **2012**, *379*, 1641–1652. [CrossRef]
25. Marmot, M.G.; Wilkinson, R.G. *Social Determinants of Health*, 2nd ed.; Oxford University Press: Oxford, UK; New York, NY, USA, 2006; p. x. 366p.
26. Fisher, M.; Baum, F. The social determinants of mental health: Implications for research and health promotion. *Aust. N. Z. J. Psychiatry* **2010**, *44*, 1057–1063. [CrossRef] [PubMed]
27. Harpham, T.; Grant, E.; Thomas, E. Measuring social capital within health surveys: Key issues. *Health Policy Plan.* **2002**, *17*, 106–111. [CrossRef] [PubMed]
28. Mammen, G.; Faulkner, G. Physical activity and the prevention of depression: A systematic review of prospective studies. *Am. J. Prev. Med.* **2013**, *45*, 649–657. [CrossRef] [PubMed]
29. McMahon, E.M.; Corcoran, P.; O'Regan, G.; Keeley, H.; Cannon, M.; Carli, V.; Wasserman, C.; Hadlaczky, G.; Sarchiapone, M.; Apter, A.; et al. Physical activity in European adolescents and associations with anxiety, depression and well-being. *Eur. Child Adolesc. Psychiatry* **2017**, *26*, 111–122. [CrossRef] [PubMed]
30. Hall, W.D.; Patton, G.; Stockings, E.; Weier, M.; Lynskey, M.; Morley, K.I.; Degenhardt, L. Why young people's substance use matters for global health. *Lancet Psychiatry* **2016**, *3*, 265–279. [CrossRef]
31. Charlet, K.; Heinz, A. Harm reduction—A systematic review on effects of alcohol reduction on physical and mental symptoms. *Addict. Biol.* **2017**, *22*, 1119–1159. [CrossRef]
32. O'Neil, A.; Quirk, S.E.; Housden, S.; Brennan, S.L.; Williams, L.J.; Pasco, J.A.; Berk, M.; Jacka, F.N. Relationship Between Diet and Mental Health in Children and Adolescents: A Systematic Review. *Am. J. Public Health* **2014**, *104*, e31–e42. [CrossRef]
33. Opie, R.S.; O'Neil, A.; Itsiopoulos, C.; Jacka, F.N. The impact of whole-of-diet interventions on depression and anxiety: A systematic review of randomised controlled trials. *Public Health Nutr.* **2015**, *18*, 2074–2093. [CrossRef]

34. Khalid, S.; Williams, C.M.; Reynolds, S.A. Is there an association between diet and depression in children and adolescents? A systematic review. *Br. J. Nutr.* **2017**, *116*, 2097–2108. [CrossRef]
35. Huppert, F.A.; Whittington, J.E. Evidence for the independence of positive and negative well-being: Implications for quality of life assessment. *Br. J. Health Psychol.* **2003**, *8*, 107–122. [CrossRef]
36. Patel, V.; Goodman, A. Researching protective and promotive factors in mental health. *Int. J. Epidemiol.* **2007**, *36*, 703–707. [CrossRef] [PubMed]
37. Hawkins, M.T.; Letcher, P.; Sanson, A.; Smart, D.; Toumbourou, J.W. Positive development in emerging adulthood. *Aust. J. Psychol.* **2009**, *61*, 89–99. [CrossRef]
38. O'Connor, M.; Sanson, A.; Hawkins, M.T.; Letcher, P.; Toumbourou, J.W.; Smart, D.; Vassallo, S.; Olsson, C.A. Predictors of positive development in emerging adulthood. *J. Youth Adolesc.* **2011**, *40*, 860–874. [CrossRef] [PubMed]
39. Lindblad, F.; Backman, L.; Akerstedt, T. Immigrant girls perceive less stress. *Acta Paediatr.* **2008**, *97*, 889–893. [CrossRef] [PubMed]
40. Whitley, R.; Wang, J.; Fleury, M.-J.; Liu, A.; Caron, J. Mental Health Status, Health Care Utilisation, and Service Satisfaction among Immigrants in Montreal: An Epidemiological Comparison. *Can. J. Psychiatry Rev. Can. Psychiatr.* **2017**, *62*, 570–579. [CrossRef] [PubMed]
41. Bas-Sarmiento, P.; Saucedo-Moreno, M.J.; Fernandez-Gutierrez, M.; Poza-Mendez, M. Mental Health in Immigrants Versus Native Population: A Systematic Review of the Literature. *Arch. Psychiatr. Nurs.* **2017**, *31*, 111–121. [CrossRef] [PubMed]
42. Harding, S.; Read, U.M.; Molaodi, O.R.; Cassidy, A.; Maynard, M.J.; Lenguerrand, E.; Astell-Burt, T.; Teyhan, A.; Whitrow, M.; Enayat, Z.E. The Determinants of young Adult Social well-being and Health (DASH) study: Diversity, psychosocial determinants and health. *Soc. Psychiatry Psychiatr. Epidemiol.* **2015**, *50*, 1173–1188. [CrossRef] [PubMed]
43. Berg, N.; Kiviruusu, O.; Karvonen, S.; Rahkonen, O.; Huurre, T. Pathways from problems in adolescent family relationships to midlife mental health via early adulthood disadvantages—A 26-year longitudinal study. *PLoS ONE* **2017**, *12*, e0178136. [CrossRef]
44. Bovier, P.A.; Chamot, E.; Perneger, T.V. Perceived stress, internal resources, and social support as determinants of mental health among young adults. *Qual. Life Res.* **2004**, *13*, 161–170. [CrossRef]
45. Cater, A.K.; Andershed, A.K.; Andershed, H. Youth victimization in Sweden: Prevalence, characteristics and relation to mental health and behavioral problems in young adulthood. *Child Abuse Negl.* **2014**, *38*, 1290–1302. [CrossRef]
46. Assari, S.; Moghani Lankarani, M. Violence Exposure and Mental Health of College Students in the United States. *Behav. Sci.* **2018**, *8*, 53. [CrossRef]
47. Kadra, G.; Dean, K.; Hotopf, M.; Hatch, S.L. Investigating Exposure to Violence and Mental Health in a Diverse Urban Community Sample: Data from the South East London Community Health (SELCoH) Survey. *PLoS ONE* **2014**, *9*, e93660. [CrossRef] [PubMed]
48. Turanovic, J.J.; Pratt, T.C. Longitudinal Effects of Violent Victimization during Adolescence on Adverse Outcomes in Adulthood: A Focus on Prosocial Attachments. *J. Pediatr.* **2015**, *166*, 1062–1069.e1. [CrossRef] [PubMed]
49. Keyes, C.L.M.; Dhingra, S.S.; Simoes, E.J. Change in Level of Positive Mental Health as a Predictor of Future Risk of Mental Illness. *Am. J. Public Health* **2010**, *100*, 2366–2371. [CrossRef]
50. Svensson, A.C.; Fredlund, P.; Laflamme, L.; Hallqvist, J.; Alfredsson, L.; Ekbom, A.; Feychting, M.; Forsberg, B.; Pedersen, N.L.; Vagero, D.; et al. Cohort Profile: The Stockholm Public Health Cohort. *Int. J. Epidemiol.* **2012**. [CrossRef] [PubMed]
51. Goldberg, D.; Williams, P. *A User's Guide to the General Health Questionnaire*; Institute of Psychiatry: London, UK, 1988.
52. Makikangas, A.; Feldt, T.; Kinnunen, U.; Tolvanen, A.; Kinnunen, M.; Pulkkinen, L. The factor structure and factorial invariance of the 12-item General Health Questionnaire (GHQ-12) across time: Evidence from two community-based samples. *Psychol. Assess.* **2006**, *18*, 444–451. [CrossRef] [PubMed]
53. Rocha, K.B.; Perez, K.; Rodriguez-Sanz, M.; Borrell, C.; Obiols, J.E. Psychometric properties and normative values of General Health Questionnaire (GHQ-12) in Spanish population. *Int. J. Clin. Health Psychol.* **2011**, *11*, 125–139.

54. Doi, Y.; Minowa, M. Factor structure of the 12-item General Health Questionnaire in the Japanese general adult population. *Psychiatry Clin. Neurosci.* **2003**, *57*, 379–383. [CrossRef] [PubMed]
55. Bowe, A. The cultural fairness of the 12-item General Health Questionnaire among diverse adolescents. *Psychol. Assess.* **2017**, *29*, 87. [CrossRef]
56. Kashyap, G.C.; Singh, S.K. Reliability and validity of general health questionnaire (GHQ-12) for male tannery workers: A study carried out in Kanpur, India. *BMC Psychiatry* **2017**, *17*, 102. [CrossRef]
57. Sconfienza, C. *Mätning av Psykiskt Välbefinnande Bland Ungdomar i Sverige: Användning av GHQ-12 [Measuring Mental Well-Being among Young People in Sweden: Application of GHQ 12]*; National Institute for Working Life: Solna, Sweden, 1998; p. 33, ISBN 91-7045-493-0.
58. Lundin, A.; Hallgren, M.; Theobald, H.; Hellgren, C.; Torgen, M. Validity of the 12-item version of the General Health Questionnaire in detecting depression in the general population. *Public Health* **2016**, *136*, 66–74. [CrossRef] [PubMed]
59. Kosidou, K.; Dalman, C.; Lundberg, M.; Hallqvist, J.; Isacsson, G.; Magnusson, C. Socioeconomic status and risk of psychological distress and depression in the Stockholm Public Health Cohort: A population-based study. *J. Affect. Disord.* **2011**, *134*, 160–167. [CrossRef] [PubMed]
60. Hawkins, M.T.; Letcher, P.; Sanson, A.; O'Connor, M.; Toumbourou, J.W.; Olsson, C. Stability and Change in Positive Development During Young Adulthood. *J. Youth Adolesc.* **2011**, *40*, 1436–1452. [CrossRef] [PubMed]
61. Hawkins, M.T.; Villagonzalo, K.-A.; Sanson, A.V.; Toumbourou, J.W.; Letcher, P.; Olsson, C.A. Associations Between Positive Development in Late Adolescence and Social, Health, and Behavioral Outcomes in Young Adulthood. *J. Adult Dev.* **2012**, *19*, 88–99. [CrossRef]
62. Conner, T.S.; Brookie, K.L.; Richardson, A.C.; Polak, M.A. On carrots and curiosity: Eating fruit and vegetables is associated with greater flourishing in daily life. *Br. J. Health Psychol.* **2015**, *20*, 413–427. [CrossRef] [PubMed]
63. Conner, T.S.; Brookie, K.L.; Carr, A.C.; Mainvil, L.A.; Vissers, M.C. Let them eat fruit! The effect of fruit and vegetable consumption on psychological well-being in young adults: A randomized controlled trial. *PLoS ONE* **2017**, *12*, e0171206. [CrossRef] [PubMed]
64. Mujcic, R.; Oswald, A.J. Evolution of Well-Being and Happiness After Increases in Consumption of Fruit and Vegetables. *Am. J. Public Health* **2016**, *106*, 1504–1510. [CrossRef]
65. Emerson, S.D.; Carbert, N.S. An apple a day: Protective associations between nutrition and the mental health of immigrants in Canada. *Soc. Psychiatry Psychiatr. Epidemiol.* **2018**. [CrossRef]
66. Paul, K.I.; Moser, K. Unemployment impairs mental health: Meta-analyses. *J. Vocat. Behav.* **2009**, *74*, 264–282. [CrossRef]
67. Cvetkovski, S.; Reavley, N.J.; Jorm, A.F. The prevalence and correlates of psychological distress in Australian tertiary students compared to their community peers. *Aust. N. Z. J. Psychiatry* **2012**, *46*, 457–467. [CrossRef]
68. Gariepy, G.; Honkaniemi, H.; Quesnel-Vallee, A. Social support and protection from depression: Systematic review of current findings in Western countries. *Br. J. Psychiatry* **2016**, *209*, 284–293. [CrossRef] [PubMed]
69. Fagg, J.; Curtis, S.; Stansfeld, S.A.; Cattell, V.; Tupuola, A.M.; Arephin, M. Area social fragmentation, social support for individuals and psychosocial health in young adults: Evidence from a national survey in England. *Soc. Sci. Med.* **2008**, *66*, 242–254. [CrossRef] [PubMed]
70. Power, M.J. Stress-buffering efffects of social support—A longitudinal study. *Motiv. Emot.* **1988**, *12*, 197–204. [CrossRef]
71. Boerma, T.; Hosseinpoor, A.R.; Verdes, E.; Chatterji, S. A global assessment of the gender gap in self-reported health with survey data from 59 countries. *BMC Public Health* **2016**, *16*, 675. [CrossRef] [PubMed]
72. Patel, V.; Saxena, S.; Lund, C.; Thornicroft, G.; Baingana, F.; Bolton, P.; Chisholm, D.; Collins, P.Y.; Cooper, J.L.; Eaton, J.; et al. The Lancet Commission on global mental health and sustainable development. *Lancet* **2018**. [CrossRef]
73. Thomas, M.L.; Kaufmann, C.N.; Palmer, B.W.; Depp, C.A.; Martin, A.S.; Glorioso, D.K.; Thompson, W.K.; Jeste, D.V. Paradoxical Trend for Improvement in Mental Health with Aging: A Community-Based Study of 1546 Adults Aged 21–100 Years. *J. Clin. Psychiatry* **2016**, *77*, e1019–e1025. [CrossRef] [PubMed]
74. Happell, B.; Koehn, S. Effect of aging on the perceptions of physical and mental health in an Australian population. *Nurs. Health Sci.* **2011**, *13*, 27–33. [CrossRef]

75. Gevaert, J.; Moortel, D.; Wilkens, M.; Vanroelen, C. What's up with the self-employed? A cross-national perspective on the self-employed's work-related mental well-being. *SSM Popul. Health* **2018**, *4*, 317–326. [CrossRef]
76. Wilkinson, R.G.; Pickett, K. *The Spirit Level: Why Greater Equality Makes Societies Stronger*, 1st ed.; Bloomsbury Press: New York, NY, USA, 2009; p. xv, 330p.
77. Fiorillo, D.; Lavadera, G.L.; Nappo, N. Social participation and self-rated psychological health: A longitudinal study on BHPS. *SSM Popul. Health* **2017**, *3*, 266–274. [CrossRef]

7

The Role of Sleep Quality in the Psychological Well-Being of Final Year Undergraduate Students in China

Keyu Zhai [1], Xing Gao [2,*] and Geng Wang [1]

[1] School of Education, University of Glasgow, Glasgow G12 8QQ, UK; k.zhai.1@research.gla.ac.uk (K.Z.); g.wang.3@research.gla.ac.uk (G.W.)

[2] The Bartlett School of Planning, University College London, London WC1E 6BT, UK

* Correspondence: xing.gao@ucl.ac.uk

Abstract: There are increasing numbers of university students in China suffering from poor sleep and psychological well-being problems. In particular, the issues are more severe among the final year undergraduate students, because they are experiencing a transitory period from university life to the workplace. However, extant research has rarely explored sleep quality and psychological well-being of final year university students. To better understand the role of sleep quality in psychological well-being, we examined the association between different sleep quality and mental health. Based on a cross-sectional survey of 2495 full-time final year university students in China, we employed multivariable logistic regression to assess association between sleep quality and psychological well-being by controlling for sociodemographic factors such as age, gender, education, marital or relationship status, household conditions, place of birth, study subjects and etc. According to the research results, we can find strong association between sleep quality and psychological well-being. Having normal sleep quality is associated with lower level of psychological well-being problems. By contrast, poor sleep quality is associated with high level of negative psychological well-being. Poor sleep quality has higher potency than normal sleep quality due to negative bias. Among covariates, age, gender and education have significant effects on psychological well-being.

Keywords: sleep quality; psychological well-being; Chinese final year university students; higher education; gender

---

1. Introduction

Psychological well-being of university students is an important research field, and thus this issue increasingly receives global concern [1]. Taking the UK as an example, the UK Psychiatric Morbidity Survey reported significant increases in anxiety and depression among the young people aged from 16 to 24 [1]. Rich research identifies positive mental health serves as a protective role against health risk behaviors, but negative mental health would result in risky behaviors among university students [2]. In addition, a large number of cross-sectional evidence shows that individual having much depression and hopeless tends to be less physically active [3] and has more negative feelings, such as suicidal thoughts [4]. Macaskill [1] studied the students from academic year for first, second and third year in the UK, and found rates of mental illness in students are same as that of the general population, whereas only 5.1% of them can receive treatment. Therefore, easier access to specialist treatment is in great need among university students. By contrast, some extant research finds that Hong Kong university students are more vulnerable than their peers regarding mental disorders, because their health is poorer and they have higher rates of getting depression and anxiety [5,6]. University students are five times more likely to be recognized with mental health issues [7]. The different context determines the different research results, and thus studying university students' sleeping quality and psychological well-being should be closely related to the specific context. There are a variety of factors influencing university students' mental health. For university students, their failure to meet basic physical activity guidelines [8] and increasing sedentary behaviors [9] are significant factors. Among a wide variety of variables, sleep quality is a significant factor [10], and sleep disorder frequently co-occurs with mental health problems.

Poor sleep quality is a symptom, and it is featured by difficulty of falling and remaining asleep [11,12]. Extensive research has shown that sleep quality has become an increasing public health focus, and poor sleep quality leads to increased risk of mental problems [13], including depression and anxiety [14]. Nowadays, poor sleep quality is a prevalent symptom among young adults, affecting over 10% of the adult population [15]. Among these young adults, there are plenty of university students [16]. Voelker [17] discussed that university students' biological sleep rhythms are disrupted, because they experience more stress regarding their futures and employment or late-night computer work. Besides, academic work, later bedtime resulted from social integration demand, environmental noise are disturbing undergraduate students' sleep quality [18,19]. In addition, a growing body of research has documented the gendered difference in mental health [20,21]. Therefore, among university students, it can be concluded that poor sleep quality is a common problem and has increased risk for their mental health [22]. In order to discover the role of sleep quality in mental health, much research has been conducted, but most of extant literature focuses on specific group such as the elderly or young adults. There is few research concentrating in studying university students [22–24]. Besides, final year university students in China are a special group, because they are undergoing a critical transitory period in which they are going from university life to adulthood and making major life decisions [25]. More importantly, Suen et al. [26] found increasing academic year in university is associated with increased rate of getting sleep problems. Last but not least, the Chinese context is very different from typical Western education systems. The common accommodation of undergraduate student in China is a special issue. In China's student accommodation, several students share a same bedroom. The relationship with roommates becomes an important factor, and it make the research of sleep problem more complicated. Facing the research background, this paper addresses what significant factors affect sleep quality, and how poor sleep quality affects psychological well-being of final year Chinese undergraduate students.

Motivated by the research question, this paper aims to examine, in a large cohort of university students, associations between sleep quality and psychological well-being of final year university students in China. We would investigate how sleep quality affects psychological well-being and compare the effects sizes associated with positive and negative quality on psychological well-being in the same statistical model.

This paper contributes to bridge two gaps. First, this paper initially explores the role of sleep quality in psychological well-being, targeting final year Chinese university students. China's is very different from the Western education system. China has the largest number of undergraduate students and the special shared student accommodation, and the fast social changes and high level of social competition dramatically influence young adults in every aspects [27]. Facing the fact that a large proportion of Chinese university students are suffering from poor sleep quality [28] and mental health problems [2], this paper is timely and necessary. Another gap that would be filled is to provide overall analysis of psychological well-being of Chinese university students. This paper would analyze a series of factors of final year university students' psychological well-being.

2. Method

The study conducted a cross-sectional data of sleep quality and psychological well-being among final year undergraduate students from large China's university. In March 2018, participants were recruited by WeChat. We invited the participants to finish an online survey to understand the effect of sleep quality on mental health. According to power calculations which depend on the prior distributions and estimates of our variables [29], our survey demanded at least 2600 participants. To be eligible, the participants must be final year undergraduate students and were expected to obtain a Bachelor degree in July 2018. There were totally 2879 eligible participants. Finally, 2495 participants provided complete results for our survey. This study was approved by the Ethics Committee of College of Social Science of University of Glasgow on 1st September 2017 (No. 400160231).

Participants provided online informed consent at the beginning of the questionnaire, and the mean survey completion time was 12.8 min. After participants finished the survey, the WeChat system would randomly generate a voucher ranging from 1 to 10 Yuan to thank them. Additionally, this could attract more participants and to some degree increase the questionnaire completion quality. Because the voucher was sent out by the WeChat software, the data was still anonymized. Collecting a voucher in WeChat does not need the participants' personal information. This study was funded by a Doctoral Fellowship from the China Scholarship Council.

2.1. *Measure of Psychological Well-Being*

In this study, we chose the K6 scale of mental well-being to measure the mental disorders, classified according to the Diagnostic and Statistical Manual of Mental Disorders, 4th Edition (DSM-IV). The K6 is the reliable and valid instrument to screen for any DSM-IV disorder [30], and additionally this measurement has been widely used to investigate the mental health of different population in China [31–33]. The K6 scale designs diagnose cases with non-specific mental illness in the general population, and is applied in national survey which is carried out by World Mental Health Initiative of World Health Organization. Regarding the K6 scale, our study took advantage of five items, including nervous, anxious, worthless, hopeless and depressed. We asked respondents how often do you feel the above five kinds of emotion within a past month. The results can range from 1 (often) to 4 (never). Thus, higher scores mean better mental health.

The results of psychological well-being were viewed as the dependent variable in the study. Due to the non-normal distribution and skewed of mental health, it cannot be served as a continuous variable [29]. Therefore, following Primack et al. [29], we processed the data of psychological well-being in the following ways to improve interpretability. Standard cutoff for depression of 11, corresponding to T-score with 60.5 [34], is first used to make the mental health based on the recommendation from American Psychiatric Association [1]. Second, because the K6 scale is for evaluating the levels of mental health, the study divided the results into three equal types—high (20); medium (17–19); low (5–16). In the first analysis, standard cutoff was applied, and three level types were used in our secondary analyses.

2.2. *Sleep Quality*

Pittsburgh Sleep Quality Index (PSQI) has been validated for application in different types of population samples [35,36]. Sleep quality in the last month was assessed via three pre-specified response categories: poor quality, impaired quality and normal quality. Guo et al. [36] indicated that poor quality means that participants have sleep deprivation symptoms, like taking sleeping peels, or insomnia; participants with normal sleep quality have the following characteristics: difficult to weak up at night, enjoying a high mood in daytime, and falling sleep within 30 min; impaired quality refers to the sleep status between poor and normal sleeping quality. However, in the process of survey, participants find it difficult to define their appropriate categories. Thus, based on the above discussions, the study divided sleep quality into two categories: normal quality and poor quality. We evaluated normal and poor sleep quality through participants' self-rated in the questionnaire. Our survey provided sliders between 0 and 100 for participants. Participants assessed the percentage of their sleep quality involved normal and poor status respectively. According to Primack et al. [29], in order to conduct logistic regression and improve results' interpretability, the study changed the participants' responses to a 10-points scale, and 1 point is equal to 10%. This transformation is based on responses' natural distribution.

2.3. Covariates

We controlled for sociodemographic factors as our covariates that are known to be related to psychological well-being and sleep quality, including education [37], household conditions [38], marital or relationship status [39], physical activity [40], and illness health [41]. In our study, education is based on the official administrative tier of China's universities, and higher level of universities means better educational quality, which may be positively related to mental health. Household conditions focus on socioeconomic status of parents. We employed Lu's division standard, which is widely used in research of socioeconomic status [42]. Regarding physical activity, following Mai et al. [43], we divided it into three types: physically inactive, less active (meaning 1–4 occasions conducted exercise or sport within a past month), and more active (meaning 5 or more). We also investigated Body Mass Index (BMI) which is derived from weight and height to measure illness health conditions [43], and the study placed it into physical activity.

In addition to above covariates, the study also asked participants to show their place of birth, subjects, gender and age. Age was treated as a continuous variable in years, ranging from 18 to 30 [29]. Place of birth was collapsed into two categories: rural and urban. Cheung [31] indicated that students from rural areas are more likely to suffer from psychological well-being problems. In our study, we were interested in questioning whether sleep quality of final year students from different subjects is different in mental health. Thus, we also investigated the subject information of participants.

2.4. Analysis Strategy

The study summarized the sample through depicting counts and percentage. According to the variables, in addition to continuous variables, there are plenty of sociodemographic variables. Multivariable models are usually preferentially selected when there are categorical variables with many categories [44]. Multivariable model has been commonly used in biometrical applications to model the associations between a result and predictor variables [44,45]. We also performed *t*-tests to evaluate the sample mean differences on continuous, and Chi-square tests for the categorical variables. The significant values of all tests were presented. In order to meet the assumptions of analytic models, the study controlled for collinearity among all covariates. The largest Pearson's correlation coefficient was 0.598, indicating that multicollinearity issues among independent variables were not a challenge. Nonsignificant *p*-values (from 0.93 to 0.98) indicated that the models using ordered logistic regression meet the proportional odds assumption [29].

Then, by employing logistic regression and ordered logistic regression, the study evaluated the effects of sleep quality on mental health. In multivariable models, the study chose a priori to adjust for all covariates. The statistical significance of a two-tailed test ($\alpha = 0.05$) was defined. Using Stata 14, we analyzed all data. Based on the method of Primack et al. [29], there were three steps of sensitivity analyses to explore results' robustness. We first used continuous variables to conduct analysis; second, extant research shows a $p < 0.20$ can avoid the overcontrolling [29]. And thus the study analyzed data by using covariates with a $p < 0.20$; third, in order to make sure that the results are consistent with the first model, we conducted the analysis by taking advantage of psychological well-being cutoffs. Due to similar results between primary models and additional analysis, this paper only demonstrated the primary results and analysis.

3. Results

Without statistically taking any confounders into account, Table 1 reports the descriptive statistics of variables. *t*-Tests and Chi-square were used to evaluate mean differences of continuous variables and the categorical variables, respectively. They indicated the variance inflation factor. The reported psychological well-being is significant. As expected, the most of final year students suffer from poor sleep quality. As shown in Table 1, gender distribution was relatively balanced. The distribution of educational background was also in line with the administrative level of Chinese universities. Household conditions were based on the father's occupation.

Table 1. Descriptive statistics (N = 2495).

Variables	Mean/Sample %	(SD)	Test Statistics [a]	p [b]
Psychological well-being	14.38	(4.02)	$t = 1.22$	$p = 0.004$
Normal sleep quality	49	(19.07)	$t = 0.56$	$p = 0.001$
Poor sleep quality	78	(32.13)	$t = 0.41$	$p = 0.002$
Gender				
Female	47%		$X^2 = 4.313$	$p = 0.036$
Male	53%			
Education				
985 project	11%		$X^2 = 1.66$	$p = 0.017$
211 project	17%			
Yi Ben	19%			
Er Ben	28%			
San Ben	25%			
Household conditions				
State & society administrator (cadre in governments), Manager (Manager or department leader in a state company, private company, foreign company and joint company)	7%		$X^2 = 4.69$	$p = 0.023$
Private enterprise owner (having large scale company), Technological specialist (teacher, engineer, doctor, academic researcher, lawyer, culture worker)	15%			
Clerk & office worker (secretary, accountant, computer operator), Individual entrepreneur (one-person company with unlimited liability)	29%			
Commercial & service worker (tertiary industry workers), Industrial worker (worker in factory, mining and transport industry)	35%			
Farmer, Unemployed	14%			
Marital or relationship status				
Yes	37%		$X^2 = 3.03$	$p = 0.002$
No	63%			
Physical activity				
Physically inactive	37%		$X^2 = 5.31$	$p = 0.000$
Less active (1–4 occasions per month)	49%			
More active (5+ occasions per month)	14%			
Body mass index; mean (SD)	26.51	(4.7)	$t = 3.08$	$p = 0.016$
Place of birth				
Rural	39%		$X^2 = 1.75$	$p = 0.015$
Urban	61%			
Subjects				
Humanities and Social Sciences	23%		$X^2 = 1.75$	$p = 0.046$
Science	35%			
Engineering	42%			
Age			$t = 4.43$	$p = 0.033$
18	2%			
19–20	3%			
21–24	85%			
25–30	10%			

[a] Test-statistics refers to t-test, assessing the two-sample mean differences of variables. Chi-tests is for assessing the categorical variables, including gender, education household conditions and household conditions. About undergraduate education, five tiers of universities were used, including 985 projects university, 211 project university, Yiben, Erben and Sanben. The tier is the basic university classification in China. [b] The p means the p-value, representing the significance in statistics.

There were 37% of students being in love or married. 37% of participants were physically inactive, whereas 14% were more active. The mean (26.51) of BMI belongs to overweight. 39% of participants lived in rural areas, and 61% were from urban areas. In terms of subjects, the majority of participants (42%) were studying Engineering, and 35% and 23% studied Science and Humanities and Social

Sciences, respectively. The age of our participant ranged from 18 to 30 years old, whose mean was 22.7 (SD = 3.2).

When psychological well-being was operationalized in tertiles, variables, including normal sleep quality, poor sleep quality and gender, show the significance relation to mental health (Table 2). Internal consistency of the four psychological well-being items is high ($\alpha = 0.90$). According to data, we found they were skewed to the right, with a mean value of 7.56 (SD = 3.6) and median of 7.1 (IQR = 5–20) on the composite scale from 5 to 20. Around 35% of sample was in the low level of mental health psychological well-being while a similar percentage was in the high level category (30%). Moreover, the distribution of all independent variables was skewed. About 11% (SD = 19) of sample reported that their sleep was normal, with a median of 63% (IQR = 27–86). Over 78% of participants reported that their sleep quality is poor, with a median of 72% (IQR = 30–95).

Table 2. Whole sample characteristics & bivariable associations (N = 2495).

Variables	Psychological Well-Being			p [b]
	High (20)	Medium (17–19)	Low (5–16)	
Normal sleep quality, mean (SD)	52 (33.07)	50 (29.45)	43 (35.51)	0.000
Normal sleep quality, median (IQR [a])	71 (30, 88)	66 (27, 87)	59 (26, 85)	0.002
Poor sleep quality, mean (SD)	77 (31)	75 (30)	80 (33)	0.001
Poor sleep quality, median (IQR)	71 (26, 97)	73 (25, 98)	74 (31, 99)	0.005
Gender, n (%) [c]				0.001
Female	347 (63)	743 (74)	812 (86)	
Male	207 (37)	259 (26)	127 (14)	
Education				0.015
985 project	121 (15)	147 (16)	115 (16)	
211 project	149 (18)	166 (18)	145 (20)	
Yi Ben	153 (19)	179 (19)	139 (19)	
Er Ben	208 (25)	224 (24)	193 (26)	
San Ben	196 (23)	219 (23)	141 (19)	
Household conditions				0.004
State & society administrator (cadre in governments), Manager (Manager or department leader in state company, private company, foreign company and joint company)	103 (16)	122 (13)	98 (13)	
Private enterprise owner (having large scale company), Technological specialist (teacher, engineer, doctor, academic researcher, lawyer, culture worker)	135 (17)	183 (19)	127 (17)	
Clerk & office worker (secretary, accountant, computer operator), Individual entrepreneur (one-person company with unlimited liability)	192 (24)	213 (22)	198 (27)	
Commercial & service worker (tertiary industry workers), Industrial worker (worker in factory, mining and transport industry)	237 (30)	269 (28)	201 (27)	
Farmer, Unemployed	133 (17)	166 (17)	118 (16)	
Marital or love status				0.016
Yes	293 (42)	377 (30)	193 (35)	
No	398 (58)	879 (70)	355 (65)	
Physical activity				0.001
Physically inactive	273 (43)	476 (36)	231 (43)	
Less active (1–4 occasions per month)	309 (49)	632 (48)	287 (53)	
More active (5+ occasions per month)	49 (8)	219 (16)	19 (4)	
Body mass index	665 (27)	1579 (63)	251 (10)	0.006
Place of birth				0.003
Rural	388 (47)	428 (38)	233 (43)	
Urban	436 (53)	698 (62)	312 (57)	
Subjects				0.020
Humanities and Social Sciences	186 (22)	253 (25)	122 (19)	
Science	252 (30)	319 (31)	165 (26)	
Engineering	403 (48)	458 (44)	339 (54)	
Age, year, n (%)				0.017
18	94 (14)	153 (12)	84 (14)	
19–20	116 (17)	179 (14)	113 (19)	
21–24	322 (48)	615 (49)	269 (46)	
25–30	135 (20)	298 (24)	117 (20)	

[a] IQR refers to inter-quartile range. [b] Significance level determined that the non-parametric Kruskal-Wallis test was used for assessing continuous independent variables, and chi-square tests for the categorical variables. [c] Column percentages, because of rounding, may not be exact 100.

The first group of multivariable models (see Table 3) explored relations with psychological well-being as a dichotomous variable. Model 1 includes normal sleep quality and the Model 2 includes poor sleep quality. Model 3 includes both of these independent variables. All relevant covariates are included in the Table 3. In models, AOR refers to adjusted odds ratio. CI represents confidence interval. In Model 1, each 10% increase in normal sleep quality would result in a 3% decrease in psychological well-being problem (AOR = 0.97; 95% CI = 0.92–1.003). In Model 2, each 10% increase in poor sleep quality was associated with a 27% increase in psychological well-being problem (AO = 1.27; 95% CI = 1.12–1.32). In Model 3, both these independent variables were in the same model, and the results were very similar. In Model 3, each 10% increase in normal sleep quality contributed to a 5% decrease in psychological well-being problem while each 10% increase in poor sleep quality was associated with 26% increase in psychological well-being problem. In the three models, covariates, including gender (male), education (211 project university) and physical activity (body mass index), significantly associated with negative mental health.

Table 3. Multivariable associations of psychological well-being as a dichotomous variable (N = 2495).

Variables	Psychological Well-Being		
	Model 1	Model 2	Model 3
	AOR (95% CI)	AOR (95% CI)	AOR (95% CI)
Normal sleep quality	0.97 (0.92–1.003)		1.05 (1.09–1.23)
Poor sleep quality		1.27 (1.12–1.32)	1.26 (1.21–1.32)
Gender			
Female	Reference	Reference	Reference
Male	1.48 (1.04–1.95)	1.56 (1.10–2.06)	1.57 (1.10–2.07)
Education			
985 project	Reference	Reference	Reference
211 project	1.84 (1.12–2.84)	1.85 (1.13–2.85)	1.85 (1.13–2.86)
Yi Ben	1.60 (0.81–2.98)	1.69 (0.84–3.17)	1.81 (0.85–3.21)
Er Ben	1.60 (0.74–3.18)	1.50 (0.69–3.01)	1.54 (0.71–3.09)
San Ben	1.57 (0.75–3.20)	1.48 (0.66–2.98)	1.53 (0.69–3.01)
Household conditions			
State & society administrator (cadre in governments), Manager (Manager or department leader in state company, private company, foreign company and joint company)	Reference	Reference	Reference
Private enterprise owner (having large scale company), Technological specialist (teacher, engineer, doctor, academic researcher, lawyer, culture worker)	1.00 (0.48–1.93)	0.93 (0.44–1.79)	0.92 (0.44–1.78)
Clerk & office worker (secretary, accountant, computer operator), Individual entrepreneur (one-person company with unlimited liability)	1.25 (0.77–1.89)	1.23 (0.76–1.85)	1.22 (0.75–1.86)
Commercial & service worker (tertiary industry workers), Industrial worker (worker in factory, mining and transport industry)	1.11 (0.62–1.84)	1.05 (0.59–1.72)	1.06 (0.60–1.73)
Farmer, Unemployed	1.13 (0.60–2.01)	1.06 (0.61–1.77)	1.07 (0.63–1.82)
Marital or relationship status			
Yes	Reference	Reference	Reference
No	1.03 (0.69–1.35)	1.05 (0.72–1.37)	1.04 (0.70–1.36)
Physical activity			
Physically inactive	Reference	Reference	Reference
Less active (1–4 occasions per month)	3.31 (1.07–2.38)	3.28 (0.99–2.27)	3.39 (1.09–3.41)
More active (5+ occasions per month)	0.74 (0.46–1.21)	1.35 (0.76–1.32)	0.63 (0.39–1.19)
Body mass index	3.07 (1.21–2.66)	3.49 (1.38–2.79)	1.96 (1.06–2.13)
Place of birth			
Rural	Reference	Reference	Reference
Urban	0.77 (0.47–1.12)	0.75 (0.45–1.10)	0.76 (0.46–1.11)
Subjects			
Humanities and Social Sciences	Reference	Reference	Reference
Science	1.31 (0.96–1.48)	1.33 (1.02–1.51)	1.27 (0.93–1.32)
Engineering	1.34 (1.03–1.56)	1.29 (0.94–1.33)	1.36 (1.05–1.41)
Age			
18	Reference	Reference	Reference
19–20	0.76 (0.49–1.24)	0.77 (0.50–1.27)	0.78 (0.51–1.28)
21–24	0.85 (0.52–1.47)	0.88 (0.54–1.52)	0.87 (0.53–1.50)
25–30	1.03 (0.50–2.17)	1.15 (0.57–2.33)	1.09 (0.54–2.25)

The second group of multivariable models explored associations with psychological well-being operationalized in tertiles. There are three models in the Table 4. Model 1 includes normal sleep quality, Model 2 includes poor sleep quality and Model 3 includes both of these independent variables. It had similar results compared with the first set of multivariable models. Model 1 in the Table 4, each 10% increase in normal sleep quality resulted in 4% decrease in negative mental health, which was of significance in statistics (AOR = 0.96; 95% CI = 0.91–0.99). In Model 2, each 10% increase in poor sleep quality contributed to a 21% increase in negative mental health. Model 3 reported the similar results compared with Model 1 and 2. In three models, gender (male), household conditions and education had significant relation with mental health. In Model 1, subject (engineering) was significantly associated with mental health. In Model 2, age (25–30) significant associated with mental health.

Table 4. Multivariable associations of psychological well-being operationalized in tertiles (N = 2495).

Variables	Mental Health		
	Model 1	Model 2	Model 3
	AOR (95% CI)	AOR (95% CI)	AOR (95% CI)
Normal sleep quality	0.96 (0.91–0.99)		1.03 (0.92–1.01)
Poor sleep quality		1.21 (1.13–1.68)	1.19 (1.09–1.57)
Gender			
Female	Reference	Reference	Reference
Male	1.71 (1.34–1.81)	1.75 (1.42–1.87)	1.79 (1.51–1.93)
Education			
985 project	Reference	Reference	Reference
211 project	1.62 (0.97–1.79)	1.50 (0.93–1.68)	1.64 (0.99–1.93)
Yi Ben	1.51 (0.94–1.69)	1.47 (0.86–1.53)	1.56 (0.97–1.71)
Er Ben	1.49 (0.89–1.57)	1.52 (0.95–1.65)	1.54 (0.96–1.67)
San Ben	1.42 (0.78–1.27)	1.45 (0.81–1.32)	1.48 (0.89–1.56)
Household conditions			
State & society administrator (cadre in governments), Manager (Manager or department leader in state company, private company, foreign company and joint company)	Reference	Reference	Reference
Private enterprise owner (having large scale company), Technological specialist (teacher, engineer, doctor, academic researcher, lawyer, culture worker)	1.36 (0.85–1.54)	1.31 (0.81–1.46)	1.29 (0.76–1.31)
Clerk & office worker (secretary, accountant, computer operator), Individual entrepreneur (one-person company with unlimited liability)	1.49 (0.93–1.72)	1.46 (0.91–1.69)	1.44 (0.89–1.63)
Commercial & service worker (tertiary industry workers), Industrial worker (worker in factory, mining and transport industry)	1.42 (0.87–1.59)	1.38 (0.86–1.55)	1.41 (0.87–1.51)
Farmer, Unemployed	1.45 (0.88–1.61)	1.32 (0.83–1.41)	1.39 (0.86–1.57)
Marital or relationship status			
Yes	Reference	Reference	Reference
No	0.92 (0.73–1.19)	0.92 (0.74–1.23)	0.92 (0.73–1.18)
Physical activity			
Physically inactive	Reference	Reference	Reference
Less active (1–4 occasions per month)	4.06 (1.49–2.88)	3.98 (1.21–2.65)	4.11 (1.53–2.92)
More active (5+ occasions per month)	1.05 (0.99–1.76)	1.57 (1.12–2.01)	0.83 (0.76–1.26)
Body mass index	3.12 (1.24–2.75)	3.57 (1.39–2.85)	2.35 (1.19–2.08)
Place of birth			
Rural	Reference	Reference	Reference
Urban	0.67 (0.79–1.03)	0.61 (0.71–0.94)	0.65 (0.75–1.01)
Subjects			
Humanities and Social Sciences	Reference	Reference	Reference
Science	1.46 (0.99–1.79)	1.51 (1.08–1.89)	1.37 (0.88–1.47)
Engineering	1.57 (1.15–1.90)	1.32 (0.79–1.38)	1.59 (1.17–1.94)
Age			
18	Reference	Reference	Reference
19–20	1.19 (0.77–1.61)	1.21 (0.78–1.63)	1.20 (0.77–1.62)
21–24	1.05 (0.63–1.50)	1.08 (0.66–1.54)	1.05 (0.63–1.52)
25–30	1.42 (0.76–2.41)	1.50 (0.79–2.54)	1.45 (0.76–2.46)

4. Discussion

This study of final year undergraduate students in China found that normal sleep quality was weakly associated with lower level of negative psychological well-being condition, but having poor sleep quality had strong association with higher level of negative mental health. The sample in this study was within age ranging from 18 to 30 years old, covering the most conditions of final year university students in China, so this study is valuable to know the associations between their sleep quality and mental health. These findings may persuade final year university students to pay attention to their sleep quality. Because final year university students in China are undergoing transitions from university to society, they have more mental disorders than their peers [25]. University, especially in the final year, is an important transient stage in which there is a variety of pressure such as academic, financial and interpersonal pressures.

One potential explanation for the effects of sleep quality on psychological well-being is that individual sleep quality is influenced by various factors in different ways, including socioeconomic factors [46], academic, financial and interpersonal pressures [25], and transitory challenges [47]. The optimistic and pessimistic perceptions of future development is different among the final year university students. Because different participants have different situations, some participants tend to have normal sleep quality based on minor pressure and promising career development while some others engage in much pressure and less support and then show poor sleep quality that may result in mental problems.

The research findings reconfirm the prevalence of poor sleep quality in university [22] and the associations between sleep quality and psychological well-being [28]. Normal sleep quality is an important physiological issue for human beings, but poor sleep quality would bring serious psychological well-being problem [48]. Depression and anxiety will appear when sleep quality becomes poor. In our model including both independent variables, each 10% increase in normal sleep quality contributed to a 5% decrease in mental problem. The result was statistically significant, and it is also consistent with studies reporting the important role of sleep quality in mental health. However, the magnitude of the results were much stronger regarding poor sleep quality. Each 10% increase in poor sleep quality would result in a 26% increase in mental problem. It is interesting that the poor sleep quality has larger effect size than normal sleep quality. One may conclude that poor sleep quality may be more potent than normal sleep quality. This reasoning conforms to negativity bias concept. This concept reports a tendency of human beings to give more emphasis to negative entities compared with positive ones [49].

In addition to normal sleep quality and poor sleep quality, there are three covariates associated with mental health. Gender, university type and age are three significant factors, and they relate mechanically each other regarding university student's sleep quality and mental health. First, gendered issue is the most significant one. Male participants had approximately 1.5-fold odds of increased mental problem than female participants. This result is divergent from plenty of extant research. Existing research reports the female university students have higher proportion of poor sleep quality [28,50,51]. It may result from China's social pressure of male university students, resulted from China's actual conditions. In Chinese society, the male has more opportunity of getting higher education and higher income than the female, but the male has lower happiness, caused by high expectation for male and huge pressure designed for Chinese male [52]. Second, participants from 211 project universities had 85% odds of increased mental problem compared with those in 985 project universities. Although it is consistent with the high level of academic pressure [25], it could also result from the fierce competition among 211 project universities. Third, participants within age ranging from 25 to 30 have 15% increase in mental problem than 18-year-old participants, which shows the increasing age is significantly associated with mental health.

Although the early findings need to be replicated, they might be useful to university students' psychological well-being practitioners. Facing the special group, the final year undergraduate students in China, specific strategies are required to improve sleep quality. In China, undergraduate students have common accommodation in which several students share one bedroom, the pressure of interpersonal communication should be paid attention to.

5. Conclusions

This study initially explores the association between sleep quality and psychological well-being among the final year undergraduate students in China. We found that having normal sleep quality is associated with lower level of mental problem. By contrast, poor sleep quality is associated with high level of negative mental health. The magnitude of effect seems to be more substantial and significant for participants having poor sleep quality. Therefore, it could be helpful to increase awareness of the importance of avoiding poor sleep quality of final year undergraduate students in China so that we can reduce the risk of mental problem. The major limitation of this study is the nature of cross-sectional data. For future study, using longitudinal data would be useful to examine the directionality of results. Additionally, we employed K6 scale to assess mental health. The measurement of sleep quality and psychological well-being is assessed by a questionnaire. Although the sample is large enough to analyze, it is a self-report scale. Instead, it is not the gold standard that involves interview under a psychiatric professional. Lastly, the lack of sleep duration metrics is also another limitation. It is very hard to measure how many sleeping hours a participant have. However, it is part of measurement of sleep quality. In future research, techniques can be used to compute sleep duration.

Author Contributions: X.G. proposed the research design. Moreover, X.G. analyzed data and then evaluated and edited the manuscript. K.Z. mainly collected data and wrote the manuscript, G.W. contributed to manuscript revision and conceptualized literature.

References

1. Macaskill, A. The mental health of university students in the United Kingdom. *Br. J. Guid. Couns.* **2013**, *41*, 426–441. [CrossRef]
2. Ma, C.M.; Lai, C. Mental health profile and health-related behavior among Hong Kong Chinese university students. *Health Psychol. Open* **2018**, *5*, 1–8. [CrossRef] [PubMed]
3. Tyson, P.; Wilson, K.; Crone, D. Physical activity and mental health in a student population. *J. Ment. Health* **2010**, *19*, 492–499. [CrossRef] [PubMed]
4. Hawton, K.; Comabella, C.C.; Haw, C. Risk factors for suicide in individuals with depression: A systematic review. *J. Affect. Disord.* **2013**, *147*, 17–28. [CrossRef] [PubMed]
5. Bayram, N.; Bilgel, N. The prevalence and socio-demographic correlations of depression, anxiety and stress among a group of university students. *Soc. Psychiatry Psychiatr. Epidemiol.* **2008**, *438*, 667–672. [CrossRef] [PubMed]
6. Wong, J.G.; Cheung, E.P.; Chan, K.K.; Ma, K.K.; Tang, S.W. Web-based survey of depression, anxiety and stress in first-year tertiary education students in Hong Kong. *Aust. N. Z. J. Psychiatry* **2006**, *40*, 777–782. [CrossRef] [PubMed]
7. Stallman, H. Psychological distress in university students: A comparison with general population data. *Aust. Psychol.* **2010**, *45*, 249–257. [CrossRef]
8. Reddy, P.; Rankins, D.; Timoshanko, A.; Dunbar, J. Life! In Australia: Translating prevention research into a large-scale intervention. *J. Diabetes Vasc. Dis.* **2011**, *11*, 193–197. [CrossRef]
9. Said, D.; Kypri, K.; Bowman, J. Risk factors for mental disorder among university students in Australia: Findings from a web-based cross-sectional survey. *Soc. Psychiatry Psychiatr. Epidemiol.* **2013**, *48*, 935–944. [CrossRef]
10. Tao, S.; Wu, X.; Zhang, Y.; Zhang, S.; Tong, S.; Tao, F. Effects of Sleep Quality on the Association between Problematic Mobile Phone Use and Mental Health Symptoms in Chinese College Students. *Int. J. Environ. Res. Public Health* **2017**, *14*, 185–195. [CrossRef]
11. Pallos, H.; Gergely, V.; Yamada, N.; Miyazaki, S.; Okawa, M. The quality of sleep and factors associated with poor sleep in Japanese graduate students. *Sleep Biol. Rhythm.* **2007**, *5*, 234–238. [CrossRef]
12. Roth, T. Insomnia: Definition, prevalence, etiology, and consequences. *J. Clin. Sleep Med.* **2007**, *3*, 7–10.

13. Glozier, N.; Martiniuk, A.; Patton, G.; Ivers, R.; Li, Q.; Hickie, I. Short sleep duration in prevalent and persistent psychological distressing young adults: The DRIVE study. *Sleep* **2010**, *33*, 1139–1145. [CrossRef] [PubMed]
14. Fleming, L.; Randell, K.; Harvey, C.J.; Espie, C.A. Does cognitive behaviour therapy for insomnia reduce clinical levels of fatigue, anxiety and depression in cancer patients? *Psychooncology* **2014**, *23*, 679–684. [CrossRef] [PubMed]
15. Gebara, M.A.; Siripong, N.; DiNapoli, E.; Maree, R.D.; Germain, A.; Reynolds, C.F.; Kasckow, J.W.; Weiss, P.M.; Karp, J.F. Effect of insomnia treatments on depression: A systematic review and meta-analysis. *Depress Anxiety* **2018**, *35*, 784–794. [CrossRef] [PubMed]
16. Xu, Z.; Su, H.; Zou, Y.; Chen, J.; Wu, J.; Chang, W. Sleep quality of Chinese adolescents: Distribution and its associated factors. *J. Paediatr. Child. Health* **2012**, *48*, 138–145. [CrossRef] [PubMed]
17. Voelker, R. Stress, sleep loss, and substance abuse create potent recipe for college depression. *J. Am. Med. Assoc.* **2004**, *291*, 2177e9.
18. Gellis, L.A.; Arigo, D.; Elliott, J.C. Cognitive refocusing treatment for insomnia: A randomized controlled trial in university students. *Behav. Ther.* **2013**, *44*, 100–110. [CrossRef]
19. Schmidt, R.E.; Gay, P.; Ghisletta, P.; Van Der Linden, M. Linking impulsivity to dysfunctional thought control and insomnia: A structural equation model. *J. Sleep Res.* **2010**, *19*, 3–11. [CrossRef]
20. Yoshioka, E.; Saijo, Y.; Kita, T.; Satoh, H.; Kawaharada, M.; Fukui, T. Gender differences in insomnia and the role of paid work and family responsibilities. *Soc. Psychiatry Psychiatr. Epidemiol.* **2012**, *47*, 651–662. [CrossRef]
21. Jaussent, I.; Dauvilliers, Y.; Ancelin, M.L.; Dartigues, J.F. Insomnia symptoms in older adults: Associated factors and gender differences. *Geriatr. Psychiatry* **2011**, *19*, 88–97. [CrossRef] [PubMed]
22. Jiang, X.; Zheng, X.; Yang, J.; Ye, C.; Chen, Y.; Zhang, Z.; Xiao, Z. A systematic review of studies on the prevalence of insomnia in university students. *Public Health* **2015**, *129*, 1579–1584. [CrossRef] [PubMed]
23. Ikeda, T.; Nagai, T.; Kato-Nishimura, K.; Mohri, I.; Taniike, M. Sleep problems in physically disabled children and burden on caregivers. *Brain Dev.* **2012**, *34*, 223–229. [CrossRef] [PubMed]
24. Bahammam, A.; Bin S., A.; Al-faris, E.; Shaikh, S. Sleep duration and its correlates in a sample of Saudi elementary school children. *Singap. Med. J.* **2006**, *47*, 875–881.
25. Chen, L.; Wang, L.; Qiu, X.; Yang, X.; Qiao, Z.; Yang, Y.; Liang, Y. Depression among Chinese University students: Prevalence and socio-demographic correlates. *PLoS ONE* **2013**, *8*, 583–588.
26. Suen, L.K.; Hon, K.L.E.; Tam, W.W. Association between sleep behavior and sleep-related factors among university students in Hong Kong. *Chronobiol. Int.* **2008**, *25*, 760–775. [CrossRef]
27. Zhao, X.; Haste, H.; Selman, L.R.; Luan, Z. Compliant, Cynical, or Critical: Chinese Youth's Explanations of Social Problems and Individual Civic Responsibility. *Youth Soc.* **2017**, *49*, 1123–1148. [CrossRef]
28. Lemma, S.; Gelaye, B.; Berhane, Y.; Worku, A.; Williams, M.A. Sleep quality and its psychological correlates among university students in Ethiopia: A cross-sectional study. *BMC Psychiatry* **2012**, *12*, 237–244. [CrossRef]
29. Primack, B.A.; Bisbey, M.A.; Shensa, A.; Bowman, N.D.; Karim, S.A.; Knight, J.M.; Sidani, J.E. The association between valence of social media experiences and depressive symptoms. *Depress Anxiety* **2018**, *35*, 784–794. [CrossRef]
30. Cornelius, B.L.R.; Groothoff, J.W.; Klink, J.J.L.; Brouwer, S. The performance of the K10, K6 and GHQ-12 to screen for present state DSM-IV disorders among disability claimants. *BMC Public Health* **2013**, *13*, 128–136. [CrossRef]
31. Cheung, N.W.T. Rural-to-urban migrant adolescents in Guangzhou, China: Psychological health, victimization, and local and trans-local ties. *Soc. Sci. Med.* **2013**, *93*, 121–129. [CrossRef] [PubMed]
32. Jin, L.; Wen, M.; Fan, J.X.; Wang, G. Trans-local ties, local ties and psychological well-being among rural-to-urban migrants in Shanghai. *Soc. Sci. Med.* **2012**, *75*, 288–296. [CrossRef] [PubMed]
33. Wen, M.; Fan, J.; Jin, L.; Wang, G. Neighborhood effects on health among migrants and natives in Shanghai, China. *Health Place* **2010**, *16*, 452–460. [CrossRef] [PubMed]
34. Cella, D.; Gershon, R.; Bass, M.; Rothrock, N. Assessment center user manual: PROMIS depression scoring manual. 2015. Available online: https://www.webcitation.org/6sDme4hlP (accessed on 9 September 2015).
35. Buysse, D.J.; Reynolds, C.F.; Monk, T.H.; Hoch, C.C.; Yeager, A.L.; Kupfer, D.J. Quantification of subjective sleep quality in healthy elderly men and women using the Pittsburgh Sleep Quality Index (PSQI). *Sleep* **1991**, *14*, 331–338. [PubMed]

36. Guo, Y.; Liu, Y.; Huang, X.; Rong, Y.; He, M.; Wang, Y.; Yuan, J.; Wu, T.; Chen, W. The Effects of Shift Work on Sleeping Quality, Hypertension and Diabetes in Retired Workers. *PLoS ONE* **2013**, *8*, 71–107. [CrossRef] [PubMed]
37. Grandner, M.A.; Ruiter Petrov, M.E.; Rattanaumpawan, P.; Jackson, N.; Platt, A.; Patel, B.P. Sleep symptoms, race/ethnicity, and socioeconomic position. *J. Clin. Sleep Med.* **2013**, *9*, 897–905. [CrossRef] [PubMed]
38. McCurry, S.M.; Song, Y.; Martin, J.L. Sleep in caregivers: What we know and what we need to learn. *Curr. Opin. Psychiatry* **2015**, *28*, 497–503. [CrossRef]
39. Chen, Y.; Kawachi, I.; Subramanian, S.V.; Acevedo-Garcia, D.; Lee, Y.J. Can social factors explain sex differences in insomnia? Findings from a national survey in Taiwan. *J. Epidemiol. Commun. Health* **2005**, *59*, 488–494. [CrossRef]
40. Magee, C.A.; Reddy, P.; Robinson, L.; McGregor, A. Sleep quality subtypes and obesity. *Health Psychol.* **2016**, *35*, 1289–1297. [CrossRef]
41. Joao, K.A.D.R.; Jesus, S.N.; Carmo, C.; Pinto, P. The impact of sleep quality on the mental health of a non-clinical population. *Sleep Med.* **2018**, *46*, 69–73. [CrossRef]
42. Lu, X. *Research Report on Social Stratum in Contemporary China*; Social Sciences Academic Press: Beijing, China, 2002.
43. Mao, Z.H.; Zhao, X.D. The effects of social connections on self-rated physical and mental health among internal migrant and local adolescents in Shanghai, China. *BMC Public Health* **2012**, *12*, 97–105. [CrossRef] [PubMed]
44. Rospleszcz, S.; Janitza, S.; Boulesteix, A. Categorical variables with many categories are preferentially selected in bootstrap-based model selection procedures for multivariable regression models. *Biom. J.* **2016**, *58*, 652–673. [CrossRef] [PubMed]
45. Royston, P.; Sauerbrei, W. *Multivariable Model-Building: A Pragmatic Approach to Regression Anaylsis Based on Fractional Polynomials for Modelling Continuous Variables*; John Wiley & Sons: Chichester, UK, 2008.
46. Anders, M.P.; Breckenkamp, J.; Blettner, M.; Schlehofer, B.; Berg-Beckhoff, G. Association between socioeconomic factors and sleep quality in an urban population-based sample in Germany. *Eur. J. Public Health* **2013**, *24*, 968–973. [CrossRef] [PubMed]
47. Stewart-Brown, S.; Evans, J.; Patterson, J.; Petersen, S.; Doll, H. The health of students in institutes of higher education: An important and neglected public health problem? *J. Public Health Med.* **2000**, *22*, 492–499. [CrossRef] [PubMed]
48. Lavie, P.; Pillar, G.; Malhotra, A. *Sleep Disorders: Diagnosis, Management & Treatment, A and Book for Clinicians*; Martin Dunitz Ltd.: London, UK, 2002.
49. Rozin, P.; Royzman, E.B. Negativity bias, negativity dominance, and contagion. *Person. Soc. Psychol. Rev.* **2001**, *5*, 296–320. [CrossRef]
50. Suen, L.K.; Tam, W.W.; Hon, K. Association of sleep hygiene-related factors and sleep quality among university students in Hong Kong. *Hong Kong Med. J.* **2010**, *16*, 180–185.
51. Lund, H.G.; Reider, B.D.; Whiting, A.B.; Prichard, J.R. Sleep patterns and predictors of disturbed sleep in a large population of college students. *J. Adolesc. Health* **2010**, *46*, 124–132. [CrossRef]
52. Li, L.; Liu, P.; Sun, H. Male or female, who is happier? *Stat. Res.* **2017**, *34*, 82–93. (In Chinese)

8

Correlation Analysis to Identify the Effective Data in Machine Learning: Prediction of Depressive Disorder and Emotion States

Sunil Kumar and Ilyoung Chong *

Department of Information and Communications Engineering, Hankuk University of Foreign Studies, Seoul 02450, Korea; sunil75umar@hufs.ac.kr

* Correspondence: iychong@hufs.ac.kr;

Abstract: Correlation analysis is an extensively used technique that identifies interesting relationships in data. These relationships help us realize the relevance of attributes with respect to the target class to be predicted. This study has exploited correlation analysis and machine learning-based approaches to identify relevant attributes in the dataset which have a significant impact on classifying a patient's mental health status. For mental health situations, correlation analysis has been performed in Weka, which involves a dataset of depressive disorder symptoms and situations based on weather conditions, as well as emotion classification based on physiological sensor readings. Pearson's product moment correlation and other different classification algorithms have been utilized for this analysis. The results show interesting correlations in weather attributes for bipolar patients, as well as in features extracted from physiological data for emotional states.

Keywords: correlation analysis; health care; machine learning; data analytics

---

1. Introduction

In order to analyze the causality in a dataset, various techniques can be used. One such technique in the domain of data analysis is frequent pattern mining. In this case, two types of analysis are widely used: identification of association rules and correlation analysis. In association rule mining, frequent pattern analysis is performed using the support count and confidence measures. An association rule will be considered strong if its support count and confidence are above some defined threshold. However, the identified rules are sometimes irrelevant and can often be misleading. This limitation can be handled by correlation analysis, which is used to determine the strength of a relationship between two item sets [1]. In this case, the strength can be identified based on three criteria: direction, form, and dispersion strength, as shown in Figure 1. The limitation of this analysis is that in the case of two independent variables, it cannot determine the causality between the two. That is, we will not have any idea which variable is affecting and which one is getting affected. Another situation that can cause distort the correlation and association results is the confounding of another attribute [2]. If this attribute is not considered in the dataset, then its effect may not be highlighted in the experimentation and thus leading to spurious analyzed correlations. In this regard, determining predictor attributes plays a very critical role, as we try to include as many relevant attributes as possible, to avoid such circumstances. Correlation analysis is a widely used statistical measure through which different studies have efficiently identified interesting collinear relations among different attributes of datasets. This study has employed correlation analysis to identify such attributes which strongly affect depressive disorder severity and emotional states.

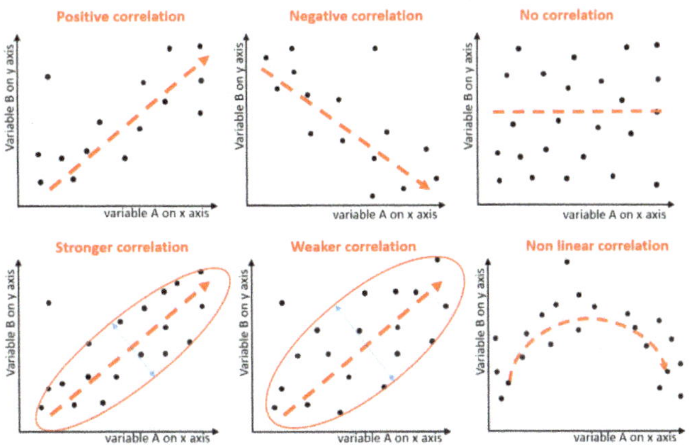

Figure 1. Correlation based on direction, form, and dispersion strength.

There are several factors that have been found leading to a higher number of depressive disorder cases in South Korea [3–5], including work pressure and overtime, loneliness, social relations, socioeconomic status, etc. However, the effect of weather conditions, which may have a considerable impact on depressive disorder, has often been overlooked in this region. With respect to emotion data analysis, the most commonly-used methodologies in practical environments and research approaches involve emotion detection through facial expressions, physiological sensor signals, speech recognition and analysis, and text analysis [6]. The former two techniques are more commonly used, because facial expressions and physiological responses are more closely related to one's emotional reactions, whereas limited information can be extracted regarding emotional reactions in the latter two techniques [7,8]. Besides, in the latter two approaches, the responses of emotional reactions can be manipulated, hence resulting in more noisy data and obstructing analysis [9,10]. This can also be the case with facial expressions, where we have a lot of noisy data, as compared to physiological responses. In this work, we have considered the first two techniques for identifying a patient's emotional state.

This work considers aspects of healthcare service provisioning using data analytics. Therefore, different challenges are addressed and overcome in this study. One of the essential problems addressed by this work is the process of identifying information that has a strong impact on depression for specified patients. Considering different studies that have identified different types of depressive disorder situations, each patient shows different behavioral trends based on his or her specific depressive disorder type and its symptoms. As there are different data sources through which we can analyze behavioral trends (facial expressions, physiological sensor signals, speech analysis, text analysis, self-reporting questionnaires, etc.), there is a strong need for mechanisms that identify such parameters with strong relationships specific to certain depressive disorder patients. Another challenge is identifying prominent and persistent relationships over longer periods of time. As there can be different levels of uncertainty in the patterns of acquired data (such as high and low levels of mood in bipolar disorder), longer periods of data are required to analyze the trends. A good prediction model requires enough data readings to acquire sufficiently steady trends to have reliable prediction results. Further, a system is required for on-demand data acquisition from different data sources based on the specific user context. Based on the above discussion, this study aims to achieve the following objectives:

- Analyzing the impact of weather on two types of depressive disorder; Bipolar and Melancholia disorder.
- Analyzing the impact of physiological data on emotions, as well as identifying patient's health status, using machine learning with strong correlated attributes.
- Experimentation for data acquisition and analysis.
- Achieving higher accuracies from the proposed methodology and discussing the results based on highly correlated data.

In this regard, the data acquisition process for the relevant information is discussed, which involves the periodic collection of multimodal data including local weather data, patient's emotional states, and depressive disorder severity information. For correlation analysis, two datasets have been considered with different characteristics. One for emotion detection application and the other is for depressive disorder situation analysis based on weather. Based on the identified correlations, strong attributes have been ranked and filtered in order to optimize the performance of the machine learning. Such attributes can be used to further analyze and predict the patient's health status.

The rest of this paper is organized as follows. Section 2 discusses the related work, which involves studies related to correlation analysis and the approaches that can be used to identify strong predictor attributes. Section 3 describes the correlation and machine learning- based methodology to identify effective datasets for predicting depressive disorder severity and emotional states. Section 4 describes the dataset description used for the data analytics. The experimental use case and results are presented in Section 5. Section 6 discusses the interpretation of results as well as provides limitations and possible direction of this research in the future works. Finally, Section 7 concludes this paper with a summary.

2. Related Works

Various techniques can be used to perform correlation analysis to identify relationships in the dataset. However, their application depends on the type of dataset. Table 1 shows the categorization of common techniques used for correlation analysis based on dataset types. However, each algorithm has its own considerations as well as limitations in identifying the relationships. For example, the Chi square test is used for determining the probability of independence in the distribution, but it does not provide the details of the relationship such as dispersion strength. Other aspects such as assumptions and hypothesis also vary from one algorithm to another. In this work, we have both quantitative and categorical data considering multimodal data. The depressive disorder severities can be represented in % as quantitative values, and can also be defined as none, mild moderate, moderately severe, and severe as categorical values.

Table 1. Correlation techniques based on data types. The highlighted Spearman's correlation shows that it considers only ordinal data in the categorical dataset type.

<table>
<tr><th colspan="3" rowspan="3">Data Types</th><th colspan="3">Dependent Variables</th></tr>
<tr><th colspan="2">Categorical</th><th rowspan="2">Quantitative</th></tr>
<tr><th>Nominal</th><th>Ordinal</th></tr>
<tr><td rowspan="3">Independent variables</td><td rowspan="2">Categorical</td><td>Nominal</td><td colspan="2">Chi square test of Independence</td><td rowspan="2">Analysis of variance (ANOVA)</td></tr>
<tr><td>Ordinal</td><td>Chi square test of Independence</td><td>Spearman's Correlation</td></tr>
<tr><td colspan="2">Quantitative</td><td colspan="2">Lift, X^2 test of Independence (Categorized Quantitative variable)</td><td>Pearson product moment correlation, Spearman's Correlation</td></tr>
</table>

Analyzing the effect of one event or occurrence on another is performed in numerous fields of research. Some research on correlation analysis has been undertaken in the financial market, agriculture sciences, imaging data analysis, signal processing, time series data analysis, statistical analysis in social and environmental data, etc. Some examples of financial market analysis include finding the relationship between stock returns in the Central and Eastern European stock market as well as identifying simultaneous trends in the world's financial markets' crises [11,12]. Inamdar et al. [13] used Pearson product moment correlation coefficient to identify the errors in hyperspectral image data. In the domain of social web content, the study [14] analyzed the prevalence and impact of different features, such as friends, views, comments, etc. in three popular websites: YouTube, Panoramio, and Epinions. The study shows the application of correlation technique in the time series data analysis [15].

The effect analysis has also been studied with respect to mental health assessment. In this regard, one application of Pearson product moment correlation is presented in emotional analysis using Electroencephalography (EEG) and speech signals [16], which observed high correlation results in the happy and sad emotional states. Huibers et al. [17] performed an association analysis on survey data collected from the south of Netherlands. The main objective of this work is to identify the environmental factors (seasons and weather) affecting mood and depressive disorders using stepwise logistic regression analysis. The environmental parameters consisted of temperature, sunshine, and rainfall, as well as the four seasonal parameters (spring, summer, fall, and winter). The questionnaire was based on the Diagnosis Inventory Depression (DID) for measuring DSM-IV (Diagnostic and Statistical Manual of Mental Disorders) symptoms of depression. The DID-based dataset was comprised of 14,478 responses collected over three years (2005 to 2007). The findings of this analysis did not show any significant effects of environmental factors on mood and depressive disorder. The seasonal changes had effects on depressive disorder and sad mood, with higher rates of both in summer and fall. These results were evaluated through univariate associations of each parameter with depression and sad mood and their odds ratios. Another study [18] that applied stepwise logistic regression studied the relationship between climate changes and depression in different regions of the United States. The data for depression monitoring was acquired from Twitter tweets. Around 600 million tweets were collected from 2013 to 2014, in which the tweets having the keyword "depress" or any of its variations were filtered and selected. Based on the data and the Koppen-Geiger climate classification system, they divided the region into seven climate zones, of which four were selected for analysis. The weather data was obtained from the National Oceanic and Atmospheric Administration (NOAA), involving the records of relative humidity, temperature, sea level pressure, precipitation, snowfall, wind speed, globe solar radiation, and length of day as independent parameters. Based on these parameters, the ratio of total tweets to tweets about depression was evaluated as a dependent variable. The results showed that summer and fall had significant effects on depression rates in all four climate zones. However, the sequence of results in summer was inverse to that of fall. With respect to weather, wind speed, snowfall, and global solar radiation had substantial effects in all zones, whereas relative humidity, precipitation, wind speed, and temperature were effective in specific areas. Sea level pressure was only effective in humid continental areas. Molin et al. [19] used Copenhagen weather data to identify the factors affecting depression. That dataset included temperature, minutes of sunshine, global radiation cloud cover, barometer pressure, precipitation, wind speed, and length of daylight. The symptom data was collected using Beck Depression Inventory (BDI) over a four-year period. The consideration criteria of patients for depressive disorder was at least three episodes in the previous five years. Spearman's method was used to identify strong relationships among entities, and the least significant parameters were identified and discarded using the backward elimination method for regression analysis. The results based on the Spearman correlation coefficient showed that global radiation, minutes of sunshine, cloud, daylight, and temperature had considerable relationships with BDI. Further, the study found that high temperature and long hours of daylight had an inverse relationship with depression score, hence they were considered to be the best predictors of depression among the parameters. The study carried out by Blanchard et al. [20] also signified another use case of correlation analysis in depressive disorder data. In that study, correlations with posttraumatic stress disorder (PTSD) and symptoms of major depression were analyzed among victims of motor-vehicle accidents. A total of 158 victims were assessed by interviews as well as psychological tests using the Beck Depression Inventory, State-Trait Anxiety Inventory, etc. In the study [20], a statistical software package LISREL (LInear Structural RELations) was used for the analysis and the evaluations scheme involved chi squared and ANOVA tests. The results showed that accident victims can develop PTSD and symptoms of major depression. However, the strength of depression symptoms had no relation with the effect of PTSD. Another study [21] identified the relationships of plasma levels of different vitamins and acids on depression severity using multiple analysis of variance (MANOVA). The results identified significant correlations between glutamate, alanine, and L-serine with patients having severe depression, as assessed by the 21-item Hamilton Rating Scale. Khalili et al. [22] adopted a similar scheme of correlation-based feature selection to improve their prediction results. Their input data included the physiological readings of galvanic skin response (GSR), respiration, blood pressure, and electroencephalography (EEG). Their results showed that the classification algorithm Quadratic Discriminant Analysis (QDA) achieved 1 to 3% increased accuracy by using the feature selection technique. Paul et al. [23] used multi regression model to analysis effect of weather on the patients' energy levels and sleep. 10 patients were involved in the study in which five were on antidepressant medication. Data regarding health conditions involved behavioral parameters which were evaluated through 1–24 Likert scale, and amount of sleep on daily basis was recorded. The weather data included temperature, sunshine, pressure and relative humidity. The overall results showed that the patients' mood and energy were highly related with season, as they showed positive mood and high energy in summer and vice versa in winter. Other weather parameters showed varied results based on patients. Besides depressive disorder, effect of weather on emotional states and mood has also been carried out in which Z. Spasova [24] has contributed. This study has evaluated emotional states and mood for 187 volunteers using 4 different psychological tests, involving self-evaluation questionnaire, and one test for the validity for responses. These volunteers were not diagnosed with any severe depressive disorder condition. The weather data involved sixteen weather types. The comparative analysis performed by *t*-test showed that emotional changes are affected by different weather types, however, the favorable weather did not always have positive effect. Besides, they also discussed the effect of abrupt weather changes with negative mood as well as the relationship between psychological behaviors and neuroticism. The study for the effect analysis of anxiety and weather is considered as a research issue. In this regard, Bulbena et al. [25] performed the analysis on emergency reports of a General Hospital in Barcelona for the year 2002. Weather data involved temperature, relative humidity, pressure, wind speed and directions, precipitation, solar radiation and rainfall. Statistical analysis involved Spearman's correlation and logistic regression. The anxiety episodes were identified as more common with hot wind, rainfall and autumn season. The occurrences of the attacks was reduced significantly on weekends.

3. Correlation Analysis Methodology

3.1. Methodology to Identify Strong Predictor Attributes

Correlation analysis determines the strength of a relationship between two item sets, which can be a dependent and an independent variable or even two independent variables [1]. In such a case, the strength can be identified based on direction, form, and dispersion strength, as shown in Figure 1. Numerically, this relationship is usually determined by a decimal value, known as the correlation coefficient. The correlation coefficient is determined under a certain predefined range (depending on the algorithm). Based on the value of the coefficient in the given range, its strength and direction can be determined. The coefficient having positive sign indicates that the two variables are positively correlated, whereas negative sign indicates negative correlation. Higher number of coefficient indicates that the two variables have strong correlation and lower value indicates otherwise. For example, Lift is one correlation measure with a coefficient ranging around one. If the value is greater than one, then the two variables are positively correlated; otherwise, they are negatively correlated. In the case of the value being 1, there is no correlation.

This relationship helps us identify which independent variables can have stronger impacts on the dependent variables, and therefore leads us to more efficiently predict the outcome of a dependent variable. Having a strong relationship, the independent variable can be considered a strong predictor for the dependent variable. The limitation of this analysis is that in the case of two independent variables, it cannot determine the causality between the two. However, in this research, we identify the correlation among independent attributes as well as between dependent and independent attributes in order to identify the strong predictor attributes.

In order to identify the data that have strong impacts on target emotion and depression state, we have adopted Pearson's product-moment correlation coefficient to study the relationship between each of the independent attributes with target classes for prediction. The product moment correlation was first proposed by Francis Galton in 1880s, then later modified by Karl Pearson in 1896, and has since been known as the Pearson product-moment correlation coefficient. It is a statistical analysis of the collinear relationship between two variables. It involves the ratio of covariance and the standard deviation of the data values between two given variables. Consider two variables A and B. Then the Pearson's correlation coefficient can be calculated using the following formula:

$$C_{A,B} = \frac{Covariance(A,B)}{\sigma_A \sigma_B} \tag{1}$$

where $C_{A,B}$ is the correlation coefficient, Covariance(A,B) is the covariance, and σ_A and σ_B are the standard deviations of A and B, respectively. In the case of a dataset involving two set, $\{a_1, a_2, \ldots, a_n\}$ and $\{b_1, b_2, \ldots, b_n\}$, the correlation coefficient can be calculated as:

$$C = \frac{\sum_{i=1}^{n}(a_i - \bar{a})\left(b_i - \bar{b}\right)}{\sqrt{\sum_{i=1}^{n}(a_i - \bar{a})^2}\sqrt{\sum_{i=1}^{n}\left(b_i - \bar{b}\right)^2}} \tag{2}$$

where n is the sample size, a_i and b_i are the ith data values, and $\bar{a}$, $\bar{b}$ are the mean values. The value of the coefficient (C) ranges between −1 and +1. Values close to +1 show strong positive correlation, those close to −1 show strong negative correlation, and those closest to 0 show no relation. Since Pearson's correlation determine linear relationship, therefore linear form is considered to be analyzed among the variables. For depressive disorder analysis, the independent attributes come from the weather dataset, and for emotion data analysis, the independent parameters come from the physiological signals dataset. In this case, the relationship is identified based on the direction, form, and strength of the dispersion of the data points between the two parameters. However, we cannot determine the strong predictor attributes based only on the correlation coefficient. Further, additional mechanisms are required to identify the combined effect of independent parameters on target classes. Therefore, in order to evaluate the correlation coefficient result, we have used stepwise selection on the applied machine learning models so that we can observe the change in accuracies that should be consistent with the result of the correlation analysis.

Figure 2 shows the steps to be performed. Machine learning and other related tasks have been performed using WEKA tool [26]. In this figure, the hypothesis emphasizes that adding features (weather parameters/physiological signal data) that have high correlation coefficients will have a positive effect on the model's accuracy, and vice versa. First, we rank the attributes based on the correlation coefficients. Then this result is used in stepwise selection, where different sets of attributes (features) are selected using the feature selection technique. The feature selection technique performs attribute evaluation, which further provides the ranks and their respective weights based on the underlying feature selection technique [27], which in our case is Pearson's correlation coefficient. Based on the selected attribute set, the machine learning model is trained and evaluated in terms of prediction accuracy. For model testing, 10-fold cross-validation scheme has been adopted. In the datasets involving multiple subjects, LOSO (Leave One Subject Out) is commonly used, however, in this study, we have considered single subject for each case. Therefore, a cross-validation scheme is considered feasible. In order to minimize the possible bias due to division of dataset applied for validation, we have performed 10-fold cross-validation five times with randomly shuffled dataset in each iteration. Finally, the average prediction accuracy is recorded of the five evaluations. This process is in compliance with existing works [28–31]. Finally, we observe the change in accuracy in order to analyze the combined effect of independent parameters set, based on correlation coefficients. For this purpose, we have used the backward elimination method. This technique is generally considered over forward selection due to some drawbacks of forward selection technique, including the fact that stepwise inclusion of features may result in reducing the significance of any feature already present in the set, i.e., p-value > 0.05. Different applications has adopted this method for feature selection [32–34].

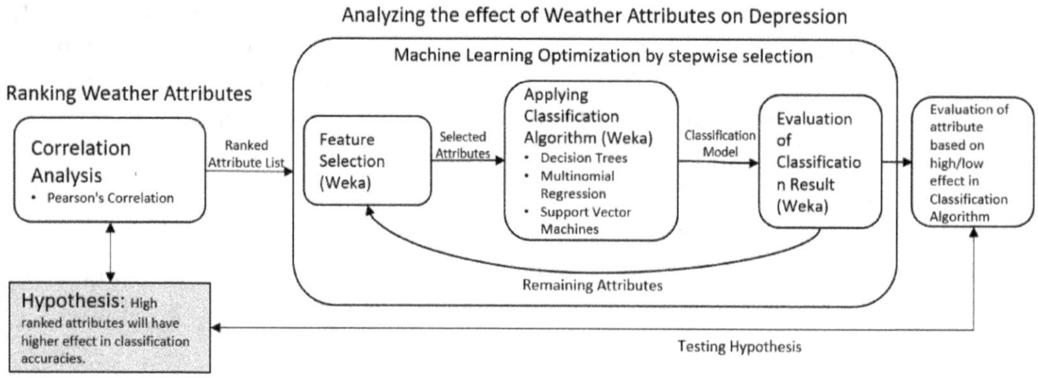

Figure 2. Methodology to identify strong predictor attributes.

3.2. Correlation-based Attribute Ranking

The Weka platform provides feature selection mechanisms which involve filtration techniques to select relevant parameters in order to optimize the machine learning model's performance. In this case, the ranking technique assigns weights to the given features based on the evaluation criteria and techniques involved in the model. Then, based on the weights, features are ranked and those features that are most suitable to be applied in the machine learning algorithm, are filtered. There are many different techniques supported in Weka for feature selection, such as Classifier subset evaluation, Chi square attribute evaluation, Relief attribute evaluation, Gain ratio attribute evaluation, etc. In our approach, we have applied Correlation attribute evaluation, in which features are weighted and ranked based on Pearson's product moment correlation. This technique has been previously described [27]. The main idea behind this approach is that the significance of a relevant feature set in a dataset can be determined by evaluating the correlation of that set with the dependent variable, as well as the correlation among the features. A feature set is considered good for a machine learning model if the features are highly correlated with the dependent class and not correlated with each other. Based on this concept, a feature set can be evaluated as follows:

$$Merit = \frac{\overline{kavg\left(corr_{fc}\right)}}{\sqrt{k + k(k-1)\overline{avg\left(corr_{ff}\right)}}} \quad (3)$$

where Merit is the correlation between the feature set and the dependent class and is the ranking criteria for evaluating the feature set, $(avg(corr_{fc}))$ is the average of the correlations between features and the dependent class, $avg(corr_{ff})$ is the average of the correlations between the features, and k is the number of features.

Here, *corr* is used in evaluating the feature set in the feature selection algorithm. Therefore, based on the above equation, a feature set can be evaluated based on the following factors:

- Higher correlations among the features indicate lower correlation between the feature set and dependent class.
- Higher correlations between the features and the dependent class indicate higher correlation between the feature set and dependent class.
- Higher number of features indicate higher correlation between the feature set and dependent class.

Based on this ranking technique, feature selection has been performed using Weka.

3.3. *Prediction based on Ranked Attributes*

For training the physiological dataset, involving highly correlated attributes, the Random Forest algorithm has been applied. The Random Forest algorithm [35] uses a bagging approach, unlike the Adaboost algorithm (Adapting boosting). In the bagging approach (Bootstrap AGGregatING), *n* different training samples are defined, and the algorithm is trained on each sample independently. The final algorithm is obtained by averaging all of the prediction results. The training subsets allows for data with replacement. The goal of this approach is to reduce the variance in the result (over fitting). In this case, the dataset is divided into randomly collected samples, and a classifier is applied to each sample. Then, based on voting, the higher occurring prediction output is selected. In Weka, the underlying decision tree algorithm for this algorithm is REPTree. In this case, the tree is generated based on information gain/variance.

Other classification algorithms that we have applied to the Depressive disorder and weather data include: Multinomial Logistic Regression, Logit Boost, Random Forest, and Support Vector Machines. Multinomial Logistic regression [36] is a classification technique that extends the capabilities of logistic regression (handling dichotomous dependent variable) to classifying nominal dependent variables. This is performed by converting a multinomial to a many binomial problem, developing a logistic regression model for each binomial category, then comparing the probability equations of the models. Another approach is to develop k-1 simultaneous models for k classes. The Logit boosting algorithm [37] adopts similar techniques as the Adaboost algorithm (Adapting boosting), by minimizing the logistic loss function of logistic regression in each iteration. Support Vector Machine [38] is another supervised learning algorithm, which creates a model based on a hyper plane. A hyper plane is a plane that best divides the classes of the dataset. An optimal hyper plane is identified by maximum margin, which defines the maximum distance between the nearest data point of each class to the hyper plane. Larger distances lead to more optimal hyper planes. In our analysis, a linear model for the hyper plane has been used in classification.

We have applied different algorithms as it is difficult to select a specific algorithm for model generation, because each algorithm may have different accuracy based on the depressive disorder severity level patterns. These algorithms have been applied without any modification in the core development of the WEKA tool. The algorithms are selected based on the prediction accuracy and compliance of their results after evaluating the models with ranked feature sets. By compliance, we mean that the model's accuracy is improved after using selected highly ranked feature set (evaluated by ranking algorithm). The prediction accuracy is calculated using following formula:

$$Accuracy = \frac{TP + TN}{TP + FP + FN + TN} \tag{4}$$

where *TP* is True Positive, *TN* is True Negative, *FP* is False Positive and *FN* is False Negative. This accuracy has been evaluated through the confusion metric in Weka. The ranking results by the correlation coefficient are evaluated with these learning algorithms using the stepwise backward elimination technique, and the accuracy for each iteration is compared.

4. Dataset Description used for Correlation Analytics

This section describes the relevant datasets which are used for correlation analysis and machine learning. In this work, three types of datasets have been considered:

- Depressive disorder symptom dataset for evaluating depression severity.
- Local weather dataset for classifying depression severity.
- Physiological sensor dataset for emotion detection.

The first two datasets have been used to determine the patient's depressive disorder situation based on the current weather. The physiological sensor data, on the other hand, is used for identifying the patient's emotional state. The description involves the metadata for understanding the dataset and data acquisition sources, as well as the preprocessing involved in extracting relevant features, if required for more refined patterns.

4.1. Depressive Disorder Symptom Dataset

There are many different types of depressive disorders, but two of them are considered depressive disorder types which are analyzed in this research: Bipolar depressive disorder and Melancholia depressive disorder [39]. Bipolar is the type of depressive disorder in which the sufferer mostly has high and low mood swings along with similar uncertainty in his energy levels. Any type of depressive disorder can be clinically identified through some predefined symptoms. These symptoms are generally the behavioral, mental, or sometimes physical effects on the patient. For Bipolar disorder, the major symptoms as listed by World Health Organization [40] as well as Smith et al. [41] are: sadness, insomnia (over-sleeping), retardation (slowed movement and working), hopelessness, worthlessness, fatigue or tiredness, elevated feeling and energy for activity, and irritation. Significantly more Bipolar disorder cases have been identified in South Korea than in other countries such as Argentina, Spain, Italy, and US [41]. Melancholia is identified as a severe form of depression where sadness and hopelessness are at their peaks. In addition, this depression has the potential to affect personal lifestyle as well as appetite and sleep [42]. In this case, the major symptoms are sadness, hopelessness, worthlessness, suicidal thoughts and suicide attempts, insomnia, lack of reactivity, loss of interest, weight loss/gain, and retardation. The clinical assessment and evaluation of depressive disorder based on symptoms is mostly done using a self-evaluation questionnaire [17,23,29,43–45]. Different studies including the ones discussed in Section 2 have also adopted this technique for obtaining depressive disorder severity information.

In this study, the depressive disorder severity is also obtained from questionnaire responses. Two main data sources are involved in the analysis of depressive disorder: the depressive disorder severity, evaluated from symptom questionnaire responses and the weather data. Two depressive disorder types have been considered in the symptom dataset: Bipolar and Melancholia. Each depressive disorder type is identified by the specified symptoms. Table 2 shows the symptom list for each depressive disorder type. These symptoms are classified as having major or minor impacts in identifying depression severity. The columns "Bipolar Disorder" and "Melancholia Disorder" shows the association of respective symptoms with them. Each symptom has a set of questions to be asked to the teen. This approach has been widely used in clinical analysis in order to identify depression. Table 3 shows the sample questions for symptoms dds.01 (refer to Table 2 for Symptom ID). The number below each response is the response score. The teen may choose any one of the responses: "Yes, always", "Yes, sometimes" and "No, never", and the corresponding score of that question will be recorded. Each symptom can have a score in a range of 0 to 100. Based on each symptom score, an aggregated depression score can be obtained. The final score for depressive disorder severity has been labeled as none, mild, moderate, moderately severe, and severe, with ranges of 0–20, 21–40, 41–60, 61–80, and 81–100, respectively. The final depressive disorder severity score has been used as a dependent variable for correlation analysis and training the dataset. One limitation of this study is that the symptom dataset is based on simulated data; that is, the questionnaire responses are generated from simulation, based on which the score is calculated.

Table 2. Depressive Disorder Symptoms for Bipolar and Melancholia disorder. The dds keyword in symptom ID (Identifier) represents Depressive Disorder Symptom, followed by the identifier number.

Symptom ID	Symptoms	Bipolar Disorder	Melancholia Disorder
dds.01	Sadness/Worthless/Hopeless	(major)	(major)
dds.02	Insomnia	(major)	(major)
dds.03	Retardation	(major)	(major)
dss.05	Elevated feelings and energy for activity	(major)	
dds.16	Isolation		(minor)
dds.12	Loss of Interest	(minor)	(major)
dds.22	Fatigue	(major)	(major)
dds.10	Anxiety	(minor)	
dds.08	Suicide		(major)
dds.11	Weight Loss/Gain	(minor)	(major)
dds.07	Irritation	(major)	(minor)

Table 3. Sample Questions for depressive disorder symptom dds.01. The dds keyword in Question ID (Identifier) represents Depressive Disorder Symptom, followed by the identifier number, followed by q, which represents Question, followed by question number.

Question ID	Question	Response and Score		
dds.01.q1	Do you consider objects and situations as unimportant as you think you are (e.g., homework, grooming, waking up in the morning etc.)?	Yes, always 30	Yes, sometimes 15	No, never 0
dds.01.q2	Do you feel that you have no value?	Yes, always 30	Yes, sometimes 15	No, never 0
dds.01.q3	Do you usually walk with you head down?	Yes, always 5	Yes, sometimes 2.5	No, never 0
dds.01.q4	Do you often have negative statements?	Yes, always 5	Yes, sometimes 2.5	No, never 0
dds.01.q5	Do you often use gestures that are dramatic and out of context?	Yes, always 5	Yes, sometimes 2.5	No, never 0
dds.01.q6	Do you feel loss of interest in doing activities?	Yes, always 5	Yes, sometimes 2.5	No, never 0
dds.01.q7	Do you often perceive your skill set as inadequate for the task at hand?	Yes, always 5	Yes, sometimes 2.5	No, never 0
dds.01.q8	Do you mostly have negative anticipation about your future?	Yes, always 5	Yes, sometimes 2.5	No, never 0
dds.01.q9	Do you feel losing affection in things?	Yes, always 5	Yes, sometimes 2.5	No, never 0
dds.01.q10	Have you ever mentioned some of the following or similar statements: • Who could ever want to be my friend? • What do my parents really think of me? • Why would anyone want to accept the love of a worthless person like me?	Yes, always 5	Yes, sometimes 2.5	No, never 0

4.2. Local Weather Dataset

The weather data consists of weather information for Suwon city in South Korea, from station 471190. This dataset is openly available online [46]. This location has been selected for being the closest to our location of observation whose data is available, at a distance of 20 km approximate. The parameters include temperature in centigrade, atmospheric pressure in hPa, humidity in %, visibility in km, wind speed in km/h, rain, snow, storm, and fog. The air quality data, for the same

Suwon city, has been collected from online repository provided by the Korean Ministry of Environment (MOE) and the Korea Environment Cooperation (KECO) [47]. The parameters include Ozone (O_3), Carbon-monoxide (CO) and Nitrogen-dioxide (NO_2), all measured in ppm. These two datasets are used for analyzing the effects of weather on depression.

The data considered is for one year of observation from January, 2017 to December, 2017. A total of 182 observations have been recorded throughout the year. The symptom data is collected after every second day and weather data has been considered for the same day. Hence, the datasets are synchronized with respect to dates. Table 4 shows the profile information of the dataset used for the analysis of depressive disorder. Here "Depression Severity" is the score evaluated from symptom questionnaire responses. This is the dependent attribute in this dataset. This dataset is used separately for Bipolar and Melancholia disorder, with their respective depressive disorder scores.

Table 4. Profile information of dataset used for depressive disorder analysis. Min Value and Max Value are the Minimum and Maximum values in the dataset. Std. Dev is the standard deviation.

Attribute	Type	Unit	Min Value	Max Value	Mean	Std. Dev
Season	Nominal	-	-	-	-	-
Temperature	Numeric	C	−8.2	31.6	12.748	10.551
Atmospheric Pressure	Numeric	hPa	998.1	1034.1	1016.88	8.083
Humidity	Numeric	%	32	99	64.621	15.665
Visibility	Numeric	km	1.8	20	12.82	5.071
Wind Speed	Numeric	km/h	1.9	15.2	6.481	2.488
Rain	Nominal	-	-	-	-	-
Snow	Nominal	-	-	-	-	-
Storm	Nominal	-	-	-	-	-
Fog	Nominal	-	-	-	-	-
Ozone	Numeric	ppm	0.006	0.044	0.027	0.012
Carbon Monoxide	Numeric	ppm	0.48	0.82	0.64	0.098
Nitrogen dioxide	Numeric	ppm	0.02	0.043	0.033	0.007
Depression Severity	Nominal	-	-	-	-	-

4.3. *Physiological Sensor Dataset*

In order to analyze the effective data in emotional states, the eight-emotion sentics dataset [48] has been adopted for correlation analysis and machine learning. This dataset consists of the physiological response data of a subject with four sensors attached to his body. The physiological signals involve: electromyogram (EMG), blood volume pulse (BVP), galvanic skin response (GSR), and respiration (Resp). The EMG sensor detects the voltage on the skin surface caused by muscle activity. In this dataset, the EMG sensor has been used to detect jaw clenching as a sign to analyze facial expressions and emotion levels at the valence and arousal scale. Its unit of measure is millivolts. A BVP sensor is used to detect heart rate variability through measuring blood volume pulse. It involves a photo sensor, which quantifies the reflected light rays from the skin's surface. Blood is pumped into the blood vessels after each heartbeat, which results in changes in colors, which then reflect the changes in reflection to the sensor. This sensor has a limitation of precision and is affected by the variability of photo sensor readings. The unit of measure is the percentage of light reflected. GSR is used for quantifying the sweat glands. This signal can be a good source for detecting anger or romantic love, as these emotions can cause skin to sweat, and hence can be identified by GSR sensor. Both the BVP and GSR sensors are attached on the left hand of the subject's body. The respiration signals are conducted through quantifying inhalation and exhalation based on chest cavity expansion and contraction, respectively. For this purpose, a Hall Effect sensor has been used. This area can monitor steady breathing and can omit gas flow due to other activities such as talking, etc. The unit of measure is the percentage stretch per seconds.

For emotion classifications, eight emotions have been considered, as proposed by Clynes [49]. These emotions and profile information used for their examination has been described in Table 5.

The emotional states have been identified and labeled as responses of physiological sensor data when the subject has been shown different images in order to trigger the respective emotional states. For example, for grief, an image of a deformed child or the thought of losing one's mother was delivered to the subject.

The experiments were performed on one single subject with all four sensors (EMG, BVP, GSR, and Respiration) attached to the subject's body. The experiment was carried out for an average of five minutes for each emotional state. The frequency of sensor data collection was 20 samples/second. The experiment was performed over 32 days with one 30-min session each day.

Table 5. Description of the eight emotional states examined.

Emotion Class	Source to Trigger	Description	Arousal and Valence Scale
No Emotion	Blank	Boredom	Low arousal and neutral valence
Anger	Images of people arousing anger	Feeling of fighting	Very high arousal and very negative valence
Hate	Image of injustice and cruelty	Anger of lesser severity	Low arousal and negative valence
Grief	Image of deformed child or thought of loss of mother	Sadness	High arousal and negative valence
Platonic Love	Images of family summer	Happiness and peace	Low arousal and positive valence
Romantic Love	Erotic imagery	Lust and feeling for romance	Very high arousal and positive valence
Joy	Song of joy	Stronger feelings of happiness	Medium high arousal and positive valence
Reverence	Images for holly places and reciting prayers	Calm and peaceful feelings	Very low arousal and neutral valence

Feature Extracted from Raw Data

Since the data collected from physiological signals show sharp peaks and irregular patterns of fluctuations, it is very difficult to find interesting relationships in the raw signal values based on this raw signal data. Therefore feature extraction is a basic requirement for extracting and analyzing meaningful information from raw signals [50]. Therefore, we have extracted six of the total features as described by Picard et al. [51], in order to normalize and smooth the dataset so as to find betters trends and correlations. Table 6 briefly describes each of these features. Feature labels are used as a short form, so that it can be referred in the rest of the paper. These features are extracted for each of the four physiological sensors, therefore a total of 24 features are extracted from the raw dataset. These features have been used in correlation analysis to identify parameters that have strong impacts on detecting emotional states. Table 7 shows the profile information of the dataset used for emotion detection. Attributes are the variables, which include feature extracted from signal data of sensors, EMG, BVP, GSR and Resp, whereas "-f1", "-f2" etc. are feature labels, described in Table 6. For example, "EMG-f1" is a variable which involves the f1 feature values extracted from raw EMG sensor data. "Emotion" is the dependent attribute in this dataset.

Table 6. Extracted features of raw physiological signals described by Picard et al. [51].

Feature Label	Description
f1	Windowed means of the raw signals.
f2	Standard deviations of the raw signals, based on windowed means.
f3	Windowed means of absolute values of the first forward differences of the raw signals.
f4	Windowed means of absolute values of the first forward differences of the normalized signals.
f5	Windowed means of absolute values of the second forward differences of the raw signals.
f6	Windowed means of absolute values of the second forward differences of the normalized signals.

Table 7. Profile information of dataset used for emotion detection. Min Value and Max Value are the Minimum and Maximum values in the dataset. Std. Dev is the standard deviation.

Attribute	Type	Min Value	Max Value	Mean	Std. Dev
EMG-f1	Numeric	1.24	329.11	3.644	6.438
EMG-f2	Numeric	0	192.05	1.147	5.582
EMG-f3	Numeric	0	50.115	0.017	0.196
EMG-f4	Numeric	0	7.29	0.003	0.022
EMG-f5	Numeric	0	50.594	0.014	0.188
EMG-f6	Numeric	0	7.29	0.003	0.021
BVP-f1	Numeric	20.717	58.378	33.545	0.82
BVP-f2	Numeric	1.002	48.439	9.023	4.736
BVP-f3	Numeric	0	36.351	0.085	0.47
BVP-f4	Numeric	0	0.493	0.008	0.022
BVP-f5	Numeric	0	37.159	0.076	0.614
BVP-f6	Numeric	0	0.417	0.007	0.018
GSR-f1	Numeric	1.41	12.996	4.905	2.318
GSR-f2	Numeric	0	0.973	0.025	0.051
GSR-f3	Numeric	0	12.108	0.002	0.071
GSR-f4	Numeric	0	3.358	0.001	0.013
GSR-f5	Numeric	0	12.113	0.002	0.1
GSR-f6	Numeric	0	3.362	0	0.018
Respiration-f1	Numeric	37.853	64.598	56.82	6.802
Respiration-f2	Numeric	0	3.252	0.297	0.319
Respiration-f3	Numeric	0	63.365	0.016	0.707
Respiration-f4	Numeric	0	3.306	0.009	0.023
Respiration-f5	Numeric	0	63.365	0.018	0.999
Respiration-f6	Numeric	0	3.33	0.001	0.016
Emotion	Nominal	-	-	-	-

5. Experimentation and Results

5.1. Experimentation Use Case: Depressive Disorder for Teens

In order to describe the applicability of the data acquisition and analysis based on the defined methodology, a use case has been designed. In this case, two depressive disorder teen-aged patients have been considered, with one suffering from bipolar disorder and the other suffering from Melancholia Disorder. The reason for considering teenagers is the prevalence of depressive disorder and suicide in teenagers [52,53]. There are other symptoms and disorder specifications as well, such as the ones existing in females (postpartum depression, baby blue, etc.) or elderly; however, these are out of the scope of this study.

Approximating depressive disorder situations close to the actual ones requires a high level of information, so that the system's decisions are justified based on analyzing the different circumstances experienced by the patient. Figure 3 shows the process flow of the use case. We have considered three types of data for the two depressive disorder cases listed above. One is emotion detection through the physiological sensor data. The second is depressive disorder symptom evaluation through the self-reporting questionnaire responses, and the third is weather information based on the patient's location. The system has three types of interactions with the environment which are related to the three different types of data acquisition. The first interaction is possible via a smartphone application, through which the teen patient provides information regarding his depression symptoms by responding to a questionnaire in the application. Bipolar and Melancholia disorder have their own defined sets of symptoms for evaluating the respective depressive disorder severities, as shown in Table 2. Therefore, each user is given a different questionnaire based on his respective disorder type. These responses are then recorded and stored by the system in the database. In the second interaction, the daily weather status has been acquired based on the teen's current location. The GPS coordinate system has been used instead of address (city, country etc.) in order to avoid naming errors. The weather information is recorded based on the city or area, covering the specified range. In this case, it is not possible to provide the data of the exact location. Therefore, the weather of the closest proximity has been used. In the third case of physiological signals, the data will be periodically collected from sensors and stored in the database. The eight emotional states have been considered for evaluation, as described in Table 5. All forms of data acquisitions are synchronized with respect to the specified date. This step is crucial for observing the patterns of depression severity, emotional states, and weather information, as well as their effects with respect to date and time.

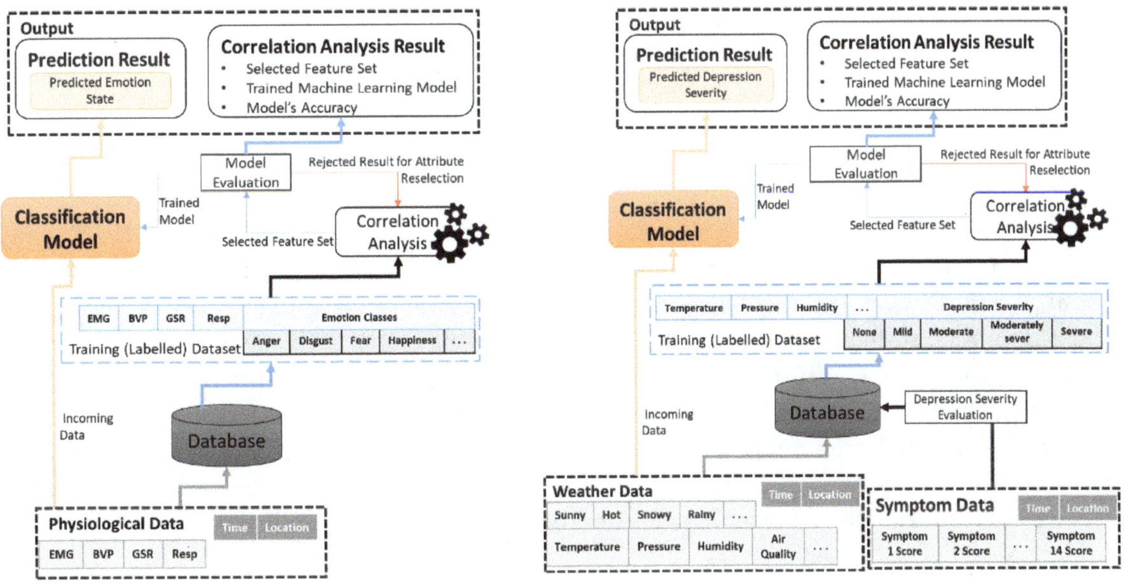

(a) (b)

Figure 3. Process flow of Data Analytics: (**a**) Emotion detection. (**b**) Identifying depressive disorder severity.

The system uses all of the collected information to analyze the health status of the teen patient. This accumulated data is used to highlight the user's status based on the collective information of weather, emotion, and depression. In this case, the analysis is performed separately for each teen profile and his depressive disorder category. The predicted emotional states are also acquired based on strong effective parameters from the physiological signals. For the machine learning and prediction, the Weka machine learning tool is used in the java platform. To begin, the system retrieves symptom response data with timestamps as the request input. It then performs calculations for depressive disorder severity. It further retrieves emotion data with timestamps as the requested input, then evaluates the depression severity level. For depression severity evaluation based on emotion score, we have referred to the valence and arousal scale described by Scherer et al. [54]. In this scale, anger is labeled as ANGRY, contempt as contemptuous, disgust as disgusted, fear as AFRAID, happiness as HAPPY, sadness as SAD, and surprise as ASTONISHED. From the scale, it can be seen that the "SAD" emotion is closest to "DEPRESSED". Therefore, it can be considered that users having high scores for sad will also have high chances of being depressed. Hence, the sad emotion score is used to evaluate the depression severity level. Then, it finally retrieves the physiological sensor data with timestamps as the requested input and sends this data to the prediction server in order to obtain the prediction result. For training the prediction model, the model creation server obtains the dataset from the database of a specified time duration. Then, based on that training dataset, it generates a prediction model beforehand. This has been tested using the WEKA tool. The prediction model is then imported in the prediction server, so that it is able to predict based on the incoming requests. The final output of the system is the health status of the particular teen based on: emotional state from Emotion API, predicted state from physiological sensor data, depression severity from questionnaire data, and predicted depression severity from weather information.

This is one component of the Web Objects-based healthcare services provisioning system [55,56]. The proposed system will be used to enhance decision-making capabilities at the Service level, which will further support applications such as forecasting, emergency detection, and notification and recommendation services [57–59]. Forecasting will involve future trends in depressive disorder levels and the number of peak levels. Emergency detection will involve suicide detection, triggers that contribute to escalating depression, notifying concerned doctors and relatives, etc. The recommendation service will involve notifying the user, based on his or her preferences [60], with such suggestions that may contribute to minimizing the severity of depression, such as recommending relaxing music, movies, food, etc.

5.2. Results of Correlation Analysis

In order to identify the strong predictor attributes for depressive disorder, the Pearson's correlation-based feature selection technique is used as described in Section 3. Table 8 shows the results of this technique for the depressive disorder symptom dataset. The ranks are ordered from most important to least important attribute for each depression type. Here "Merit" is the weight calculated for each attribute based on the correlation coefficient, which is the ranking criteria described in Equation (3). For bipolar disorder, it can be seen that temperature, atmospheric pressure, season and ozone lie in the top four ranking, and can, therefore, be considered as strong predictors for this disorder severity. The temperature, season and ozone lie in the top four in both depressive disorder categories. In contrast, wind speed, rain, and visibility are evaluated among the lowest ranks in both categories. Storm and Humidity are among the bottom-ranked factors in Bipolar and Melancholia disorder, respectively.

Table 8. Ranking of attributes based on Correlation Coefficient.

Rank	Bipolar-Disorder	Merit	Melancholia-Disorder	Merit
1	Temperature	0.526	Season	243.18
2	Atmospheric Pressure	0.421	Ozone	182.8
3	Season	0.38	Carbon-monoxide	155.3
4	Ozone	0.31	Temperature	102.6
5	Nitrogen-dioxide	0.29	Nitrogen-dioxide	94.4
6	Carbon-monoxide	0.264	Atmospheric Pressure	33.6
7	Snow	0.204	Fog	15.2
8	Humidity	0.179	Snow	10.2
9	Fog	0.13	Storm	6.5
10	Rain	0.125	Humidity	2.43
11	Visibility	0.122	Visibility	1.7
12	Storm	0.105	Wind speed	0.008
13	Wind speed	0.07	Rain	0.003

In case of Melancholia disorder, the coefficients' values are very low, i.e., near zero, therefore showing overall very weak correlation. This can contribute to the fact that the merit is higher than that of the usual case. Hence, it is difficult to determine the effect of weather parameters on Melancholia disorder based on collinear relationship analysis.

This ranking is an important finding, as it has helped enhance the accuracies of prediction algorithms by applying the stepwise selection technique. This finding has also provided support to the analysis of factors affecting depression. Figure 4 shows the scatter plot in Weka, of the top-ranked weather parameters with bipolar depression severity. The strength of correlation can be related to the results in Table 8. Temperature has the strongest negative correlation with bipolar depression severity, followed by atmospheric pressure, which is positively correlated, and then ozone, which also has a positive correlation with depression.

In order to identify the correlation of each physiological sensor data with emotion, Pearson correlation has been used. Table 9 shows the correlation result and the p-value for significance. It can be seen from the result that Pearson's correlation does not provide any significant result, as all of the correlation coefficients are near zero, and the p-value also shows no significance.

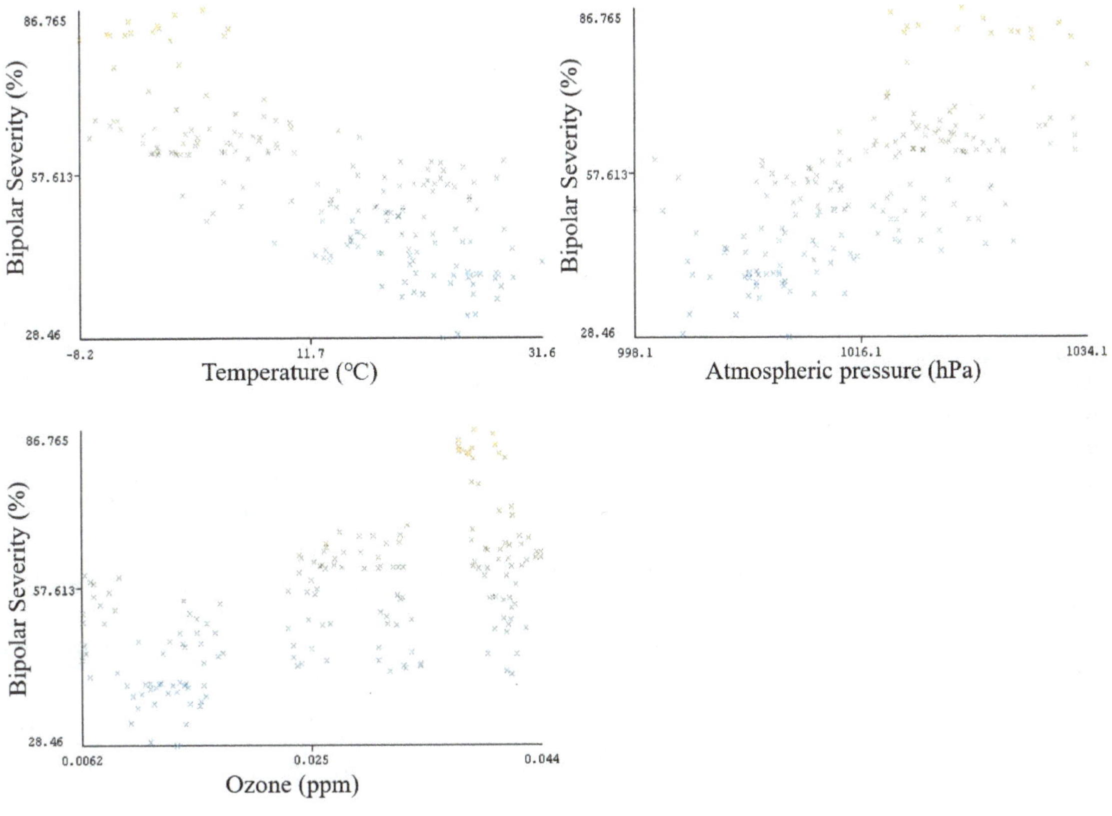

Figure 4. Scatter plot in Weka, of top-ranked weather parameters for Bipolar disorder.

Furthermore, we have also analyzed the correlation results among the sensor data with respect to each emotion class. Here, the results also show no or very minimum correlation among the sensor data. Only the readings under "No Emotion" and "Anger" class have small factors of positive correlation between GSR and Respiration sensors, which are 0.325 and 0.456, respectively.

This correlation signifies an inverse effect in analyzing the sensor data attributes. In this case, weaker correlation means that there is less similarity in the patterns of the sensed data. This indicates that each sensor data has unique patterns, which can be an important factor in identifying emotional states. In the case of strong correlation, it would indicate that the strongly-correlated attributes can have the same impact in predicting the emotional states, and hence one of them can be considered a redundant attribute and discarded.

Table 9. Correlation-based ranking for physiological dataset.

Physiological Sensor	Emotion	p-Value
EMG	−0.085599801	<0.001
BVP	−0.001507079	0.39
GSR	−0.073850046	<0.001
RESP	−0.023263153	<0.001

After applying the feature extraction described in Section 3, we applied the correlation over the extracted features and found significant results. Table 10 shows the correlation among the extracted features. Having 24 features makes the correlation table very large, therefore we have selected and shown only the highly-correlated parameters. Here the highest correlations are observed between EMG-f1 and EMG-f2, BVP-f5 and Resp-f5, GSR-f3 and Resp-f3, and GSR-f5 and Resp-f5, each having coefficients around 0.9, followed by correlations between BVP-f5 and GSR-f5 and between BVP-f3 and Resp-f3, each having coefficients around 0.8. In the case of correlation with emotion class, only BVP-f2 showed a small negative coefficient value of -0.38021. Here, we can observe that most of the coefficient values are positive. This is due to two factors: one is that there is no negative signal reading in the dataset, and the second is that very few signal readings show the inverse trend related to the other trend. The difference is only based on the amplitude of the observed signal with respect to the others in the respective emotional state. The ones having negative coefficient values are close to zero.

Table 10. Correlation-based ranking for physiological dataset.

Feature	EMG-f1	EMG-f3	EMG-f5	BVP-f3	BVP-f5	GSR-f3	GSR-f4	GSR-f5	Resp-f3
EMG-f1	1								
EMG-f2	0.9095								
EMG-f4	0.0200	0.6472							
EMG-f6	−0.0219	0.2994	0.6227						
BVP-f5	4.09×10^{-5}	0.16253	0.336666	0.647586	1				
GSR-f3	0.0037	0.2420	0.2529	0.7875	0.6084	1			
GSR-f5	0.0001	0.1733	0.3592	0.5576	0.8610	0.7066	0.3286	1	
GSR-f6	0.0002	0.0867	0.1793	0.1491	0.2309	0.333	0.6973	0.4712	
Resp-f3	0.0006	0.2431	0.25349	0.86176	0.66583	0.90413	0.23156	0.64011	1
Resp-f5	6.76×10^{-5}	0.17323	0.35939	0.609938	0.941885	0.639795	0.163974	0.905452	0.706954

The ranking of extracted features has been performed using Weka, based on the approach described in Section 3.2. Table 11 shows the 24 features sorted based on the rank and the respective weight. Here it is observed that f5 and f6 of all four physiological signals are ranked least by the Weka feature selection algorithm. One possible reason for this is that these features involve first and second forward differences of the raw signal readings, which are smaller based on the scale of the values. Therefore, no significant correlation is found in these features.

Table 11. Correlation-based ranking for physiological dataset.

Rank	Feature	Weight for Ranking	Rank	Feature	Weight for Ranking
1	BVP-f2	0.12407258	13	BVP-f3	5.1806×10^{-4}
2	GSR-f1	0.09261232	14	Resp-f5	6.639×10^{-5}
3	EMG-f1	0.07958459	15	BVP-f5	5.092×10^{-5}
4	GSR-f2	0.0676282	16	GSR-f5	3.489×10^{-5}
5	EMG-f2	0.0629491	17	Resp-f3	3.022×10^{-5}
6	Resp-f2	0.05206328	18	Resp-f6	2.369×10^{-5}
7	Resp-f1	8.8696×10^{-3}	19	EMG-f3	2.314×10^{-5}

5.3. Machine Learning Results

For predicting the depressive disorder severity levels based on the weather dataset, four classification techniques have been applied as described in Section 3.3. Each of these algorithms has been evaluated with the backward elimination technique in order to analyze the effects of the predictors (the weather attributes) on the dependent variable (the depression severity levels), based on the proposed ranking technique. Each of the classification algorithms has been evaluated with the 10 folds cross-validation scheme in WEKA.

Table 12 shows the classification results for Bipolar disorder, using the backward elimination process. Each row contains the accuracy of each classification algorithm based on the specified number of attributes. These numbers of attributes are decreasing based on the ranking output from Table 8. For example, 13 predictors contain all of the 13 weather parameters used for classification, 12 predictors contain all parameters except for wind speed, 11 predictors also exclude storm, and so on. The other values are the accuracies for each algorithm. Here it can be seen that, as the weak predictors are removed, the overall accuracies of the algorithms increase until around 40–50% of predictor attributes remain. LogitBoost show higher accuracies with up to nine attributes. Therefore, nine parameters from Table 8 are sufficient for predicting depression severity. Support Vector Machine (SVM) shows higher accuracies until four predictors. Random forest shows higher accuracy until eight predictors, and Logistic regression until nine. The highest accuracy in all 44 evaluations is of Random Forest with eight predictors, at 89.01%. Therefore, Random Forest is the most suitable model for prediction in this depression type. From both the observations of feature selection and the classification results, it can be seen that wind speed, storm, visibility, rain, and fog have degraded effects or no effect on training the prediction models. In the case of SVM, its accuracy is highest with only three predictors: temperature, atmospheric pressure, and ozone. With these observations, we have evaluated temperature, atmospheric pressure, and ozone to be the strong predictors for depression severity.

Table 12. Classification Results for Bipolar Disorder. SVM is abbreviation for Support Vector Machines.

Number of Predictors	Logit Boost (%)	SVM (%)	Random Forest (%)	Logistic Regression (%)
13	85.16	80.77	87.36	79.12
12	85.16	80.77	87.91	80.22
11	86.26	81.32	88.46	83.52
10	86.26	82.42	89.01	84.07
9	86.26	81.32	88.46	85.16
8	85.71	84.07	89.01	84.62
7	85.71	84.62	87.91	84.07
6	84.62	84.62	87.91	81.87
5	85.71	84.62	85.16	84.07
4	82.42	84.62	84.07	81.87
3	74.18	72.53	67.58	72.53

In the case of Melancholia disorder, there is no significant overall change in accuracies, as compared to the results for Bipolar disorder. The main reason for this noncompliance with the correlation result is that the coefficient values are closer to zero than in other depressive disorder types. Therefore, correlation analysis is not effective in this case, and a more complex algorithm is needed to identify relevant relationships.

For the prediction of emotional states, we have applied the tree-based approach for the classification of emotions. For this purpose, the Random Forest algorithm has been applied for classification based on the 24 features set. In this regard, the training set consists of 66% of the total dataset, whereas the remaining 34% has been used for evaluations. Figure 5 shows the graph of accuracies with respect to selected features based on the ranking result displayed in Table 11. The features are selected such that the lowest ranked features are eliminated one by one in each step. The first value in Figure 5 is the accuracy of the learning algorithm when all 24 features are selected, and the last value shows the accuracy when the top four features are selected from the ranked list in Table 11. The results show 85.7936% accuracy at 24 features selected for classification. This result is also in compliance with the results in related studies. This learning model is optimized up to 91.1511% with top 9 ranked features. After that, the accuracy reduces as the features with lower ranks are removed.

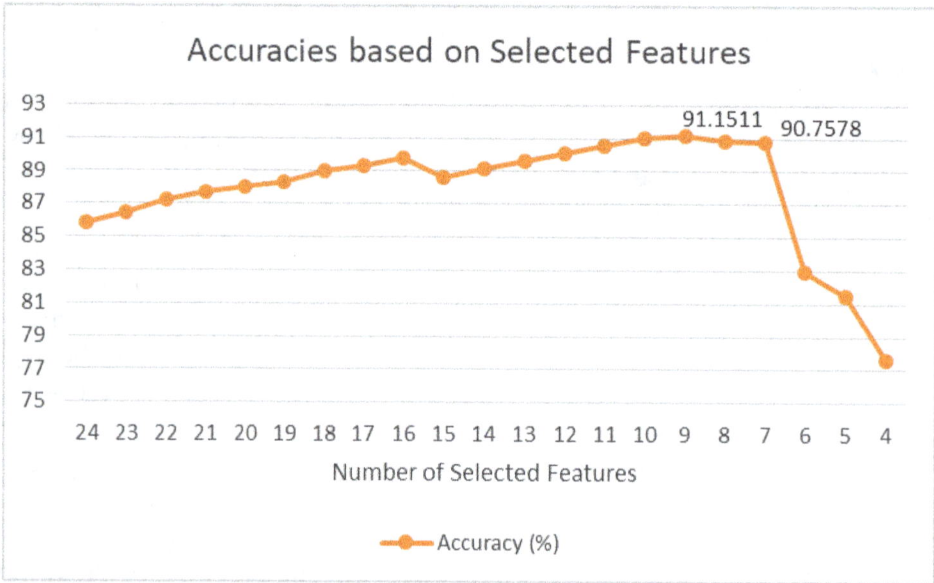

Figure 5. Accuracies of prediction models with respect to stepwise feature selection.

From these results, it can be concluded that the nine top-ranked features from Table 11 provide the optimum results in the case of using Random Forest as the classification model. In this case, f5 and f6 of all the sensors are eliminated, as they provided lower rankings based on the correlation algorithm.

According to the results shown by Picard et al. [51], the highest accuracy achieved is around 88% using the K Nearest Neighbors (kNN) classifier with only the selected emotional states of Anger, Joy, and Reverence. The accuracy of the trained classifier is much lower in the case considering all emotional states. In our results, the dataset involving all eight emotions has been used; however, only the top-ranked features are selected based on the correlation results. By using a tree-based learning algorithm, Random Forest, the accuracy is improved to 91.511% in our approach. We have also applied the kNN algorithm to train the model at $k = 10$. However, the accuracy is not optimized as well as it takes more time to train and cross-validate the model based on kNN than the Random Forest model.

6. Discussions

The results show different characteristics of the dataset as well as different situations are debatable in this aspect. In Bipolar case, temperature, pressure, season and ozone show strong relationship with depression severity. The effect of temperature on depression was also identified by Molin et al. [19]. Whereas the study carried out by Yang et al. [18], identified pressure as effective only in humid areas. Also in other studies, the season was observed as important parameter [17,18], specifically considering peaks of summer and winter. If we consider the machine learning results, when trained and tested excluding wind speed, storm, visibility, rain and fog, showed increase in the accuracies of all the models except SVM. Hence it can be considered that these attributes have least or no relationship with respect to this dataset. In case of rain, storm and fog, one reason for this lack of relationship can be the limited number of observations. Korea is one of those countries where rain is often observed throughout the year, but even then one year is not sufficient for expecting steady trends. Another reason can be the nominal data type. Continuous or ratio based data type may be able to provide more information, for example, mm of rain per minute. In case of Ozone, we cannot be certain of this relationship as the data scatter shows signs of heteroscedasticity. Although, we can apply different tests to identify heteroscedasticity, but still we need larger number of observations for certainty. In case of Melancholia disorder, no significant results were obtained. One of the factor can be the lack of similarity in the dataset as compared to the one acquired from real test subject. Second reason can be the limited number of observations which then fails to provide any steady trends. Third reason can be the limitation of correlation to only collinear relationships. This dataset is required to be analyzed with other techniques to indicate possible relationship with weather. Feature selection technique also plays an important role in filtering out non-relevant features extracted from physiological signals. Using correlation-based feature selection, we observed that f1 and f2 (Table 6) are important features for detecting emotional states. In this study, we have extracted only 6 features, whereas, different other features can also be extracted to analyze new interesting trends, for example, Z-score, local maxima, local minima etc. In this study, we have referred to the valence and arousal scale in [54] to highlight the possible relationship of emotion with depression. However, other possible emotional states can also be mapped at symptom level to have more descriptive relationships. For example, "Elevated feelings and energy for activity" (symptom dds.05 in Table 2) can be mapped to "elated", "EXCITED", "adventurous" and "aroused" in the valance and arousal scale. In another way, it is also possible to analyze the depressive disorder situation through physiological sensors. In particular, different studies have utilized EEG sensor for analyzing brain signal to analyze depressive disorder situations [61–63]. In other case, studies have proved that the stress can be detected using physiological sensors which is an initial state of depression, therefore, it can be easily implied that the monitoring of long term stress using physiological signals can help us in detecting depression [64].

This research has used correlation measure to identify relationships of different parameters affecting mental health situations, specifically the bipolar and melancholia disorder and emotion states. In this regard, there are some limitations that are highlighted with respect to statistical measures, data characteristics and scope. Correlation measure is used to identify the strength of a relationship between two variables. But, it cannot determine the causality between the two variables. In case of independent and dependent variable, this causality covers the aspects of analysis. In case of two independent variables, there can be a possibility of spurious relationship, where the correlation has been produced by extraneous third factor and neither of the variables involved in the correlation has influenced the other. Different tests are used in order to identify such relationship, such as Breusch-Pagan test [65] and White test [66]. In this research, by performing these test we still cannot validate the presence of heteroscedasticity due to limited set of observations. The expected results may also have some uncertain discovered trend or some unidentified relationship due to the limited observations in datasets. As indicated in other studies, the dataset considered usually involves more than one year of observations or higher number of subjects [17–19]. Therefore, involving more observations may form steady trends and thus lead to identifying new relationships that are not discovered in the current dataset size. Another point of concern, which requires discussion, is the high correlation values observed in Table 10 (for example: $C > 0.9$). We have considered this problem and have tested PCA (Principal Component Analysis) with physiological dataset using Weka. It was observed that none of the Eigen values were exactly zero, implying that high correlation in the employed dataset does not cause singularity. Nonetheless, similar datasets yielding higher correlation values may cause singularity and result in zero determinant of the feature matrix, which can further lead to issues when modeling different feature selection techniques, such as Principal Component Analysis (PCA). As our future work, we intend to perform comparative analysis amongst various feature selection techniques on physiological dataset to highlight such issues.

7. Conclusions

This research aimed to analyze the effects of certain data features on depression severities and the emotional states, in order to predict patient's current situations. In this case, correlation and machine learning-based data analysis has been performed using different data sources considering specified depressive disorder patients. Based on the correlation and classification results, the parameters that have a strong effect on depression are: temperature, atmospheric pressure, and ozone. In the emotion dataset, the first and second extracted features of all four sensor signals (based on the means and standard deviations of the raw signals) showed a high effect in classifying the emotional states.

Identifying a patient's health status using data analysis is a very complicated research issue as it involves various aspects, such as work and peer pressure, loneliness and social isolation, conflict in social relations, socioeconomic status, medications, physical impairment and disability, environmental effect, location, incident-based trauma, and so on. This research carries the main assumption which does not consider these situations. In the future, analyzing the impacts of these related factors on our results and also based on real test environment cases will be considered the focal point of the research. Further, longer periods of observation will provide stable and more prominent results in correlation and trend analysis. In this study, a linear correlation model has been used for identifying relationships. However, some weather parameters have complex patterns, so this model could not identify certain relationships. Hence, different correlation models must be analyzed in identifying nonlinear and other relevant relationships in the future.

Author Contributions: Conceptualization, S.K. and I.C.; Formal analysis, S.K.; Methodology, S.K.; Project administration, I.C.; Supervision, I.C.; Writing–original draft, S.K.; Writing– review & editing, S.K.

References

1. Han, J.; Kamber, M. *Data Mining: Concepts and Techniques*, 2nd ed.; University of Illinois at Urbana-Champaign: Champaign, IL, USA, 2006; ISBN 9781558609013.
2. Bauman, A.E.; Sallis, J.F.; Dzewaltowski, D.A.; Owen, N. Toward a better understanding of the influences on physical activity: The role of determinants, correlates, causal variables, mediators, moderators, and confounders. *Am. J. Prev. Med.* **2002**, *23*, 5–14. [CrossRef]
3. Park, J.N.; Han, M.A.; Park, J.; Ryu, S.Y. Prevalence of Depressive Symptoms and Related Factors in Korean Employees: The Third Korean Working Conditions Survey (2011). *Int. J. Environ. Res. Public Health* **2011**, *13*, 424. [CrossRef] [PubMed]
4. Choi, K.-S.; Kang, S.-K. Occupational Psychiatric Disorders in Korea. *J. Korean Med. Sci.* **2010**, *25*, 87–93. [CrossRef] [PubMed]
5. Jeong, B.G.; Veenstra, G. The intergenerational production of depression in South Korea: Results from a cross-sectional study. *Jeong Veenstra Int. J. Equity Heal.* **2017**, *16*, 13. [CrossRef] [PubMed]
6. Jarwar, M.A.; Abbasi, R.A.; Mushtaq, A.; Maqbool, O.; Aljohani, N.R.; Daud, A.; Alowibdi, J.S.; Cano, J.R.; García, S.; Chong, I. Undefined CommuniMents: A Framework for Detecting Community Based Sentiments for Events. 2017. Available online: https://www.igi-global.com (accessed on 19 July 2018).
7. Pantic, M.; Patras, I. Dynamics of facial expression: Recognition of facial actions and their temporal segments from face profile image sequences. *IEEE Trans. Syst. Man Cybern. Part B* **2006**, *36*, 433–449. [CrossRef]
8. El Ayadi, M.; Kamel, M.S.; Karray, F. Survey on speech emotion recognition: Features, classification schemes, and databases. *Pattern Recognit.* **2011**, *44*, 572–587. [CrossRef]
9. Kessous, L.; Castellano, G.; Caridakis, G. Multimodal emotion recognition in speech-based interaction using facial expression, body gesture and acoustic analysis. *J. Multimodal User Interfaces* **2010**, *3*, 33–48. [CrossRef]
10. Batliner, A.; Seppi, D.; Steidl, S.; Schuller, B. Segmenting into Adequate Units for Automatic Recognition of Emotion-Related Episodes: A Speech-Based Approach. *Adv. Hum.-Comput. Interact.* **2010**, *2010*, 1–15. [CrossRef]
11. Syllignakis, M.N.; Kouretas, G.P. Dynamic correlation analysis of financial contagion: Evidence from the Central and Eastern European markets. *Int. Rev. Econ. Financ.* **2011**, *20*, 717–732. [CrossRef]
12. Sandoval Junior, L. Correlation of financial markets in times of crisis. *Phys. A Stat. Mech. Appl.* **2012**, *391*, 187–208. [CrossRef]

13. Inamdar, D.; Leblanc, G.; Soffer, R.J.; Kalacska, M. The correlation coefficient as a simple tool for the localization of errors in spectroscopic imaging data. *Remote Sens.* **2018**, *10*, 231. [CrossRef]
14. Vavliakis, K.N.; Gemenetzi, K.; Mitkas, P.A. A Correlation Analysis of Web Social Media. In Proceedings of the International Conference on Web Intelligence, Mining and Semantics, Sogndal, Norway, 25–27 May 2011.
15. Erdem, O.; Ceyhan, E.; Varli, Y. A new correlation coefficient for bivariate time-series data. *Phys. A* **2014**, *414*, 274–284. [CrossRef]
16. Abhang, P.A.; Gawali, B.W. Correlation of EEG Images and Speech Signals for Emotion Analysis. *Br. J. Appl. Sci. Technol.* **2015**, *10*, 1–13. [CrossRef]
17. Huibers, M.J.H.; de Graaf, L.E.; Peeters, F.P.M.L.; Arntz, A. Does the weather make us sad? Meteorological determinants of mood and depression in the general population. *Psychiatry Res.* **2010**, *180*, 143–146. [CrossRef] [PubMed]
18. Yang, W.; Mu, L.; Shen, Y. Effect of climate and seasonality on depressed mood among twitter users. *Appl. Geogr.* **2015**, *63*, 184–191. [CrossRef]
19. Molin, J.; Mellerup, E.; Bolwig, T.; Scheike, T. The influence of climate on development of winter depression. *J. Affect. Disord.* **1996**, *37*, 151–155. [CrossRef]
20. Blanchard, E.B.; Buckley, T.C.; Hickling, E.J.; Taylor, A.E. Posttraumatic Stress Disorder and Comorbid Major Depression: Is the Correlation an Illusion? *J. Anxiety Disord.* **1998**, *12*, 21–37. [CrossRef]
21. Mitani, H.; Shirayama, Y.; Yamada, T.; Maeda, K.; Ashby, C.R.; Kawahara, R. Correlation between plasma levels of glutamate, alanine and serine with severity of depression. *Prog. Neuro-Psychopharmacol. Biol. Psychiatry* **2006**, *30*, 1155–1158. [CrossRef]
22. Khalili, Z.; Moradi, M.H. Emotion recognition system using brain and peripheral signals: Using correlation dimension to improve the results of EEG. In Proceedings of the 2009 International Joint Conference on Neural Networks, Atlanta, GA, USA, 14–19 June 2009; pp. 1571–1575.
23. Albert, P.S.; Rosen, L.N.; Alexander, J.R., Jr.; Rosenthal, N.E. Effect of daily variation in weather and sleep on seasonal affective disorder. *Psychiatry Res.* **1991**, *36*, 51–63. [CrossRef]
24. Spasova, Z. The effect of weather and its changes on emotional state—Individual characteristics that make us vulnerable. *Adv. Sci. Res.* **2012**, *6*, 281–290. [CrossRef]
25. Bulbena, A.; Pailhez, G.; Acena, R.; Cunillera, J.; Rius, A.; Garcia-Ribera, C.; Gutiérrez, J.; Rojo, C. Panic anxiety, under the weather? *Int. J. Biometeorol.* **2005**, *49*, 238–243. [CrossRef] [PubMed]
26. Frank, E.; Hall, M.A.; Witten, I.H. *The WEKA Workbench. Online Appendix for "Data Mining: Practical Machine Learning Tools and Techniques"*; Morgan Kaufmann: Burlington, MA, USA, 2016.
27. Hall, M.A. *Correlation-Based Feature Selection for Machine Learning*; The University of Waikato: Hamilton, New Zealand, 1999.
28. Sun, F.-T.; Kuo, C.; Cheng, H.-T.; Buthpitiya, S.; Collins, P.; Griss, M. *Activity-Aware Mental Stress Detection Using Physiological Sensors*; Springer: Berlin/Heidelberg, Germany, 2012; pp. 282–301.
29. Burns, M.N.; Begale, M.; Duffecy, J.; Gergle, D.; Karr, C.J.; Giangrande, E.; Mohr, D.C. Harnessing context sensing to develop a mobile intervention for depression. *J. Med. Internet Res.* **2011**, *13*, e55. [CrossRef] [PubMed]
30. Zeng, L.-L.; Shen, H.; Liu, L.; Wang, L.; Li, B.; Fang, P.; Zhou, Z.; Li, Y.; Hu, D. Identifying major depression using whole-brain functional connectivity: A multivariate pattern analysis. *Brain* **2012**, *135*, 1498–1507. [CrossRef] [PubMed]
31. Van der Gaag, M.; Hoffman, T.; Remijsen, M.; Hijman, R.; de Haan, L.; van Meijel, B.; van Harten, P.N.; Valmaggia, L.; de Hert, M.; Cuijpers, A.; et al. The five-factor model of the Positive and Negative Syndrome Scale II: A ten-fold cross-validation of a revised model. *Schizophr. Res.* **2006**, *85*, 280–287. [CrossRef]
32. Wählby, U.; Jonsson, E.N.; Karlsson, M.O. Comparison of stepwise covariate model building strategies in population pharmacokinetic-pharmacodynamic analysis. *AAPS PharmSciTech* **2002**, *4*, 68–79. [CrossRef] [PubMed]
33. Li, J.; Zhang, Z.; Rosenzweig, J.; Wang, Y.Y.; Chan, D.W. Proteomics and bioinformatics approaches for identification of serum biomarkers to detect breast cancer. *Clin. Chem.* **2002**, *48*, 1296–1304.
34. Ambroise, C.; McLachlan, G.J. Selection bias in gene extraction on the basis of microarray gene-expression data. *Proc. Natl. Acad. Sci. USA* **2002**, *99*, 6562–6566. [CrossRef]
35. Breiman, L. Random Forests. *Mach. Learn.* **2001**, *45*, 5–32. [CrossRef]

36. Le Cessie, S.; Van Houwelingen, J.C.; Le Cessiet, S.; Van Houwelingen, J.C. Ridge Estimators in Logistic Regression. *Source J. R. Stat. Soc. Ser. C (Appl. Stat. Appl. Stat.)* **1992**, *41*, 191–201. [CrossRef]
37. Friedman, J.; Hastie, T.; Tibshirani, R. Additive logistic regression: A statistical view of boosting (With discussion and a rejoinder by the authors). *Ann. Stat.* **2000**, *28*, 337–407. [CrossRef]
38. Manzalawy, Y.; Weka, V.H. LibSVM (WLSVM): Integrating LibSVM into Weka Environment. Available online: http://ailab.ist.psu.edu/yasser/wlsvm.html (accessed on 29 May 2018).
39. American Psychiatric Association. *Diagnostic and Statistical Manual of Mental Disorders*; American Psychiatric Association: Philadelphia, PA, USA, 2013; ISBN 089042554X.
40. World Health Organization. *The ICD-10 Classification of Mental and Behavioural Disorders Clinical Descriptions and Diagnostic Guidelines*; World Health Organization: Geneva, Switzerland, 1992.
41. Smith, M.; Segal, J. "Bipolar Disorder Signs and Symptoms: Recognizing and Getting Help for Mania and Bipolar Depression". Available online: https://www.helpguide.org/articles/bipolar-disorder/bipolar-disorder-signs-and-symptoms.htm (accessed on 18 December 2018).
42. Kerr, M. Melancholic Depression: Symptoms, Treatment, Tests and More. Available online: https://www.healthline.com/health/depression/melancholic-depression#symptoms (accessed on 15 June 2018).
43. Doryab, A.; Min, J.K.; Wiese, J.; Zimmerman, J.; Hong, J.I. Detection of Behavior Change in People with Depression. In AAAI Workshop: Modern Artificial Intelligence for Health Analytics. June 2014. Available online: https://www.aaai.org/ocs/index.php/WS/AAAIW14/paper/viewFile/8850/8303 (accessed on 29 May 2018).
44. Helm, S.V.; Pollitt, A.; Barnett, M.A.; Curran, M.A.; Craig, Z.R. Differentiating environmental concern in the context of psychological adaption to climate change. *Glob. Environ. Chang.* **2018**, *48*, 158–167. [CrossRef]
45. Chattopadhyay, S.; Rabhi, F.A.; Bhanjachaudhuri, S.; Jena, S.K. Mining important symptoms of adult depression. *Int. J. Comput. Appl.* **2012**, *57*. Available online: https://www.ijcaonline.org/archives/volume57/number5/9108-3258 (accessed on 29 May 2018).
46. Climate SUWON-Climate Data (471190). Available online: https://en.tutiempo.net/climate/ws-471190.html (accessed on 29 May 2018).
47. Airkorea. Available online: http://www.airkorea.or.kr/eng/index (accessed on 4 December 2018).
48. Vyzas, E. *Recognition of Emotional and Cognitive State Using Physiological Data*; Massachusetts Institute of Technology: Cambridge, MA, USA, 1999.
49. Ortony, A.; Clore, G.L.; Collins, A. *The Cognitive Structure of Emotions*; Cambridge University Press: Cambridge, UK, 1988; ISBN 0521386640.
50. Wagner, J.; Kim, J.; Andre, E. From Physiological Signals to Emotions: Implementing and Comparing Selected Methods for Feature Extraction and Classification. In Proceedings of the 2005 IEEE International Conference on Multimedia and Expo, Amsterdam, The Netherlands, 6–8 July 2005; pp. 940–943.
51. Picard, R.W.; Vyzas, E.; Healey, J. Toward machine emotional intelligence: Analysis of affective\nphysiological state. *IEEE Trans. Pattern Anal. Mach. Intell.* **2001**, *23*, 1175–1191. [CrossRef]
52. Zong, S. A study on adolescent suicide ideation in South Korea. *Procedia-Soc. Behav. Sci.* **2015**, *174*, 1949–1956. [CrossRef]
53. Park, H.Y.; Heo, J.; Subramanian, S.V.; Kawachi, I.; Oh, J. Socioeconomic Inequalities in Adolescent Depression in South Korea: A Multilevel Analysis. *PLoS ONE* **2012**, *7*, e47025. [CrossRef] [PubMed]
54. Scherer, K.R. What are emotions? and how can they be measured? *Soc. Sci. Inf.* **2005**, *44*, 695–729. [CrossRef]
55. Ali, S.; Kibria, M.G.; Jarwar, M.A.; Kumar, S.; Chong, I. Microservices Model in WoO based IoT Platform for Depressive Disorder Assistance. In Proceedings of the International Conference on Information and Communication Technology Convergence (ICTC 2017), Jeju Island, Korea, 18–20 October 2017.
56. Jarwar, M.A.; Ali, S.; Chong, I.Y. Exploring Web Objects enabled Data-Driven Microservices for E-Health Service Provision in IoT Environment. In Proceedings of the 9th International Conference on Information and Communication Technology Convergence (ICTC 2018), Jeju Island, Korea, 17–19 October 2018; pp. 112–117. [CrossRef]
57. Kumar, S.; Kibria, M.G.; Ali, S.; Jarwar, M.A.; Chong, I. Smart spaces recommending service provisioning in WoO platform. In Proceedings of the 2017 International Conference on Information and Communications (ICIC), Hanoi, Vietnam, 26–28 June 2017; pp. 311–313.
58. Jarwar, M.; Kibria, M.; Ali, S.; Chong, I. Microservices in Web Objects Enabled IoT Environment for Enhancing Reusability. *Sensors* **2018**, *18*, 352. [CrossRef]

59. Ali, S.; Kim, H.-S.; Chong, I. Implementation model of WoO based smart assisted living IoT service. In Proceedings of the 2016 International Conference on Information and Communication Technology Convergence (ICTC), Jeju Island, Korea, 19–21 October 2016; pp. 816–818.
60. Ali, S.; Kibria, M.G.; Chong, I. WoO enabled IoT service provisioning based on learning user preferences and situation. In Proceedings of the 2017 International Conference on Information Networking (ICOIN), Da Nang, Vietnam, 11–13 January 2017; pp. 474–476.
61. Hosseinifard, B.; Moradi, M.H.; Rostami, R. Classifying depression patients and normal subjects using machine learning techniques and nonlinear features from EEG signal. *Comput. Methods Progr. Biomed.* **2013**, *109*, 339–345. [CrossRef]
62. Khodayari-Rostamabad, A.; Reilly, J.P.; Hasey, G.M.; de Bruin, H.; MacCrimmon, D.J. A machine learning approach using EEG data to predict response to SSRI treatment for major depressive disorder. *Clin. Neurophysiol.* **2013**, *124*, 1975–1985. [CrossRef]
63. Knott, V.; Mahoney, C.; Kennedy, S.; Evans, K. EEG power, frequency, asymmetry and coherence in male depression. *Psychiatry Res. Neuroimaging* **2001**, *106*, 123–140. [CrossRef]
64. Khowaja, S.A.; Prabono, A.G.; Setiawan, F.; Yahya, B.N.; Lee, S.-L. Contextual activity based Healthcare Internet of Things, Services, and People (HIoTSP): An architectural framework for healthcare monitoring using wearable sensors. *Comput. Netw.* **2018**, *145*, 190–206. [CrossRef]
65. Breusch, T.S.; Pagan, A.R. A Simple Test for Heteroscedasticity and Random Coefficient Variation. *Econometrica* **1979**, *47*, 1287. [CrossRef]
66. White, H. A Heteroskedasticity-Consistent Covariance Matrix Estimator and a Direct Test for Heteroskedasticity. *Econometrica* **1980**, *48*, 817. [CrossRef]

9

Perceptions of Fetal Alcohol Spectrum Disorder (FASD) at a Mental Health Outpatient Treatment Provider in Minnesota

Jerrod Brown [1,2,3,*] and Diane Harr [4]

1 Pathways Counseling Center, Inc., St. Paul, MN 55104, USA
2 Department of Human Services, College of Humanities and Social Sciences, Concordia University, St. Paul, MN 55104, USA
3 American Institute for the Advancement of Forensic Studies, St. Paul, MN 55104, USA
4 Department of Graduate Teacher Education, College of Education, Concordia University, St. Paul, MN 55104, USA; dharr@csp.edu
* Correspondence: jerrod01234brown@live.com,

Abstract: Resulting from prenatal exposure to alcohol, Fetal Alcohol Spectrum Disorder (FASD) is characterized by deficits in adaptive and cognitive functioning. This disorder is typically accompanied by co-occurring disorders and conditions (e.g., mood, anxiety, psychosis, and substance use disorders). This complicated presentation of diverse symptoms makes the process of screening, assessing, and diagnosing FASD very difficult, limiting the likelihood that clients receive the treatment and services that they need. Although mental health care providers have an opportunity to intervene on behalf of clients with FASD, professionals may not be very familiar or comfortable with this complicated and life-altering disorder. The present study explores the familiarity of 79 mental health outpatient treatment professionals' personal knowledge and training about FASD. Findings suggest that the majority of respondents had received at least some FASD training, understood the basic symptoms of FASD, and were realistic about FASD's impact on treatment.

Keywords: fetal alcohol spectrum disorder; education; mental health; training

---

1. Introduction

Estimates of Fetal Alcohol Spectrum Disorder's (FASD) prevalence in the United States range from 3% to 5% [1]. Disorders that fall under the FASD umbrella include fetal alcohol syndrome (FAS), alcohol related neurodevelopmental disorder (ARND), and alcohol related birth defects (ARBD). This irreversible affliction is caused by prenatal exposure to alcohol [2]. FASD is characterized by deficits in cognitive (e.g., executive function, information processing, short- and long-term memory, and attentional control), social (e.g., immaturity and verbal and non-verbal communication skills), and adaptive functioning [3–7]. In a minority of cases, physical impairments like dysmorphia and musculoskeletal conditions are even present [6,8–10]. These diverse and ranging symptoms often have devastating consequences on an individual's functioning at school and work along with independent living skills such as managing a household and financial responsibilities [11–13].

In addition to the symptoms of FASD, the disorder is typically accompanied by co-occurring disorders and conditions. In fact, researchers have estimated that nearly 90% of those with FASD also exhibit at least one comorbid condition [14,15]. These co-occurring conditions are often mood (i.e., depression and bipolar), anxiety, psychosis (i.e., schizophrenia), behavioral (e.g., ADHD and conduct disorder), attachment (e.g., reactive), or substance use disorders [15–17]. As such, the presentation of FASD symptoms and co-occurring disorders can present in vastly different combinations on a client-by-client basis [15,18,19]. The wide array of symptoms from both FASD and any co-occurring conditions make the process of screening, assessing, and diagnosing FASD very difficult. This contributes to the frequent missed diagnosis and misdiagnosis of the disorder [2,18,20]. A consequence of these difficulties is that those with FASD are less likely to receive the treatment and services that they need [21].

In an effort to improve identification and diagnosis, FASD was included in the Diagnostic and Statistical Manual, Fifth Edition [22]. This is called Neurodevelopmental Disorder Associated with Prenatal Alcohol Exposure (ND-PAE) and is considered a condition in need of further study. Diagnostic criteria include the presence of prenatal alcohol exposure along with impairments in neurocognitive, self-regulation, and adaptive functioning. While these diagnostic criteria undergo clinical and scientific evaluation, FASD must still be diagnosed by medical professionals in the meantime.

When not accurately diagnosed and properly treated and supported, individuals with FASD are prone to negative life outcomes including involvement in the criminal justice system [23–25]. For example, Streissguth, Barr, Kogan, and Bookstein [15] estimate that approximately 60% of individuals with FASD enter into the criminal justice system at some point in their lives. This legal involvement could be the direct consequence of the cognitive, social, and adaptive functioning impairments of FASD [26]. Unfortunately, these FASD symptoms also limit an individual's capacity to function in the criminal justice system. Specifically, individuals with FASD could have difficulty making important legal decisions (e.g., waiving Miranda rights), participating in police interviews and interrogations, and being competent to stand trial [27–31].

Although mental health care providers have an opportunity to intervene on behalf of clients with FASD, professionals may not be very familiar with this devastating disorder [32]. This concern is emphasized by the findings of a survey about psychologists' knowledge of FASD from 2007 of 447 doctoral-level American Psychological Association members [33]. This questionnaire was designed to gauge a respondent's knowledge of alcohol's effects during pregnancy and FASD. The results indicated that these professionals generally had limited familiarity with the prevention, diagnosis, and treatment of prenatal alcohol exposure [33]. Further, a 2003 study of 391 Canadian psychiatrists found approximately half of respondents felt unprepared to assist patients in the management of alcohol misuse and its consequences [34].

The present study, focused specifically on FASD, was developed to explore the generalizability of previous research and any changes over the last decade. Specifically, mental health outpatient treatment providers in a Midwestern state were surveyed about their training and knowledge of FASD. We have three hypotheses. First, we expect that professionals will have had at least some training on FASD. Second, we predict these professionals will have a strong grasp of foundational knowledge in the area of FASD. Third, we anticipate that professionals will believe additional training and the availability of FASD screening tools would be beneficial.

2. Materials and Methods

The survey titled Perceptions of Fetal Alcohol Spectrum Disorder (FASD) at a Mental Health Outpatient Treatment Provider in Minnesota was constructed and administered using Google Forms. The mental health outpatient treatment provider sampled for this survey was Headway Emotional Health Services (HEHS). This organization has provided care and services in the Twin Cities Minnesota community for over 40 years. Headway treats children, adolescents, adults, couples, and families across a wide range of circumstances. This organization was selected specifically because it has many years of experience treating individuals with either suspected or confirmed FASD. The anonymous survey was distributed electronically by a representative of Headway to the staff of the organization ($n = 189$). After the initial recruitment email, two subsequent reminder emails were sent out between 20 August 2018, and 20 September 2018, requesting participation. Prior to completing the survey, participants were prompted with an informed consent page. Participants were required to select the "Agree" option to begin the survey. Responses were stored in a Google Sheets document for later analysis. This study was approved by the Institutional Review Board at Concordia University, St. Paul, Minnesota (Study Number: 2017_103).

Of 189 potential participants, 42% (n = 79) at least partially completed the survey submission. The respondents were mostly women (82%; n = 65) and between the ages of 25–34 (49%, n = 32) or 35–44 (33%, n = 26). Although all respondents earned at least an undergraduate degree, such as an Associate of Arts (AA), Bachelor of Arts (BA), 65% (n = 51) had a graduate degree, including Master of Arts (MA) or other Master's level degrees, and 6% (n = 5) had a doctorate degree. The majority of respondents had 10 years or less of experience in the field of mental health, with 41% (n = 32) having less than 5 years of experience and 37% (n = 29) having between 5 and 10 years of experience.

The survey consisted of 30 closed-ended response questions and two open-ended long answer questions. Of these 32 items, 25 items were specific to FASD (e.g., familiarity with FASD symptoms, impact of FASD on treatment, and FASD training received) and seven items pertained to demographic information (i.e., age, gender, education history, and job position). Each survey question can be reviewed in Appendix A.

3. Results

3.1. Training

To explore the level, recency, and quality of FASD training among respondents, a series of questions were asked. First, participants were asked if they had ever received FASD training. Almost two-thirds of participants (62%, n = 49) indicated that they had received FASD training in the past, whereas 38% (n = 30) had never received FASD.

Second, among those who had received FASD training, participants were asked about how long ago the FASD training took place. For most respondents, the training was between 1 and 5 years ago (61%, n = 31). The next most common responses were that the training took place between 5 and 10 years ago (18%, n = 9), within the last 12 months (16%, n = 8), and more than 10 years go (4%, n = 2). Of interest, a participant who indicated never having had a training did select between 1 and 5 years ago.

Third, the participants were asked if FASD training was helpful in determining the presence of FASD. Of those that received training, most found the training "Helpful" (33%, n = 26). The other responses were "Somewhat Helpful" (10%, n = 8), "Somewhat Unhelpful" (9%, n = 7), and "Not Helpful at All" or "Extremely Helpful" (4%, n = 3). Nonetheless, a substantial proportion of the group, consistent with above, still had not received FASD training (41%, n = 32).

Fourth, the participants were asked if they felt education/training in the identification of FASD should occur regularly. The most common responses were that training should occur every 2 years on a recurring basis (47%, n = 37) or every 12 months on a recurring basis (33%, n = 26). Fewer respondents endorsed having training every 5 years on a recurring basis (13%, n = 10), every 6 months on a recurring basis (6%, n = 5), or not having regular training at all (1%, n = 1).

Finally, the participants were asked if a continuing education course that addresses the interaction between FASD and the mental health system would be beneficial. The response was overwhelmingly positive. The vast majority responded "Yes" (96%, n = 76), whereas only 4% (n = 3) responded "No."

3.2. Diagnostic Knowledge

To better understand the knowledge of mental health practitioners in the area of FASD, a range of questions were asked about the disorder and its presentation. First, the participants were asked to select all of the consequences associated with FASD from a list of 15 choices, with those selected by 90% or more of all study participants shown in Figure 1 below. This included Impulse Control Problems (96%), Social Skill Deficits (95%), Poor judgment (95%), Attention Deficits (94%), Executive Function Deficits (92%), Learning Disabilities (91%), Adaptive Functioning Deficits (91%), and Concentration

Deficits (90%). These findings indicate that the mental health professionals were very familiar with many of the most commonly associated consequences of FASD.

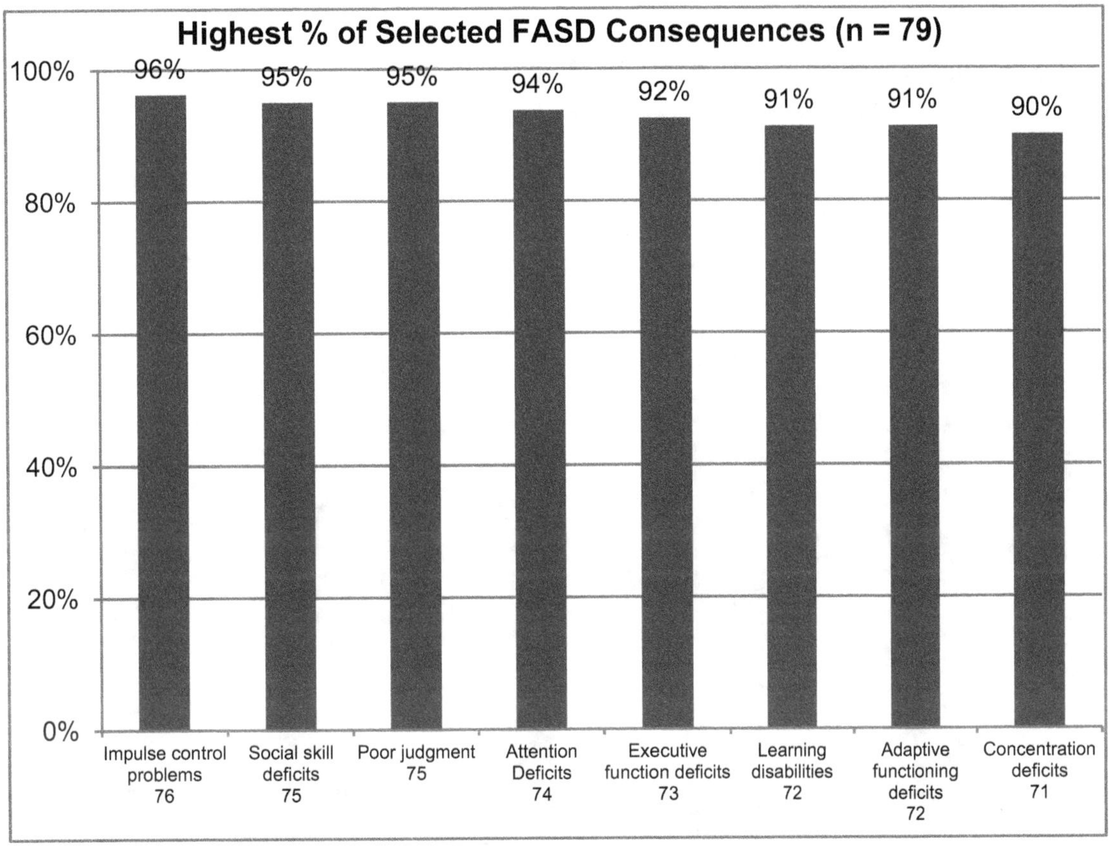

Figure 1. Highest % of selected Fetal Alcohol Spectrum Disorder (FASD) consequences.

Similarly, participants were asked to identify any mental health disorders that commonly co-occur with FASD from a list of 22 choices with those selected by 50% or more of all study participants shown in Figure 2 below. The most common co-occurring mental health disorders were Attention Deficit/Hyperactivity Disorder (87%), Oppositional Defiant Disorder (75%), Learning Disorder (70%), Reactive Attachment Disorder (61%), and Conduct Disorder (54%). Less commonly endorsed disorders included Post-Traumatic Stress Disorder (33%), Autism Spectrum Disorder (28%), Sleep disorders (22%), and Anti-Social Personality Disorder (19%).

Another important topic of consideration is how often individuals with FASD present with facial abnormalities. This includes physical features like wideset eyes, thin upper lip, smooth philtrum, upturned nose, epicanthal folds, and small head size. The majority of respondents selected that facial features were present in 1% to 25% (53%, *n* = 42). Others responded that facial features were present in 26% to 50% (32%, *n* = 25), 51% to 75% (9%, *n* = 7), or 76% to 100% (6%, *n* = 5) of FASD cases.

In light of these ranging diagnostic features and co-occurring disorders, the participants were asked about the potential utility of a FASD screening tool or application. The overwhelming response was that a screening tool or application would be helpful (97%, *n* = 76). Only 3% (*n* = 2) of respondents did not believe such an instrument would be helpful.

The knowledge of mental health professionals on the impacts of FASD on the various facets of everyday life was also explored. When asked if FASD significantly impacts the social skills of the client, most participants "Agreed" that social skills were impaired (62%, *n* = 49) and a substantial proportion of participants even "Strongly Agreed" (28%, *n* = 22). Fewer participants endorsed the options of "Neither Disagree nor Agree" (8%, *n* = 6) or "Strongly Disagree" (3%, *n* = 2). Similarly, participants were asked if FASD significantly impairs parenting ability. This notion was "Agreed" with by just under half of the participants (42%, $n = 33$). However, others responded "Neither Disagree nor Agree" (33%, $n = 26$), "Strongly Agree" (23%, $n = 18$), "Disagree" (1%, $n = 1$), or "Strongly Disagree" (1%, $n = 1$).

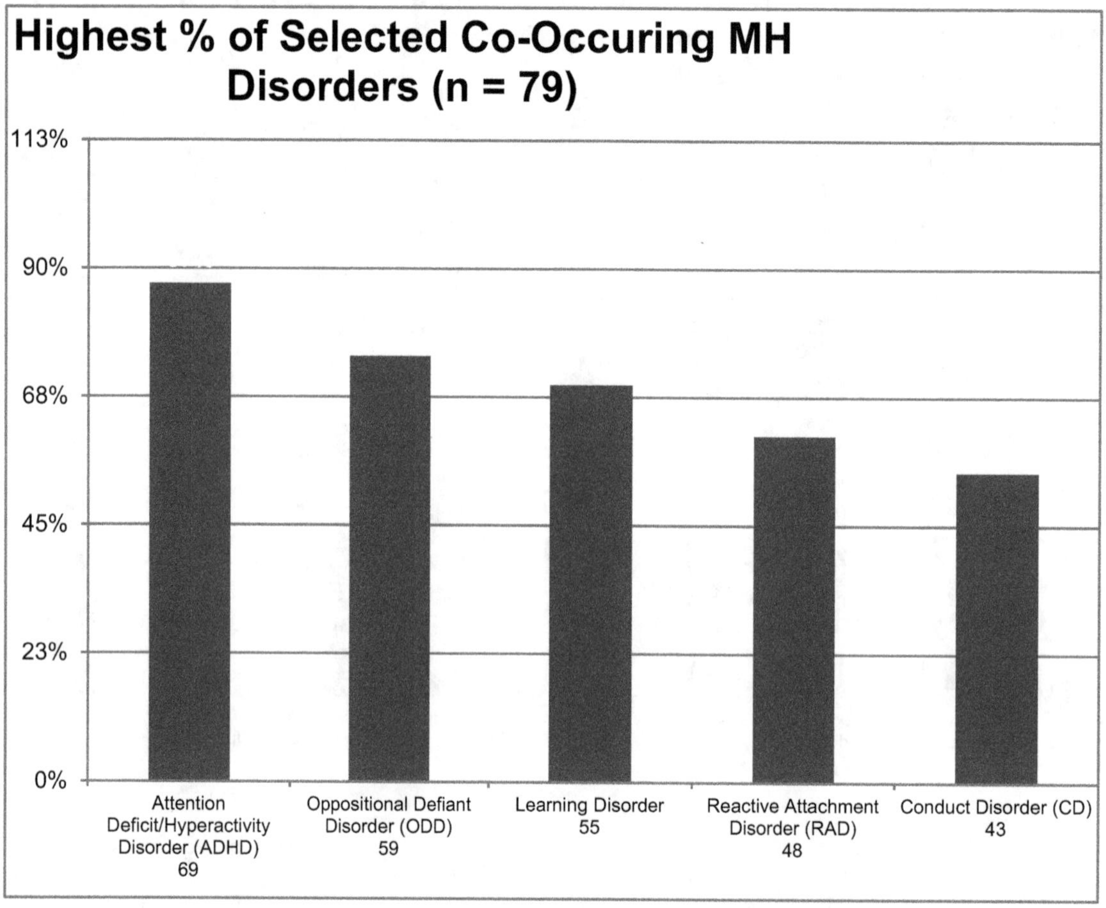

Figure 2. Highest % of selected co-occurring mental health disorders.

3.3. Treatment

To explore the perceptions of mental health professionals on the impact of FASD on treatment, a series of questions were developed and asked. First, the participants were asked if FASD plays a role in patient adherence to a treatment plan. A majority of the participants "Agree" that FASD impacts adherence (57%, $n = 45$). That said, others responded "Neither Disagree nor Agree" (20%, $n = 16$), "Strongly Agree" (13%, $n = 10$), "Disagree" (6%, $n = 5$), or "Strongly Disagree" (4%, $n = 3$). Second, the participants were asked if the duration of treatment increases for patients with FASD. Again, a majority of the participants "Agree" that FASD increases treatment duration (53%, $n = 42$). However, others responded "Neither Disagree nor Agree" (28%, $n = 22$), "Strongly Agree" (16%, $n = 13$), "Disagree" (1%, $n = 1$), and "Strongly Disagree" (1%, $n = 1$). Third, the participants were asked if FASD adversely impacts the effectiveness of services provided. The most common responses were "Neither Disagree nor Agree" (48%, $n = 38$) and "Agree" (41%, $n = 32$). Very few participants endorsed either "Disagree" (6%, $n = 5$) or "Strongly Agree" (5%, $n = 4$). Fourth, the participants were asked how likely they would be to refer a client with FASD to an outside mental health provider. The most common responses were "I do not have clients with FASD" (29%, $n = 23$), "76% to 100%" (23%, $n = 18$), and "26% to 50%" (20%, $n = 16$). Less commonly endorsed options included "51% to 75%" (15%, $n = 12$) and "0% to 25%" (13%, $n = 10$).

Lastly, to identify the respondents' preferred treatment strategies, the survey asked, "What interventions and strategies have you found most helpful when treating this population within the context of outpatient mental health treatment?" In this optional response, some respondents opted to identify specific interventions whereas others identified techniques and strategies. Interventions identified included cognitive behavioral therapy, behavioral therapy, family therapy, and applied behavioral analysis. Approaches and strategies identified included using concrete answers, emphasizing repetition, maintaining consistency and structure, working towards goals, developing social skills, and coordinating services. For a complete summary of responses, please see Table 1.

Table 1. Summary of responses.

Responses
Coordinated services
Black and white and concrete answers
Repetition
Impulse control related strategies such as: "Stop and think about the consequences before acting"
Narrative-based approaches
Increase social supports and services provided; repetitive and simplified Cognitive Behavioral Therapy (CBT) and interpersonal interventions; social skills training and practice (repetitive)
Client centered therapy
ABA therapy (Applied Behavioral Analysis)
Repetition of strategies, using visuals, parent education and support, connecting behavior to consequences and if it is a situation where we are discussing their behavior then discussing it without blame. For younger clients, token reinforcements seem to work well. For older clients, focusing on transition planning and ensuring continued support once they turn 18
Coordinating care with residential mental health support whenever possible (if client receives these services too, of course)
Depends on the client
Repetition, consistency, and mindfulness / coping skills
Behavioral interventions, helping them express their feelings, skills related work
Behavioral therapy
Consistency, clear and concrete expectations and communication with client and/or parent or guardian. Use of visuals definitely help
More in depth with questions and explanations. Working with the client on goals and treatment instead of choosing and having client adapt to my goals
Repetitive social skill training. one on one discussion, in order to gain insight into an issue, discuss something in multiple pieces, building on the information until the perspective is seen differently with empathy
SKILLS work, brain scanning and neurocognitive testing
Repetition, basic skills, Independent Living Skills (ILS)
Psych-education, slower pace of therapy, reducing own expectations, being flexible with strategies, exploring/developing support systems for client.
Emotional regulation through body relaxation and awareness. Social skills
CBT and skills-based supports

3.4. Suggestibility and Crime

To explore the less explored consequences of FASD, three additional questions were administered in relation to suggestibility and crime. First, the participants were asked if FASD increased an individual's susceptibility to suggestion. The vast majority of respondents believed that FASD increased the risk of suggestibility (75%, *n* =59). Only 25% (*n* = 20) of participants responded that this was not the case. Further, the participants were asked if FASD increased an individual's susceptibility to the unintentional creation of false memories (confabulation). Again, the majority of respondents believed that FASD increased the risk of confabulation (61%, *n* = 48). However, approximately 39% (*n* = 31) did not believe that FASD increased the risk of confabulation. Finally, the participants were also asked what percentage of individuals impacted by FASD become involved in the criminal justice system. The most common responses were that "26% to 50%" (37%, *n* = 39) and "51% to 75%" (30%, *n* = 24) of individuals with FASD become involved in the criminal justice system. Fewer respondents endorsed "1% to 10%" (16%, *n* = 13) or "11% to 25%" (16%, *n* = 13).

4. Discussion

FASD is a devastating condition that can be challenging for mental health professionals to deal with in clinical settings. There are FASD diagnostic clinics in many states. Additional information can be found at the websites of the National Organization on Fetal Alcohol Syndrome (NOFAS), which includes the Minnesota Organization on Fetal Alcohol Syndrome (MOFAS). The Minnesota Organization on Fetal Alcohol Syndrome recently renamed itself as Proof Alliance, additional information can be found at proofalliance.org. This study sought to better understand how professionals understood and serve clients with FASD. This study has four key findings. First, the majority of respondents (76%) had at least some FASD training within the last 5 years. Second, the vast majority of respondents could demonstrate basic knowledge of FASD. For example, respondents were able to identify key symptoms of FASD including deficits in cognitive function (e.g., executive function and attention), social skills, and adaptive functioning. Third, respondents typically recognized the impact of FASD of treatment length, effectiveness, and adherence. Fourth, the majority of respondents recognized FASD's impact on suggestibility and crime. Together, these findings suggest that mental health professionals may be better equipped to understand and treat FASD than professionals over a decade ago. Nonetheless, future research is needed to better understand if and how these findings may generalize from the staff members of this facility to other settings across the United States.

Limitations

This study had several limitations. Less than half the sampled population responded to complete the entire survey. Overall, participants totaled 79 individuals, which limited the power of the study. The participants that did complete the survey were overwhelmingly female with approximately four female participants for each male participant. Some of the research reported on crime involvement is somewhat dated and reinforces the need for more current studies in light of the changing legal landscape. The present study was unable to ascertain the sources participants utilized to obtain FASD training. Understanding where professionals are obtaining training on FASD would be substantially beneficial to the field's efforts to increase knowledge about FASD in general.

5. Conclusions

FASD is a disorder which causes cognitive, social, and adaptive challenges throughout a person's life. It is, therefore, imperative that mental health professionals remain cognizant of both the identification and treatment of clients with FASD. It must be recognized, however, that such identification is challenging due to misdiagnosis and undiagnosed situations. FASD does have a large scope of symptoms, some of which present physically and some without. There are often comorbid or secondary disabilities that affect the clients as well. Due to the executive and adaptive functioning deficits, assessment can be complicated with this population. Contributing to this, there is a lack of standardized and established FASD screening and assessment tools available to professionals. For these reasons, and more, mental health professionals require on-going training and education specific to working with individuals with FASD. This allows for continued growth in knowledge and understanding focused on the effects and impact of prenatal exposure to alcohol. With such awareness, individuals with FASD are more likely to receive support and servicing from mental health professionals.

Author Contributions: Conceptualization, J.B. and D.H.; Methodology, J.B.; Software, J.B.; Validation, J.B. and D.H.; Formal Analysis, J.B. and D.H.; Investigation, J.B.; Resources, J.B.; Data Curation, J.B.; Writing-Original Draft Preparation, J.B.; Writing-Review & Editing, D.H.; Visualization, J.B. and D.H.; Supervision, J.B.

Appendix A

Survey Questions

1. Please describe the consequences associated with FASD? Choose all that apply.
2. Overall, what percentage of individuals (clients) impacted by FASD become involved in the criminal justice system? Choose one response.
3. Based on your knowledge, what percentage of individuals diagnosed with Fetal Alcohol Spectrum Disorder have facial abnormalities such as wideset eyes, thin upper lip, smooth philtrum, upturned nose, epicanthal folds, or small head size? Choose one response.
4. What are the most common co-occurring Mental Health Disorders amongst your clients with FASD? Choose all that apply.
5. Have you ever received training (education) related to FASD? Choose one response.
6. If you had training, how long ago was this training/education? Choose one response.
7. If you have received training on the recognition of FASD, how useful was it in helping you decide if someone has FASD? Choose one response.
8. Do you think having an FASD screening tool/app would help you screen more often for FASD? Choose one response.
9. How many years have you been working in the field of mental health? Choose one response.
10. In a typical month how many individuals do you interact with who are impacted by FASD as part of your duties as a mental health worker? Choose one response.
11. What % of your client's with FASD also have a history of suicidal behaviors? Choose one response.
12. What % of your client's with FASD also have (a) separate, one or more, co-occurring mental health disorder(s)? Choose one response.
13. What % of your client's with FASD demonstrate impulse control issues? Choose one response.
14. FASD significantly impacts the accuracy of the data gathered from the patient during intake. Choose one response.
15. FASD significantly impacts the diagnostic data gathering process. Choose one response.
16. FASD plays a role in misdiagnosing of new patients. Choose one response.
17. FASD plays a role in patient compliance with keeping their scheduled mental health appointments. Choose one response.
18. FASD plays a role in patient adherence to a treatment plan. Choose one response.
19. The duration of treatment increases for patients with FASD. Choose one response.
20. FASD significantly impacts the social skills of the patient. Choose one response.
21. FASD significantly impairs the parenting ability of the patient. Choose one response.
22. FASD significantly adversely impacts the effectiveness of services provided. Choose one response.
23. How likely are you to refer a patient with FASD to an outside mental health provider? Choose one response.
24. Do you believe FASD increases an individual's susceptibility to suggestion? Choose one response.
25. Do you believe FASD increases an individual's susceptibility to the unintentional creation of false memories (confabulation)? Choose one response.
26. What interventions and strategies have you found most helpful when treating this population within the context of outpatient mental health treatment? Answering is optional.
27. What is your gender? Choose one response.
28. What is your age range? Choose one response.
29. Do you feel education/training in the identification of FASD should occur regularly? Choose one response.
30. Would you benefit from a continuing education course that addresses the interaction between FASD and the mental health system? Choose one response.
31. What is your highest completed level of education? Choose one response.

32. What is your role at Headway? Please list your title and a brief job description. Answering is optional.

References

1. May, P.A.; Chambers, C.D.; Kalberg, W.O.; Zellner, J.; Feldman, H.; Buckley, D.; Taras, H. Prevalence of fetal alcohol spectrum disorders in 4 U.S. communities. *JAMA* **2018**, *319*, 474–482. [CrossRef] [PubMed]
2. Benz, J.; Rasmussen, C.; Andrew, G. Diagnosing fetal alcohol spectrum disorder: History, challenges and future directions. *Paediatr. Child Health* **2009**, *14*, 231–237. [CrossRef] [PubMed]
3. Fuglestad, A.J.; Whitley, M.L.; Carlson, S.M.; Boys, C.J.; Eckerle, J.K.; Fink, B.A.; Wozniak, J.R. Executive functioning deficits in preschool children with Fetal Alcohol Spectrum Disorders. *Child Neuropsychol.* **2015**, *21*, 716–731. [CrossRef] [PubMed]
4. Hofer, R.; Burd, L. Review of published studies of kidney, liver, and gastrointestinal birth defects in fetal alcohol spectrum disorders. *Birth Defects Res. Part A Clin. Mol. Teratol.* **2009**, *85*, 179–183. [CrossRef] [PubMed]
5. Kingdon, D.; Cardoso, C.; McGrath, J.J. Research Review: Executive function deficits in fetal alcohol spectrum disorders and attention-deficit/hyperactivity disorder—A meta-analysis. *J. Child Psychol. Psychiatry* **2016**, *57*, 16–131. [CrossRef]
6. Manning, M.A.; Hoyme, H.E. Fetal alcohol spectrum disorders: A practical clinical approach to diagnosis. *Neurosci. Biobehav. Rev.* **2007**, *31*, 230–238. [CrossRef] [PubMed]
7. Wheeler, S.M.; Stevens, S.A.; Sheard, E.D.; Rovet, J.F. Facial memory deficits in children with fetal alcohol spectrum disorders. *Child Neuropsychol.* **2012**, *18*, 339–346. [CrossRef]
8. Spohr, H.L.; Willms, J.; Steinhausen, H.C. Prenatal alcohol exposure and long-term developmental consequences. *Lancet* **1993**, *341*, 907–910. [CrossRef]
9. Spohr, H.L.; Willms, J.; Steinhausen, H.C. The fetal alcohol syndrome in adolescence. *Acta Paediatr.* **1994**, *404*, 19–26. [CrossRef]
10. Steinhausen, H.C.; Willms, J.; Spohr, H.L. Long-term psychopathological and cognitive outcome of children with fetal alcohol syndrome. *J. Am. Acad. Child Adolesc. Psychiatry* **1993**, *32*, 990–994. [CrossRef]
11. Denys, K.; Rasmussen, C.; Henneveld, D. The effectiveness of a community-based intervention for parents with FASD. *Community Ment. Health J.* **2011**, *47*, 209–219. [CrossRef]
12. Jirikowic, T.; Olson, H.C.; Kartin, D. Sensory processing, school performance, and adaptive behavior of young school-age children with fetal alcohol spectrum disorder. *Phys. Occup. Ther. Pediatr.* **2008**, *28*, 117–136. [CrossRef]
13. Sanders, J.L.; Buck, G. A long journey: Biological and non-biological parents' experiences raising children with FASD. *J. Popul. Ther. Clin. Pharmacol.* **2010**, *17*, e308–e322.
14. Famy, C.; Streissguth, A.P.; Unis, A.S. Mental illness in adults with fetal alcohol syndrome or fetal alcohol effects. *Am. J. Psychiatry* **1998**, *155*, 552–554. [CrossRef]
15. Streissguth, A.P.; Barr, H.M.; Kogan, J.; Bookstein, F.L. *Understanding the Occurrence of Secondary Disabilities in Clients with Fetal Alcohol Syndrome (FAS) and Fetal Alcohol Effects (FAE)*; Final report to the Centers for Disease Control and Prevention (CDC); University of Washington School of Medicine: Seattle, WA, USA, 1996; pp. 96–106.
16. Crocker, N.; Vaurio, L.; Riley, E.P.; Mattson, S.N. Comparison of verbal learning and memory in children with heavy prenatal alcohol exposure or attention-deficit/hyperactivity disorder. *Alcohol. Clin. Exp. Res.* **2011**, *35*, 1114–1121. [CrossRef] [PubMed]
17. Green, C.R.; Mihic, A.M.; Nikkel, S.M.; Stade, B.C.; Rasmussen, C.; Munoz, D.P.; Reynolds, J.N. Executive function deficits in children with fetal alcoholspectrum disorders (FASD) measured using the Cambridge Neuropsychological Tests Automated Battery (CANTAB). *J. Child Psychol. Psychiatry* **2009**, *50*, 688–697. [CrossRef] [PubMed]
18. Clarren, S.K.; Lutke, J. Building clinical capacity for fetal alcohol spectrum disorder diagnoses in western and northern Canada. *Can. J. Clin. Pharmacol.* **2008**, *15*, e223–e237.
19. Popova, S.; Lange, S.; Shield, K.; Mihic, A.; Chudley, A.E.; Mukherjee, R.A.; Rehm, J. Comorbidity of fetal alcohol spectrum disorder: A systematicreview and meta-analysis. *Lancet* **2016**, *387*, 978–987. [CrossRef]

20. Morleo, M.; Woolfall, K.; Dedman, D.; Mukherjee, R.; Bellis, M.A.; Cook, P.A. Under-reporting of fetal alcohol spectrum disorders: An analysis of hospital episode statistics. *BMC Pediatr.* **2011**, *11*, 14. [CrossRef]
21. Mills, R.M.; McLennan, J.D.; Caza, M.M. Mental health and other service use by young children with fetal alcohol spectrum disorder. *J. FAS Int.* **2006**, *4*, 1–11.
22. American Psychiatric Association. *Diagnostic and Statistical Manual of Mental Disorders*, 5th ed.; American Psychiatric Association: Washington, DC, USA, 2013; ISBN 978-0-89042-555-8.
23. Brown, N.N.; Wartnik, A.P.; Connor, P.D.; Adler, R.S. A proposed model standard for forensic assessment of Fetal Alcohol Spectrum Disorders. *J. Psychiatry Law* **2010**, *38*, 383–418. [CrossRef]
24. Murawski, N.J.; Moore, E.M.; Thomas, J.D.; Riley, E.P. Advances in diagnosis and treatment of fetal alcohol spectrum disorders: From animal models to human studies. *Alcohol Res. Curr. Rev.* **2015**, *37*, 97–108.
25. Olson, H.C.; Oti, R.; Gelo, J.; Beck, S. "Family matters:" fetal alcohol spectrum disorders and the family. *Dev. Disabil. Res. Rev.* **2009**, *15*, 235–249. [CrossRef]
26. LaDue, R.; Dunne, T. Legal issues and the fetal alcohol syndrome. *FEN Pen* **1995**, *3*, 6–7.
27. Brown, J.M.; Haun, J.; Zapf, P.A.; Brown, N.N. Fetal Alcohol Spectrum Disorders (FASD) and competency to stand trial (CST): Suggestions for a 'best practices' approach to forensic evaluation. *Int. J. Law Psychiatry* **2017**, *52*, 19–27. [CrossRef]
28. Conry, J.L.; Fast, D.K.; Loock, C.A. *Youth in the Criminal Justice System: Identifying FAS and Other Developmental Disabilities*; Final Report to the Ministry of the Attorney General; Province of British Columbia, Ministry of the Attorney General: Vancouver, BC, Canada, 1997.
29. Conry, J.L.; Lane, K.A. *Characteristics of Youth with FASD on Adjudicated Probation Orders*; Final report to the Department of Justice Canada and British Columbia Ministry of Children and Family Development; Ministry of Child and Family Development: Vancouver, BC, Canada, 2009.
30. Roach, K.; Bailey, A. The relevance of fetal alcohol spectrum disorder in Canadian criminal law from investigation to sentencing. *UBCL Rev.* **2009**, *42*, 1–68.
31. Verbrugge, P. *Fetal Alcohol Spectrum Disorder and the Youth Criminal Justice System: A Discussion Paper*; Youth Justice Research; Department of Justice Canada: Ottawa, ON, Canada, 2003.
32. Brown, J.; Harr, D.; Morgan, S.; Varga, S.; Fenrich, A. Fetal Alcohol Spectrum Disorder (FASD): A call on mental health treatment professionals to become informed. *J. Psychol. Psychiatry* **2017**, *1*, 1–3. [CrossRef]
33. Wedding, D.; Kohout, J.; Mengel, M.B.; Ohlemiller, M.; Ulione, M.; Cook, K.; Rudeen, K.; Braddock, S. Psychologists' knowledge and attitudes about fetalalcohol syndrome, fetal alcohol spectrum disorders, and alcohol use during pregnancy. *Prof. Psychol. Res. Pract.* **2007**, *38*, 208–213. [CrossRef]
34. Tough, S.C.; Clarke, M.; Hicks, M. Knowledge and attitudes of Canadian psychiatrists regarding fetal alcohol spectrum disorders. *Can. Child Adolesc. Psychiatry Rev.* **2003**, *12*, 64–71.

10

Four Wellbeing Patterns and their Antecedents in Millennials at Work

Tariku Ayana Abdi [1], José M. Peiró [2], Yarid Ayala [3,*] and Salvatore Zappalà [4,5]

1 Department of Psychology, University of Campania, 8100 Caserta, Italy; tarikuayana.abdi@unicampania.it
2 IVIE & IDOCAL, University of Valencia, 46010 Valencia, Spain; jose.m.peiro@uv.es
3 Department of Economics and Management, Pontificia Universidad Javeriana, 110111 Bogotá, Colombia
4 Department of Psychology, University of Bologna, 40126 Bologna, Italy, salvatore.zappala@unibo.it
5 Department of Human Resource Management and Psychology, Financial University under the Government of the Russian Federation, 125993 Moscow, Russia
* Correspondence: ayala.christianyarid@javeriana.edu.co;

Abstract: Literature suggests that job satisfaction and health are related to each other in a synergic way. However, this might not always be the case, and they may present misaligned relationships. Considering job satisfaction and mental health as indicators of wellbeing at work, we aim to identify four patterns (i.e., satisfied-healthy, unsatisfied-unhealthy, satisfied-unhealthy, and unsatisfied-healthy) and some of their antecedents. In a sample of 783 young Spanish employees, a two-step cluster analysis procedure showed that the unsatisfied-unhealthy pattern was the most frequent (33%), followed by unsatisfied-healthy (26.6%), satisfied-unhealthy (24.8%) and, finally, the satisfied-healthy pattern (14.3%). Moreover, as hypothesized, discriminant analysis suggests that higher levels of job importance and lower levels of role ambiguity mainly differentiate the satisfied-healthy pattern, whereas overqualification and role overload differentiate, respectively, the unsatisfied-healthy and satisfied-unhealthy patterns. Contrary to our expectations, role conflict also characterizes the satisfied-unhealthy pattern. We discuss the practical and theoretical implications of these findings.

Keywords: health; job satisfaction; wellbeing; wellbeing misalignment; Millennials

---

1. Introduction

Employee wellbeing is a multidimensional construct covering various facets and experiences, and it has no single definition [1–3]. However, probably the most influential narrative on wellbeing and health in the workplace is the seminal review by Danna and Griffin [4]. After a thorough synthesis of the literature, these authors propose a theoretical framework to organize and direct future theory, research, and practice focused on wellbeing and health in the workplace. In their model, wellbeing is proposed as the broader, encompassing construct that includes two main elements of the organizational research arena. First, the model suggests including both generalized job-related experiences (e.g., job satisfaction) and more facet-specific dimensions (satisfaction with co-workers). Second, the model also suggests including general health as a sub-component of wellbeing, including mental (e.g., anxiety) or physical indicators (e.g., blood pressure). Based on this model, we study wellbeing at work by focusing on job satisfaction and mental health as main indicators of employees' wellbeing.

Ceteris paribus, researchers often assume that job satisfaction and mental health are associated with each other in a harmonious way, and this assumption is solidly based on previous meta-analytical evidence. For instance, a meta-analysis of 22 studies of over 4000 workers in Hong Kong [5] and another meta-analysis of 485 studies of over 250,000 individuals [6] show that employees with high job satisfaction also show high levels of mental health. Thus, there is strong evidence that these two indicators of wellbeing may have a harmonious association in which high job satisfaction is correlated with high mental health [5,6], and the opposite may be true, that is, low job satisfaction would be associated with low mental health [6]. However, in this study we consider cases where job satisfaction and mental health are associated in misaligned ways; i.e., high job satisfaction could be associated with low mental health, and vice-versa. We first provide some examples of previous research describing these paradoxical patterns, and then we propose and clarify the aim of this study.

The first misaligned wellbeing pattern is characterized by high levels of job satisfaction and low mental health. For instance, an employee may be satisfied with his/her contribution to a new program launch and, at the same time, stressed because the program unfolds more slowly than expected [7]. Another example of this type of misalignment is an employee who occupies a high-level job position who, although enjoying greater job satisfaction, might also experience low mental health in the form of high levels of job-related anxiety [8]. This type of wellbeing misalignment may also be present when high performing employees with higher-than-average salaries have high job satisfaction but also higher levels of job-demands, leading to emotional exhaustion and low mental health [2].

The second misaligned wellbeing pattern is characterized by low levels of job satisfaction and high mental health. A situation illustrating this second scenario might be the case of overqualification. Researchers have shown that overqualified employees, although reporting low levels of job satisfaction in terms of payment, growth, and promotion opportunities or incentives, also report high levels of life satisfaction, which is an indicator of mental health [9–11]. As such, this is a counterintuitive situation and contrasts with the concept of wellbeing spillover, which suggests that the work-domain and family-domain have similar effects on each other [12], and that low levels of job satisfaction should be related to low levels of life satisfaction or mental health.

Together, these two misaligned wellbeing patterns challenge the concept of wellbeing spillover. At the same time, they also challenge the idea that wellbeing at work should be more responsive to conditions and activities in the work-domain, and that context-free wellbeing should be more responsive to health or family-domains [13]. Paradoxically, what these misaligned wellbeing patterns suggest is that specific conditions, activities, or situations at work may simultaneously and independently impact several work-domain (e.g., job satisfaction) or context-free (e.g., mental health) aspects of wellbeing.

Therefore, the main aim of this study is to make a theoretical contribution to the understanding of misaligned wellbeing patterns. To accomplish this research aim, we propose two specific research objectives. The first objective involves the empirical identification of four wellbeing patterns. We argue that we can identify the four just mentioned wellbeing patterns by combining job satisfaction and mental health; they are: the satisfied-healthy pattern (both job satisfaction and mental health are optimized); the unsatisfied-unhealthy pattern (neither job satisfaction nor mental health are optimized); the satisfied-unhealthy pattern (job satisfaction is optimized, but not mental health); and the unsatisfied-healthy pattern (job satisfaction is not optimized, but mental health is). The second specific research objective involves identifying organizational and personal antecedents that characterize and differentiate each of the four patterns. Based on the model of health and wellbeing in the workplace, proposed by Danna and Griffin [4], we consider organizational stress (in terms of role stress and overqualification) and personal factors (in terms of job importance) as possible antecedents of the four wellbeing patterns. In Table A1, we list the constructs definitions and their relationship with employees' wellbeing. In the following, we argue on the role they may have on the mis/aligned wellbeing patterns.

1.1. Role Stress

Job-related role stress has been a topic of concern across multiple disciplines [14]. Role stress can involve role conflict, role ambiguity, and role overload. Here, we briefly introduce how these components are related to job satisfaction and mental health at work.

Role conflict occurs when an employee receives contradictory or incompatible requests from different parties, or when an employee needs to produce results in different contradictory aspects. Role ambiguity occurs when employees may not have clear information about tasks required by their roles, which makes them feel uncertain about what actions to take. In today's workplace context, role conflict and role ambiguity are salient characteristics in organizational settings. For instance, in complex organizational environments (e.g., digitalization, job redesign, multicultural works), employees are constantly required to fulfill multiple expectations and organizational roles that are ambiguous and/or contradict each other [15–17]. Meta-analytic evidence shows that conflicting and ambiguous roles correlate with low job satisfaction and low health [18], corroborating the role theory, which states that role conflict and role ambiguity will lead to job dissatisfaction and anxiety [19]. However, the strength of the effects of role ambiguity and role conflict on job satisfaction and mental health, although significant, may not be same. Miles [20] indicated that role ambiguity has stronger effects than role conflict on job satisfaction and mental health. Consistent with this finding, we argue that the stronger effect of role ambiguity, compared to role conflict, on the unsatisfied-unhealthy pattern is still pending confirmation. However, we do know that both role ambiguity and role conflict are significantly and negatively related to job satisfaction and mental health.

Role overload occurs when employees have too much work to do within a limited time or with limited resources, which increases the demands they must deal with. Role expansion theory states that multiple roles are beneficial for the individual because the positive effects of strong engagement in both paid work and family life outweigh the possible stressful effects on wellbeing [21]. Thus, engaging in various roles (role overload), although depleting mental health, might have positive outcomes for employee job satisfaction in terms of earning extra income, privilege, and status security [21,22], which would be related to the satisfied-unhealthy wellbeing pattern. However, further research is needed to empirically confirm whether role overload is positively related to job satisfaction, but negatively related to mental health wellbeing.

1.1.1. Job Importance

Some scholars have shown that job importance, as an antecedent of employee wellbeing patterns, is associated with high job satisfaction and life satisfaction [23]. Being satisfied with life may also be related to positive mental health [10], which may predict the satisfied-healthy wellbeing pattern. More specifically, studies have shown that jobs that provide employees with job facets that are important to them can enhance their job satisfaction and decrease stress [24]. Therefore, we argue that jobs that provide employees with intrinsic, extrinsic, and social job importance facets enhance job satisfaction and mental health. Accordingly, based on role theory and empirical evidence on job importance, we hypothesize that:

H1: *Role conflict, role ambiguity, and job importance will mainly differentiate between the unsatisfied-unhealthy and the satisfied-healthy patterns.*

H2: *High role overload will characterize employees with the satisfied-unhealthy wellbeing pattern.*

1.1.2. Overqualification

Nowadays, overqualification is ubiquitous across European job markets, especially in Italy and Spain, and even more so among younger employees [25–27]. Beyond its ubiquity, overqualification raises concerns due to its negative effects on job satisfaction. For instance, studies conducted on young Spanish and Italian employees show that overqualified employees have lower job satisfaction [9,26,28].

Some scholars explain the negative effect of overqualification on job satisfaction based on equity theory. According to equity theory, employees compare the resources they put into work (such as level of education, skills, knowledge, experience) to what they receive in return (e.g., payment, recognition, or responsibility), in order to determine their sense of fairness [9]. When they perceive that their input is greater than what they receive, they develop a sense of unfairness, and as a result, they experience dissatisfaction with their job. However, some studies have shown that, although overqualification has a negative relationship with job satisfaction, at the same time, it has a null or positive indirect relationship with mental health [10,26]. Therefore, we argue that overqualification might negatively affect employees' job satisfaction, but not necessarily their mental health. Furthermore, a study in German firms on the effects of overeducation on productivity, comparing employees working in jobs with similar levels of requirements, observed that overqualified employees are found to be healthier and strongly work- and career-minded [29]. Therefore, we also hypothesize that:

H3: *Overqualification will mainly discriminate employees with the unsatisfied-healthy pattern from the rest of the patterns.*

We test our hypotheses in a sample composed of young employees born between 1980 and 2000, typically called Millennials [30]. Knowledge about individual key outcomes such as wellbeing and health in young employees is still limited and deserves the attention of researchers and practitioners [31]. At the same time, there are approximately 1.8 billion millennials around the world. In 2018, they represent nearly 50% of the global workforce [32]. Therefore, improving outcomes for youth is fundamental to building more inclusive and sustainable societies [33], and one way to this is by promoting full and productive employment and decent work for all [...] including young people [...], which is part of the global agenda of the Sustainable Development Goals [34]. Figure 1 summarizes the four wellbeing patterns resulting from job satisfaction and mental health and the five antecedents we are considering.

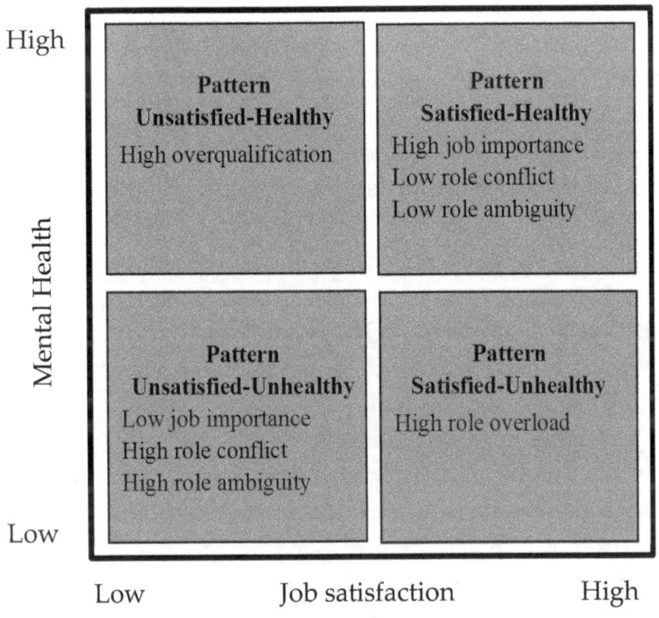

Figure 1. Research Model.

2. Materials and Methods

2.1. Study Design and Procedure

Data were collected from a survey on the transition of young employees to the labor market, which is part of the Valencian Institute of Economic Research (IVIE in Spanish). The survey was designed to facilitate the socioeconomic and psychosocial analysis of young employees' transition to the labor market. Participants between 16 and 30 years old who had been looking for or had found a job in the past 5 years were randomly selected for this study and then contacted by telephone. After two attempted contacts, the researchers replaced non-respondents with a randomly chosen substitute of the same age and gender. Considering the aims of this study, we focused only on respondents who were currently employed. Employees contacted by telephone were always informed of the purpose of the study and assured of the confidentiality of the data. Those who gave their consent to take part in the research were interviewed in their homes using a structured face-to-face procedure.

2.2. Participants

In all, 783 young Spanish respondents were selected for this study. This sample is representative of all the regions in Spain. As mentioned above, the ages of the participants ranged from 16 to 30 years old (M_{age} = 25.21, *SD* = 3.40), with slightly more females (52%). Most of the participants worked in the private sector (82%), and most of them had a temporary contract (58%).

2.3. Variables/Instruments

Job satisfaction was assessed as the composite of extrinsic, intrinsic, and social job satisfaction [35]. This measure can be applied to a wide range of jobs. Extrinsic job satisfaction was measured with seven items. A sample item is: "Indicate your level of satisfaction with your schedule". Intrinsic job satisfaction was measured with seven items. A sample item is: "Indicate your level of satisfaction with the variety of tasks to perform". Finally, social job satisfaction was measured with five items. A sample item is: "Indicate your level of satisfaction with your coworkers". All items were scored on a 5-point Likert scale (from 1 = *not at all* to 5 = *very much*). The three subscales had good reliability, $\alpha = 0.86$ (extrinsic job satisfaction), $\alpha = 0.91$ (intrinsic job satisfaction), $\alpha = 0.80$ (social job satisfaction), and $\alpha = 0.94$ (for the composite of the three subscales).

Items measuring health belong to the scale of the General Health Questionnaire, developed by Banks [36] in young community sample. The reliability of the 12 items reported by Banks [36] was $\alpha = 0.76$. In the current study, we applied four items with higher factor loadings to measure employees' health. A sample item is: "In the last few weeks I have noticed being constantly overwhelmed and under stress". The respondents answered on a 5-point Likert scale (from 1 = *strongly disagree* to 5 = *strongly agree*). The scale showed good reliability ($\alpha = 0.76$).

Job importance was assessed as the composite of extrinsic, intrinsic, and social job importance [37]. We chose 19 items to measure job importance provided by England and Harpaz [37]. Items were preceded by the phrase "Please, indicate the importance that each of the following aspects of the work has for you"; sample items for each facet are: "Security at work"; "Useful work for society"; "Meaningful work that makes sense to do." The respondents answered on a 5-point Likert scale (from 1 = *nothing* to 5 = *a lot*). The scale showed good reliability ($\alpha = 0.89$).

Role ambiguity was measured with the scale provided by Rizzo et al. [19]. The original reliabilities, reported by Rizzo and colleagues in two different samples were good ($\alpha = 0.82$). In the current study, we selected three items with higher factor loadings to measure role ambiguity. A sample item is: "I know how and what my responsibilities and competencies are at work". The respondents answered on a 5-point Likert scale (from 1 = *strongly disagree* to 5 = *strongly agree*). We performed reverse-scoring of the three items. This scale showed good reliability ($\alpha = 0.80$).

Role conflict was measured with the scale provided by Rizzo et al. [19]. The original reliabilities in two different samples were $\alpha = 0.82$. In this study, we selected three items with higher factor loadings to measure role conflict. A sample item is: "I receive incompatible requests from two or more people". The respondents answered on a 5-point Likert scale (from 1 = *strongly disagree*, to 5 = *strongly agree*). This scale also showed a good reliability ($\alpha = 0.75$).

Role overload was measured with the scale of perceived work overload, proposed by Cooke and Rousseau [38]. In the current study, we selected three items with higher factor loadings. A sample item is: "I have too much work to do everything well". The respondents answered on a 5-point Likert scale (from 1 = *strongly disagree* to 5 = *strongly agree*). This scale showed a good reliability score in this study ($\alpha = 0.82$).

Overqualification was measured with the item: "If an individual had to perform your job, what level of education would you recommend him or her to have?" Participants responded on a 12-point scale of the International Standard Classification of Education—ISCED ((from 1 = no studies (ISCED level 1) to Doctorate (ISCED level 12)). We also considered the individual level of education and transformed both the recommended level of education and the individual level of education into years of education. To determine whether an employee was overqualified, the recommended level of education was subtracted from the level of education achieved. Negative and zero scores were considered indicators of education under-qualification and match, respectively, and positive scores were considered indicators of overqualification [25]. In our study, 21.7% of the participants were overqualified, which is similar to the rate (21.5%) of overqualification across Europe [25].

To eliminate some alternative explanations, we considered some variables that could affect our outcome variables and therefore we controlled for gender (0 = male, 1 = female), type of sector (0 = private, 1 = public), type of employment/contract (0 = temporal, 1 = permanent), and age (in years). We describe in detail the choices and procedures related to the control variables in order to ensure transparency and facilitate the reproducibility of the results [39].

In terms of gender, previous studies show that relatively to men, women tend to report higher levels of depression, but that the positive relationship between the efforts to fulfill work role demands (which interfere with employee's ability to fulfill family demands) and depression is stronger among men [40]. In terms of type of sector and age, previous studies also show that public organizations are good in fulfilling their promises to young employees i.e., their psychological contract, and that this is translated into improved job satisfaction [41]. Considering the type of contract, previous studies also suggest that permanents as compared with temporaries engage more in relational psychological contracting, therefore, when this is violated (e.g., by producing job insecurity), this compromises more the job satisfaction for permanents than for temporaries [42]. Finally, previous research [43] also shows that temporary employees report higher wellbeing (e.g., mental health).

2.4. Data Analysis

To identify the four wellbeing patterns, we performed cluster analyses. One of the advantages of using cluster analysis is that unlike other methods that emphasize the relationship among variables, clustering involves sorting cases or variables according to their similarity in one or more dimensions and producing groups that maximize within-group similarity and minimize between-group similarity [44]. Therefore, to identify the four groups of wellbeing patterns, the 783 employees were clustered based on their individual levels of job satisfaction and mental health, applying a two-step cluster analysis procedure. Loglikelihood measured the distance between job satisfaction and mental health. The clustering criterion was Schwarz's Bayesian Criterion (BIC). Finally, to balance the distribution of responses on the job satisfaction and mental health variables, we standardized these two variables to Z-scores ($M = 0$, $SD = 1$) before performing the cluster analyses.

To test our hypotheses, we employed discriminant analysis to test the unique differentiating role of stress (role ambiguity, role conflict, and role overload), job importance, and overqualification across the four patterns. We conducted a stepwise solution to remove variables that did not make a unique contribution to the predictive and discriminatory function at a probability of 0.05 or less. The stepwise criterion was minimization of Wilks' lambda. Similar studies analyzing wellbeing profiles [45] applied discriminant analysis considering Wilks' lambda stepwise minimization criteria, as we did in the current study. Discriminant analysis is a method used in a multi-group setting to find out if a set of independent variables (nominal and/or continuous) are related to group membership and how they are combined to better understand group differences [46]. In fact, various authors suggest the use of cluster analysis in combination with discriminant analysis for further validation of clusters [47].

3. Results

3.1. Descriptive and Preliminary Analyses

We present the summary of descriptive statistics and bivariate correlations for all the variables included in this research in Table 1. Considering preliminary analyses, missing data, which can occur due to nonresponse to some questions, are a common problem in organizational research [48]. Fichman and Cummings [48] argue that improper treatment of missing data (e.g., listwise deletion, mean imputation) could lead to biased statistical inference using complete case analysis statistical techniques. However, given that we have a reasonably large sample size ($n = 783$), and considering that the percentage of missing data was rather small (less than 1%), we concluded that the missing data had no effect on the results of our study [46].

3.2. Cluster Analysis

With five cases identified as outliers and six cases registered as missing from the system, the two-step cluster analysis efficiently and automatically formed four clusters. Following the recommendations of Aguinis, Gottfredson, and Joo [49] about the best practices for defining, identifying, and handling outliers, we defined them as cluster analysis outliers. We handled them by performing the rest of the analyses (e.g., discriminant) with and without them. We found that they were non-influential outliers because they did not significantly change the rest of our results. Figure 2 depicts the centroids (means) of each cluster, expressed in standardized scores of job satisfaction and mental health measures. The silhouette coefficient (which was approximately 0.5) suggested that a four-cluster solution had fair levels of cohesion and separation. We named the four clusters, considering the centroids of job satisfaction and mental health. Cluster 1 was called unsatisfied-unhealthy and comprised 33% of the sample (258 employees), showing the lowest means on job satisfaction (−0.62) and mental health (−0.97). Cluster 2 was called unsatisfied-healthy and comprised 26.6% of the sample (208 employees), showing low levels of job satisfaction standardized means (−0.56), but high levels of mental health (0.76). Cluster 3 was called satisfied-unhealthy and comprised 24.8% of the sample (194 employees), in this case showing high levels of job satisfaction (0.83), but low levels of mental health (−0.15). Finally, Cluster 4 was called satisfied-healthy and comprised only 14.3% of the sample (112 employees), showing the highest levels of both job satisfaction (1.11) and mental health (1.24). To test whether the clusters were significantly different from one another, we conducted an analysis of variance (ANOVA). The results suggested that there were significant differences in job satisfaction ($F_{(4, 772)} = 276.41, p < 0.01$) and health ($F_{(4, 772)} = 477.93, p < 0.01$) among the four patterns. Tukey post-hoc analyses also suggested that all the clusters were significantly different from each other. Together, these results reflect different patterns of the relations between job satisfaction and mental health.

3.3. Discriminant Analysis

We present the summary of the results of the discriminant analysis in Table 2. The results show that employees with the unsatisfied–unhealthy pattern (Cluster 1) have systematically higher means on role ambiguity and lower means on job importance, compared to employees with the satisfied-healthy wellbeing pattern (Cluster 4) and the rest of the patterns. Therefore, we partially confirmed hypothesis 1. Thus, role ambiguity and job importance strongly differentiated between the unsatisfied-unhealthy and satisfied-healthy patterns, but we failed to confirm role conflict. Contrary to our expectations, role conflict mainly characterized satisfied-unhealthy employees. Discriminant results also show that employees with the satisfied-unhealthy pattern (Cluster 3), systematically had significantly higher means on role overload (and role conflict), compared to employees with the satisfied-healthy pattern (Cluster 4). Therefore, we confirmed hypothesis 2, which stated that role overload characterized employees with the satisfied-unhealthy pattern. Finally, employees with the unsatisfied-healthy pattern (Cluster 2) have significantly higher means on overqualification (in comparison with the rest of the patterns) and lower means on role conflict, compared to the satisfied-unhealthy pattern (Cluster 3). Therefore, we also confirmed our hypothesis 3; thus, employees with the unsatisfied-healthy pattern perceived themselves as more overqualified for the job/position compared to their satisfied-unhealthy counterparts and the rest of the patterns.

Table 1. Bivariate correlations and descriptive statistics of the job satisfaction-mental health pattern predictors.

Variables	*M*	*SD*	1	2	3	4	5	6	7	8	9	10	11
1. Age	25.21	3.40	-	−0.02	0.21 **	−0.00	0.02	0.09 *	0.08 *	0.02	0.07	0.12 **	−0.03
2. Gender	0.48	0.50		-	0.11 **	0.06	−0.09 *	0.04	0.08 *	0.07 *	−0.08 *	0.02	0.00
3. Type of contract	0.58	0.50			-	−0.01	−0.05	0.02	0.01	−0.09 *	0.05	0.14 **	0.05
4. Type of sector	0.18	0.38				-	−0.13 **	0.03	0.01	−0.00	0.07 *	0.09 *	−0.04
5. Overqualification	0.22	0.41					-	−0.02	0.09 *	0.04	−0.03	−0.20 **	-0.04
6. Role overload	2.91	0.97						(0.82)	0.37 **	0.07	0.06	0.05	−0.15 **
7. Role conflict	2.78	0.99							(0.75)	0.25 **	−0.06	−0.12 **	−0.29 **
8. Role ambiguity	2.05	0.80								(0.80)	−0.28 **	−0.46 **	−0.25 **
9. Job importance	4.14	0.51									(0.89)	0.50 **	0.16 **
10. Job satisfaction	3.68	0.73										(0.94)	0.26 **
11. Mental health	3.67	0.83											(0.76)

Internal alpha estimates are in parenthesis * $p = 0.05$; ** $p < 0.01$. (two-tailed).

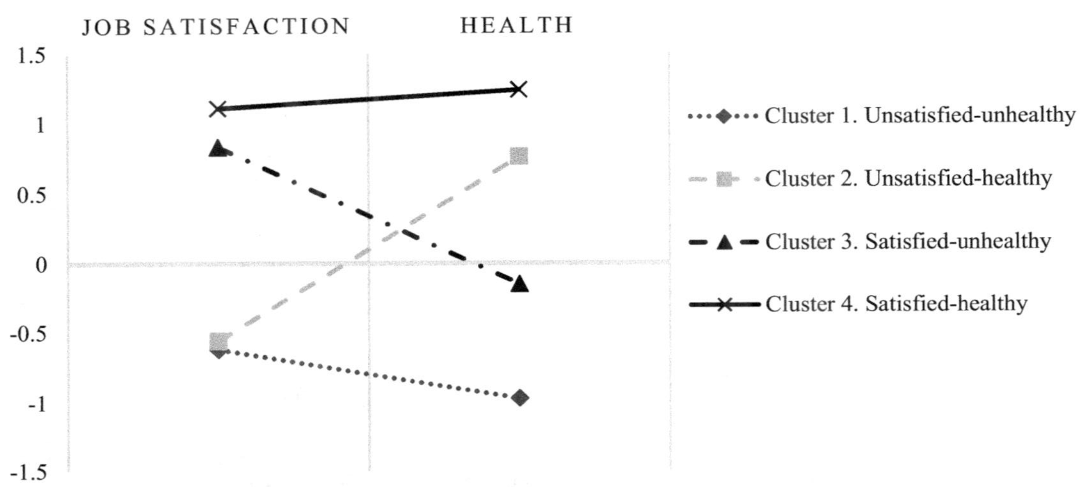

Figure 2. Four-cluster solution: standardized cluster means.

Table 2. Discriminant analysis of the four patterns of relations between job satisfaction and mental health with job importance, role ambiguity, role conflict, role overload, and overqualification as discriminant variables.

Variables/Discriminant Function Statistics	Means (Standard Deviations) of Wellbeing Patterns				Standardized Discriminant Function Coefficients [a]		
	Cluster 1	Cluster 2	Cluster 3	Cluster 4			
	Unsatisfied-Unhealthy (n = 258)	Unsatisfied-Healthy (n = 208)	Satisfied-Unhealthy (n = 194)	Satisfied-Healthy (n = 112)	Function 1	Function 2	Function 3
Covariates							
Gender [b,c]	0.48 (0.50)	0.44 (0.50)	0.52 (0.50)	0.45 (0.50)	0.10	0.07	−0.03
Sector [c,d]	0.21 (0.41)	0.13 (0.33)	0.17 (0.38)	0.22 (0.42)	−0.07	0.06	−0.04
Type of contract [c,e]	0.54 (0.50)	0.58 (0.50)	0.61 (0.49)	0.64 (0.48)	−0.06	0.08	0.15
Age	24.96 (3.43)	24.99 (3.33)	25.85 (3.31)	24.81 (3.56)	−0.07 (−0.09)	0.21 (0.12)	0.77 (**0.77**)
Discriminant variables							
Job importance	3.96 (0.48)	3.97 (0.50)	4.29 (0.44)	4.52 (0.33)	−0.79 (**−0.73**)	0.25 (0.24)	−0.07 (−0.17)
Role ambiguity	2.33 (0.77)	2.12 (0.78)	1.86 (0.66)	1.51 (0.64)	0.65 (**0.50**)	0.17 (0.03)	−0.12 (−0.13)
Role conflict	3.09 (0.88)	2.53 (0.97)	2.82 (0.93)	2.39 (1.12)	0.29 (0.13)	0.84 (**0.78**)	−0.16 (**−0.43**)
Role overload	3.03 (0.88)	2.77 (0.97)	3.03 (0.93)	2.59 (1.07)	0.14 (0.14)	0.54 (0.23)	0.48 (**0.59**)
Overqualification	0.23 (0.42)	0.30 (0.46)	0.17 (0.38)	0.13 (0.34)	0.19 (0.22)	−0.32 (**−0.41**)	0.15 (0.18)
Significance of function					0.01	0.01	0.05
Canonical correlation					0.50	0.26	0.13
Eigenvalue					0.32	0.07	0.02
Explained variance					79.1%	17.1%	3.9%
Centroid of:							
Cluster 1					0.52	0.20	−0.09
Cluster 2					0.27	−0.39	0.06
Cluster 3					−0.42	−0.22	0.16
Cluster 4					−1.15	−0.13	−0.20

Note: n = 772 after listwise deletion of cases with missing data. [a] In parentheses are the coefficients of a stepwise solution that included only variables entered at the 0.05 significance level (coefficients higher than 0.30 are in boldface). The stepwise criterion was minimization of the overall Wilks' lambda. [b] Gender: Coded 0 = male, 1 = female. [c] The group mean of the dichotomous/dummy variables indicates the proportion of the higher coded category. [d] Sector: Coded 0 = private, 1 = public. [e] Type of Contract: Coded 0 = temporary, 1 = permanent.

Together, the results of the discriminant analyses suggest that job importance, role ambiguity, role conflict, role overload, and overqualification help to differentiate among the four patterns of relations between job satisfaction and mental health. When comparing these variables, job importance and role ambiguity were better at differentiating employees with the unsatisfied-unhealthy pattern from those with the satisfied-healthy pattern. Overqualification and role conflict were better at differentiating between employees with the unsatisfied-healthy and satisfied-unhealthy patterns.

4. Discussion

The main aim of this study was to contribute to the theoretical understanding of misaligned wellbeing patterns by considering the profiles emerging from the combination of different levels of job satisfaction and mental health. To accomplish this aim, we pursued two research objectives. The first was to identify four patterns of employee wellbeing based on a configurational variable that combines job satisfaction and mental health. Second, we examined some antecedents that can discriminate each of the four patterns. The antecedents we considered were role stress (role ambiguity, role conflict, and role overload), job importance, and overqualification.

Results showed that hypothesis 1 was partially confirmed. We confirmed that role ambiguity and job importance strongly differentiate between the unsatisfied-unhealthy and satisfied-healthy patterns and the rest of the patterns. On the one hand, our findings are aligned with previous studies on role ambiguity showing that the strength of relationships between role ambiguity, and job dissatisfaction and tension/anxiety are generally stronger than those for role conflict [20], whereas other studies have also shown that role ambiguity has adverse effects on employee job satisfaction and mental health [18,19,50]. On the other hand, with this hypothesis, we also confirmed that employees who perceive various facets of job importance, such as intrinsic (e.g., learning opportunity), extrinsic (e.g., job security), and social (e.g., societal contribution) facets, have optimal job satisfaction and mental health, compared to employees who have high role ambiguity. This result is consistent with previous studies [24].

Contrary to our expectation that role conflict would differentiate employees with the unsatisfied-unhealthy pattern from those with the satisfied-healthy pattern, our results instead showed that role conflict, along with role overload, characterized employees with the satisfied-unhealthy pattern. This result partly supports our hypothesis 2, confirming that role overload characterizes the satisfied-unhealthy pattern. Thus, role conflict and role overload had negative consequences on mental health, but less on job satisfaction. These results corroborate role expansion theory, which asserts that employees who engage in multiple roles at the same time receive incentives, status security, and position increments, which in turn have a positive effect on job satisfaction [21,22]. Furthermore, this study also confirms that focusing only on negative consequences of role stress is just one side of the issue, as asserted by McGowan et al. [50]. As the Job-Demand Control model indicates, highly demanding jobs can provide high decision latitude, control, and autonomy for employees, which, in turn, may decrease the negative effects of job demands on job satisfaction, although they can still produce negative effects on health [50].

Finally, we confirmed our hypothesis 3. Our argument was that overqualification would characterize employees with the unsatisfied-healthy wellbeing pattern. Results show that employees with higher levels of overqualification were characterized by job dissatisfaction and, at the same time, showed optimal levels of mental health. They may perceive that the salary, incentives, and other resources they receive from their work are not fair, given their qualifications. This argument substantiates equity theory. According to equity theory, employees compare the resources they put into the work (such as level of education, skills, knowledge, experience, etc.) to what they receive in return (such as payment, recognition, responsibility, etc.) in order to determine their sense of fairness [9]. If they perceive unfairness in what they receive, they may be dissatisfied with their job. Previous studies also have shown that overqualified employees have low job satisfaction [9,26] but higher satisfaction with their life and better mental health [6,10].

We also accomplished our first specific research objective, which was to identify these four wellbeing patterns involving job satisfaction and mental health. Surprisingly, the most populated cluster was the unsatisfied-unhealthy pattern, and more than half of our sample had a misaligned pattern i.e., either satisfied-unhealthy or unsatisfied-healthy. Traditionally, job satisfaction and mental health are believed to be harmoniously and positively correlated, with high (or low) job satisfaction positively correlated with high (or low) mental health. However, this might not always be the case. In this research, we focused on a new research paradigm by studying the combinations of different levels of job satisfaction and mental health. By combining different levels of job satisfaction and health, we identified four important wellbeing patterns and their antecedents. We especially focused on the anomalous or misaligned wellbeing patterns (satisfied-unhealthy or unsatisfied-healthy) as new typologies. Therefore, we believe that our research findings may motivate scholars to investigate the wellbeing patterns by using the current model as a framework. Furthermore, future studies could also combine the effects of role ambiguity, role conflict, role overload, job importance, and overqualification to move towards more generalizable empirical findings and theory development.

The results that job satisfaction and mental health together form four wellbeing patterns, indicate the need for theoretical precision; it is in fact important to integrate this complexity into the harmonious relationship between job satisfaction and mental health in order to study a broader taxonomy of relations and the conditions in which these patterns are elicited. For instance, our study questions the model of health and wellbeing in the workplace by Danna and Griffin [4], suggesting that it should be integrated with the four patterns of wellbeing and mental health described here. At the same time, our study questions whether wellbeing spillover always happens. Wellbeing spillover proposes that work and family domains of wellbeing have similar effects on one another [12]; therefore, we would expect low levels of job satisfaction to be related to low levels of mental health. Although our study suggests that this may be the case for the satisfied-healthy and unsatisfied-unhealthy patterns, and their antecedents in terms of role ambiguity and role importance, our results also suggest that this spillover may not always take place because spillover may not be present in the misaligned patterns. The results on their antecedents also suggest that work-related conditions and activities may affect work-domain (e.g., job satisfaction) and context-free (mental health) wellbeing at the same time, which challenges the idea that context-free wellbeing should be more responsive to health or family-domains [13]. We have already described why role conflict, role overload, and overqualification are separately related to the misaligned patterns, but we identified an alternative interaction explanation. For instance, in the introduction of this paper we argued that young employees who are overqualified may not have worse mental health because they may have jobs that do not stress them and that are viewed as stepping-stones to help them achieve higher goals (such as finishing college), all of which lead to the unsatisfied-healthy pattern. Aligned with this idea is that these employees also showed lower levels of job importance, thus confirming previous studies that showed that overqualified employees are more cynical about the meaningfulness of their job [51] and such reduce task importance, or significance, depends on how many other overqualified peers work in the same context [52]. We believe that low levels of importance to one's job may be, for young overqualified employees, a way to reduce the cognitive dissonance between their qualification and skill's usage and this may help in maintaining higher level of mental health. Therefore, future research should study the boundary conditions of the relationship between the antecedents here described (role conflict, role overload, and overqualification) and the misaligned wellbeing patterns.

Future studies might also investigate other potentially relevant antecedents, or moderators, of the mis/alignment between job satisfaction and mental health. In particular, following Danna and Griffin [4] and Nielsen et al. [53], it might be interesting to examine the sector of employment, in particular if it involves hazardous and stressful work settings (requiring for instance, night shifts or traveling), job resources as job autonomy, and also HR practices and social support. Literature has in fact showed that such factors may increase or decrease job satisfaction and wellbeing [4,53], but it should be examined if they differentially affect job satisfaction and mental health, also in relation to the family status of the employees (single, married, with children) and family history of mental health.

Finally, another major point concerns the sample being studied. The sample is composed of so-called millennials, thus, a very specific subgroup. These employees might differ in their general health (both mental and physical), wellbeing, satisfaction, etc., from other employees. As a group, millennials are in between twenties and late thirties, thus they do have a better physical health than older generations. Nevertheless, their lower tolerance to frustrations and their need to deal and face the economic crisis (initiated on 2008), which results in fewer career opportunities, may have as an effect a poorer level of mental health, especially in minor symptoms such as anxiety, life dissatisfaction, etc. Another specific situation of the millennials is that they face the transition from school to work in a situation that is in many cases not favorable. The support from their families, the resignation to have precarious/flexible jobs, to get incomes for subsistence or searching for jobs abroad, are some of the different ways of coping with the complex and difficult situation that millennials are facing during the actual economic crisis period.

5. Limitations and Practical Implications

One of the potential limitations of the current study is related to the sample, which is limited to young Spanish employees. To make better generalizations about the four wellbeing patterns, it is necessary to document their occurrence in other contexts. However, the sample was representative of all the regions of Spain, and the independent variables (role stress, job importance, and overqualification) that we tested in this research might be applicable to millennials in other contexts, which could make the generalization of these research findings more robust. Therefore, this limitation may be at least partially neutralized because the procedures and variables we used are applicable to millennials in other contexts. In addition, to test the external validity of the study, it would be useful to replicate it with millennials in other countries.

Another limitation is related to the measurement of job satisfaction and mental health. In job satisfaction measurement, cognitive/subjective biases may affect employees' evaluations of their satisfaction. Similarly, we assessed mental health by using the General Health Questionnaires (GHQ) in terms of a specific time period: '*during the past few weeks* ... '. However, events occurring "weeks ago" may be poorly recalled, and, therefore, induce some possible inaccuracy in mental processing [3]. However, the measurements of both job satisfaction and mental health are based on well validated and accepted instruments, and so we expect cognitive/personal biases and inaccuracy in mental processing to have little or no impact on the validity of the current research findings.

One of the main aims of organizational psychology is to improve employees' wellbeing. In this regard, our taxonomical approach provides relevant empirical evidence, facilitating the achievement of this endeavor. First, by combining job satisfaction and mental health, this study maps synergistic but also misaligned wellbeing patterns. Second, our study also provides valuable information of some personal and organizational variables related to them. In this way, our study informs organizational psychologists of when they may be improving at the same time job satisfaction and mental health, but also when this might not happen, creating misaligned wellbeing patterns instead. Thus, an important implication of our study is the provision of a useful wellbeing-pattern taxonomy from where to study and improve employees' wellbeing.

We also identify implications for other stakeholders. For instance, our results show that it would be worthwhile for organizations to find mechanisms to track and ensure the fulfillment of their commitments to millennials. Our results show, in fact, that only a small portion of employees are in the optimal job satisfaction and mental health category, whereas larger portions are in the unsatisfied-unhealthy and misaligned patterns. At the same time, organizations should carefully consider HR policies, such as staffing, to establish mechanisms to avoid phenomena such as role ambiguity, role conflict, role overload, and overqualification. These organizational and personal phenomena have been shown to have toxic effects on both job satisfaction and mental health.

Third, the results show that job importance is an important mechanism for a sustainable young workforce. In our study, young employees who reported having high job importance were characterized by being satisfied and healthy. Therefore, we argue that managers and employers should increase job importance by providing incentives related to job satisfaction and mental health. Often the jobs available for youngsters are "poor" overqualified and in some cases precarious. Thus, it is important that the companies enhance the meaning of work for youngsters offering jobs that are valuable and meaningful. This is the type of "incentives" that may make work more meaningful for youth and less toxic, dissatisfying and unhealthy.

6. Conclusions

At the beginning of this paper, we noted that the relationship between job satisfaction and mental health is mainly considered harmonious, and that there is scarce research about the anomalous/misaligned patterns between these two variables. The main aim of this study was to extend the relationship between job satisfaction and mental health by identifying four patterns: satisfied-healthy, satisfied-unhealthy, unsatisfied-healthy, and unsatisfied-unhealthy. This taxonomy seems to provide a valid, interesting, and useful way to study employees' wellbeing by considering their job satisfaction and mental health. It is our hope that addressing this more extended pattern of relationships between the two variables will lead to a possible resolution of the satisfied-healthy conundrum. Thus, the unsatisfied-healthy or satisfied-unhealthy profiles should be the targets of future research. Moreover, this research has contributed to identifying some organizational and personal antecedents that influence and differentiate the four patterns. Future research will need to study how stable or dynamic these patterns are over time, and what their consequences are in the long run. This knowledge will help us to create more effective interventions so that organizations can assist millennials in moving toward a more positive and optimal job satisfaction level and assess its contribution to health and vice-versa.

Author Contributions: T.A.A. performed formal analyses, visualization, and writing–original draft; Y.A. was responsible for the study conception, design, data curation, and writing–review & editing; J.M.P and S.Z. contributed to the conceptualization, project administration, supervision, and writing–review & editing.

Acknowledgments: The authors also thank the IVIE for the authorization to use the database from the Spanish Observatory of Youth Labor Market Entry and Employment.

Appendix A

Table A1. Constructs Definitions and their relationship with employees' wellbeing.

Constructs	Definitions	Relationships with Employees' Wellbeing
Job satisfaction	Job satisfaction is an individual's attitude toward the job, that is, an overall evaluative judgment about one's job that is caused by affective experiences on the job and (cognitive) beliefs about the job [54].	A recent review of quantitative studies show that job satisfaction is the most common conceptualization of employee wellbeing [55]
Mental health	We operationalize the definition of the health sub-dimension of wellbeing proposed by Danna and Griffin [4] in terms of general positive mental health self-reported by employees [36].	Danna and Griffin [4] consider mental health to be a sub-component of wellbeing at work
Role conflict Role ambiguity	We define role conflict as parties' contradictory expectations about aspects of a single role or between different roles [15,56]. We define *role ambiguity* as lack of sufficient information or uncertainty about expectations and actions to fulfill a role/job [15,56]	Studies indicate that when employees are exposed to conflicting and ambiguous roles, they experience job dissatisfaction and low mental health [18,19].
Role overload	We define *role overload* as lack of the personal resources that an individual needs to fulfill multiple roles, commitments, obligations, or requirements demanded by the work [15]	Research findings on the impact of role overload on employee job satisfaction and mental health are inconsistent. Some scholars, for instance, show that role overload correlates with low job satisfaction [57] and low mental health (such as experiencing fatigue and tension) [38]. However, in other research, Cooke and Rousseau [38] indicate that role overload does not affect the job satisfaction of employees engaged in multiple roles.
Job importance	Job importance refers to the level of personal significance and value an employee associates with various facets of the job (extrinsic, intrinsic and social) [23,58].	We argue that jobs that provide employees with intrinsic, extrinsic, and social job importance facets enhance job satisfaction and mental health.
Overqualification	We define overqualification as employees' perceptions of having excess education, knowledge, abilities, and skills, compared to the requirements of the job [59]	Scholars indicate that overqualified employees enjoy greater satisfaction with life [28], which correlates with better mental health [10].

References

1. Grant, A.M.; Christianson, M.K.; Price, R.H. Happiness, health, or relationships? managerial practices and employee well-being tradeoffs. *Acad. Manag. Perspect.* **2007**, *21*, 51–63. [CrossRef]
2. Van De Voorde, K.; Boxall, P. Individual well-being and performance at work in the wider context of strategic HRM. In *Well-Being and Performance at Work: The Role of Context, 95–111*; Psychology Press: New York, NY, USA, 2014.
3. Sinclair, R.R.; Wang, M.; Tetrick, L.E. *Research Methods in Occupational Health Psychology: Measurement, Design, and Data Analysis*; Routledge: Abington Thames, UK, 2012.
4. Danna, K.; Griffin, R.W. Health and well-being in the workplace: A review and synthesis of the literature. *J. Manag.* **1999**, *25*, 357–384. [CrossRef]
5. Cass, M.H.; Siu, O.L.; Faragher, E.B.; Cooper, C.L. A meta-analysis of the relationship between job satisfaction and employee health in Hong Kong. *Stress Health* **2003**, *19*, 79–95. [CrossRef]
6. Faragher, E.B.; Cass, M.; Cooper, C.L. The relationship between job satisfaction and health: A meta-analysis. *Occup. Environ. Med.* **2005**, *62*, 105–112. [CrossRef] [PubMed]
7. Fong, C.T. The effects of emotional ambivalence on creativity. *Acad. Manag. J.* **2006**, *49*, 1016–1030. [CrossRef]
8. Warr, P. *Work, Happiness, and Unhappiness*; Psychology Press: New York, NY, USA, 2011.
9. Erdogan, B.; Bauer, T.N.; Peiró, J.; Truxillo, D.M. Overqualified employees: Making the best of a potentially bad situation for individuals and organizations. *Ind. Organ. Psychol.* **2011**, *4*, 215–232. [CrossRef]

10. Headey, B.; Kelley, J.; Wearing, A. Dimensions of mental health: Life satisfaction, positive affect, anxiety and depression. *Soc. Indic. Res.* **1993**, *29*, 63–82. [CrossRef]
11. Johnson, G.J.; Johnson, W.R. Perceived overqualification and dimensions of job satisfaction: A longitudinal analysis. *J. Psychol.* **2000**, *134*, 537–555. [CrossRef]
12. Ilies, R.; Schwind, K.M.; Heller, D. Employee well-being: A multilevel model linking work and nonwork domains. *Eur. J. Work. Organ. Psychol.* **2007**, *16*, 326–341. [CrossRef]
13. Warr, P. How to think about and measure psychological well-being. In *Research Methods in Occupational Health Psychology*; Wang, M., Sinclair, R.R., Tetrick, L.E., Eds.; Psychology Press/Routledge: New York, NY, USA, 2013; Volume 1, pp. 76–91.
14. Babin, B.J.; Boles, J.S. The effects of perceived co-worker involvement and supervisor support on service provider role stress, performance and job satisfaction. *J. Retail.* **1996**, *72*, 57–75. [CrossRef]
15. Peterson, M.F.; Smith, P.B.; Akande, A.; Ayestaran, S.; Bochner, S.; Callan, V.; Francois, P. Role conflict, ambiguity, and overload: A 21-nation study. *Acad. Manag. J.* **1995**, *38*, 429–452.
16. Ashforth, B.E.; Rogers, K.M.; Pratt, M.G.; Pradies, C. Ambivalence in organizations: A multilevel approach. *Organ. Sci.* **2014**, *25*, 1453–1478. [CrossRef]
17. Keller, R.T. Role conflict and ambiguity: Correlates with job satisfaction and values. *Pers. Psychol.* **1975**, *28*, 57–64. [CrossRef]
18. Jackson, S.E.; Schuler, R.S. A meta-analysis and conceptual critique of research on role ambiguity and role conflict in work settings. *Organ. Behav. Hum. Decis. Process.* **1985**, *36*, 16–78. [CrossRef]
19. Rizzo, J.R.; House, R.J.; Lirtzman, S.I. Role conflict and ambiguity in complex organizations. *Adm. Sci. Q.* **1970**, *15*, 150–163. [CrossRef]
20. Miles, R.H. A comparison of the relative impacts of role perceptions of ambiguity and conflict by role. *Acad. Manag. J.* **1976**, *19*, 25–35.
21. Nordenmark, M. Multiple social roles and well-being: A longitudinal test of the role stress theory and the role expansion theory. *Acta Sociol.* **2004**, *47*, 115–126. [CrossRef]
22. Sieber, S.D. Toward a theory of role accumulation. *Am. Sociol. Rev.* **1974**, *39*, 567–578. [CrossRef]
23. Iris, B.; Barrett, G.V. Some relations between job and life satisfaction and job importance. *J. Appl. Psychol.* **1972**, *56*, 301–304. [CrossRef]
24. Thompson, C.A.; Prottas, D.J. Relationships among organizational family support, job autonomy, perceived control, and employee well-being. *J. Occup. Health Psychol.* **2006**, *11*, 100–118. [CrossRef]
25. Agut, S.; Peiró, J.M.; Grau, R. The effect of overeducation on job content innovation and career-enhancing strategies among young Spanish employees. *J. Career Dev.* **2009**, *36*, 159–182. [CrossRef]
26. Di Pietro, G.; Urwin, P. Education and skills mismatch in the Italian graduate labour market. *Appl. Econ.* **2006**, *38*, 79–93. [CrossRef]
27. Pouliakas, K. *Safeguarding Education Investments: Mitigating Overqualification in the EU*; Cedefop: Thessaloniki, Greece, 2015.
28. Peiró, J.M.; Agut, S.; Grau, R. The relationship between overeducation and job satisfaction among young Spanish workers: The role of salary, contract of employment, and work experience. *J. Appl. Soc. Psychol.* **2010**, *40*, 666–689. [CrossRef]
29. Büchel, F. The effects of overeducation on productivity in Germany—The firms' viewpoint. *Econ. Educ. Rev.* **2002**, *21*, 263–275. [CrossRef]
30. De Hauw, S.; De Vos, A. Millennials' career perspective and psychological contract expectations: Does the recession lead to lowered expectations? *J. Bus. Psychol.* **2010**, *2*, 293–302. [CrossRef]
31. Akkermans, J.; Brenninkmeijer, V.; Blonk, R.W.B.; Koppes, L.L.J. Fresh and healthy? Well-being, health and performance of young employees with intermediate education. *Career Dev. Int.* **2009**, *14*, 671–699. [CrossRef]
32. International Labour Organization. *Global Employment Trends for Youth 2013: A Generation at Risk*; International Labour Organization: Geneva, Switzerland, 2013.
33. International Labour Organization (ILO). *World Employment and Social Outlook: Trends 2015*; International Labour Office: Geneva, Switzerland, 2015.
34. Transforming Our World: The 2030 Agenda for Sustainable Development. A/RES/70/1, 70Cong. 2015. Available online: http://research.un.org/en/docs/ga/quick/regular/70 (accessed on 24 October 2018).
35. Warr, P.; Cook, J.; Wall, T. Scales for the measurement of some work attitudes and aspects of psychological well-being. *J. Occup. Organ. Psychol.* **1979**, *52*, 129–148. [CrossRef]

36. Banks, M.H. Validation of the general health questionnaire in a young community sample. *Psychol. Med.* **1983**, *13*, 349–353. [CrossRef]
37. England, G.W.; Harpaz, I. Some methodological and analytic considerations in cross-national comparative research. *J. Int. Bus. Stud.* **1983**, *14*, 49–59. [CrossRef]
38. Cooke, R.A.; Rousseau, D.M. Stress and strain from family roles and work-role expectations. *J. Appl. Psychol.* **1984**, *69*, 252–260. [CrossRef]
39. Bernerth, J.B.; Aguinis, H. A critical review and best-practice recommendations for control variable usage. *Pers. Psychol.* **2016**, *69*, 229–283. [CrossRef]
40. Frone, M.R.; Russell, M.; Barnes, G.M. Work–family conflict, gender, and health-related outcomes: A study of employed parents in two community samples. *J. Occup. Health Psychol.* **1996**, *1*, 57–69. [CrossRef] [PubMed]
41. Ayala, Y.; Silla, J.M.P.; Tordera, N.; Lorente, L.; Yeves, J. Job Satisfaction and Innovative Performance in Young Spanish Employees: Testing New Patterns in the Happy-Productive Worker Thesis—A Discriminant Study. *J. Happiness Stud.* **2017**, *18*, 1377–1401. [CrossRef]
42. Cuyper, N.; Witte, H. The impact of job insecurity and contract type on attitudes, well-being and behavioural reports: A psychological contract perspective. *J. Occup. Organ. Psychol.* **2006**, *79*, 395–409. [CrossRef]
43. Dawson, C.; Veliziotis, M.; Hopkins, B. Temporary employment, job satisfaction and subjective well-being. *Econ. Ind. Democr.* **2017**, *38*, 69–98. [CrossRef]
44. Henry, D.B.; Tolan, P.H.; Gorman-Smith, D. Cluster analysis in family psychology research. *J. Fam. Psychol.* **2005**, *19*, 121–132. [CrossRef] [PubMed]
45. Keyes, C.L.; Shmotkin, D.; Ryff, C.D. Optimizing well-being: The empirical encounter of two traditions. *J. Pers. Soc. Psychol.* **2002**, *82*, 1007–1022. [CrossRef] [PubMed]
46. Raykov, T.; Marcoulides, G.A. *An Introduction to Applied Multivariate Analysis*; Routledge: Abington Thames, UK, 2012.
47. McIntyre, R.M.; Blashfield, R.K. A nearest-centroid technique for evaluating the minimum-variance clustering procedure. *Multivar. Behav. Res.* **1980**, *15*, 225–238. [CrossRef]
48. Fichman, M.; Cummings, J.N. Multiple imputation for missing data: Making the most of what you know. *Organ. Res. Methods* **2003**, *6*, 282–308. [CrossRef]
49. Aguinis, H.; Gottfredson, R.K.; Joo, H. Best-Practice Recommendations for Defining, Identifying, and Handling Outliers. *Organ. Res. Methods* **2013**, *16*, 270–301. [CrossRef]
50. McGowan, J.; Gardner, D.; Fletcher, R. Positive and negative affective outcomes of occupational stress. *N. Z. J. Psychol.* **2006**, *35*, 92–98.
51. Luksyte, A.; Spitzmueller, C.; Maynard, D.C. Why do overqualified incumbents deviate? Examining multiple mediators. *J. Occup. Health Psychol.* **2011**, *16*, 279–296. [CrossRef] [PubMed]
52. Hu, J.; Erdogan, B.; Bauer, T.N.; Jiang, K.; Liu, S.; Li, Y. There are lots of big fish in this pond: The role of peer overqualification on task significance, perceived fit, and performance for overqualified employees. *J. Appl. Psychol.* **2015**, *100*, 1228–1238. [CrossRef] [PubMed]
53. Nielsen, K.; Nielsen, M.B.; Ogbonnaya, C.; Känsälä, M.; Saari, E.; Isaksson, K. Workplace resources to improve both employee well-being and performance: A systematic review and meta-analysis. *Work. Stress* **2017**, *31*, 101–120. [CrossRef]
54. Ziegler, R.; Hagen, B.; Diehl, M. Relationship between job satisfaction and job performance: Job ambivalence as a moderator. *J. Appl. Soc. Psychol.* **2012**, *42*, 2019–2040. [CrossRef]
55. Peiró, J.M. Employees' hedonic and eudemonic well-being and their performance. Do results matter for professional practice? In Proceedings of the 29th International Conference of Applied Psychology (ICAP), Montreal, Canada, 26–30 June 2018.
56. Behrman, D.N.; Perreault, W.D., Jr. A role stress model of the performance and satisfaction of industrial salespersons. *J. Mark.* **1984**, *48*, 9–21. [CrossRef]
57. Beehr, T.A.; Walsh, J.T.; Taber, T.D. Relationships of stress to individually and organizationally valued states: Higher order needs as a moderator. *J. Appl. Psychol.* **1976**, *61*, 41–47. [CrossRef]

58. McFarlin, D.B.; Rice, R.W. The role of facet importance as a moderator in job satisfaction processes. *J. Organ. Behav.* **1992**, *13*, 41–54. [CrossRef]
59. Maynard, D.C.; Joseph, T.A.; Maynard, A.M. Underemployment, job attitudes, and turnover intentions. *J. Organ. Behav.* **2006**, *27*, 509–536. [CrossRef]

11

Prevalence and Risk Factors of Depression, Anxiety, and Stress in a Cohort of Australian Nurses

Shamona Maharaj, Ty Lees and Sara Lal *

Neuroscience Research Unit, School of Life Sciences, University of Technology Sydney, 15 Broadway, Ultimo, Sydney, NSW 2007, Australia; shamona.maharaj@uts.edu.au (S.M.); ty.lees@uts.edu.au (T.L.)

* Correspondence: sara.lal@uts.edu.au

Abstract: Nurses remain at the forefront of patient care. However, their heavy workload as a career can leave them overworked and stressed. The demanding nature of the occupation exposes nurses to a higher risk of developing negative mental states such as depression, anxiety, and stress. Hence, the current study aimed to assess the prevalence and risk factors of these mental states in a representative sample of Australian nurses. The Depression Anxiety Stress Scale was administered to 102 nurses. Information about demographic and work characteristics were obtained using lifestyle and in-house designed questionnaires. Prevalence rates of depression, anxiety, and stress were found to be 32.4%, 41.2%, and 41.2% respectively. Binominal logistic regressions for depression and stress were significant ($p = 0.007$, $p = 0.009$). Job dissatisfaction significantly predicted a higher risk of nurses developing symptoms of depression and stress respectively ($p = 0.009$, $p = 0.011$). Poor mental health among nurses may not only be detrimental to the individual but may also hinder professional performance and in turn, the quality of patient care provided. Further research in the area is required to identify support strategies and interventions that may improve the health and wellbeing of nursing professionals and hence the quality of care delivered.

Keywords: mental health; nursing; depression; anxiety; stress

---

1. Introduction

The health workforce in Australia is dominated by nurses, making them indispensable to the healthcare sector [1,2]. Nurses not only provide care and assistance to patients, but also participate in their rehabilitation, provide support to patients and their families, and advocate health education [3], playing an important role in improving and promoting health services in the community [4]. Their broad and multifaceted workload presents them with the largest amount of time spent with patients and allows them to cover all areas of the healthcare network [3]. Yet, the profession is invariably recognised as a stressful and demanding occupation.

Nurses regularly experience a variety of work-related stressors including but not limited to: long work hours, time constraints, meeting patients' needs, irregular schedules, and lack of professional support [2,5–7]. With such demanding occupations, the ongoing strain faced by healthcare professionals could have a severe impact on their mental health and quality of life [8,9]. Previous studies have shown that the ongoing stress faced by these professionals can have negative effects on their psychological well-being [10,11]. Poor mental health among health care providers may also hinder their professional performance and have a considerable effect on the quality of care they provide to patients [2,10] (inevitably impacting negatively on patients' health). Therefore, administrators and nursing managers are becoming increasingly interested in the health status of nurses.

Psychological indicators for distress include but are not limited to, low self-esteem, fatigue, and sleep/appetite disturbances [12]; while physical impacts may include the increased risk of cardiovascular disease, high blood pressure, decreased immunity, migraines, muscle aches, and chronic fatigue [13]. Additionally, high levels of stress may lead to or exacerbate maladaptive behaviours, such as smoking, over/under eating, excessive alcohol consumption, and substance abuse [14,15]. Depression and anxiety also remain two of the most prevalent mental disorders in Australia with 12-month prevalence rates of approximately 4% and 14% respectively [16]. Investigating depression, anxiety, and stress levels in nurses and identifying predictors for these mental states is crucial for future health systems to provide safer and more amenable workplaces while promoting the well-being of its employees.

The prevalence of depressive symptoms among nurses in the USA was between 35–41%, but another study reported it to be 18% [7,10], 11%–80% in Iranian nurses [17,18], 35% in Chinese nurses [19], 17% in Australian Midwives [20], and 51% in Brazilian nurses [21]. Additionally, approximately 33% of French nurse managers and 10% Canadian nurses were found to suffer from depressive symptoms as well [22,23]. A high incidence of anxiety in nursing professionals is also evident, with studies stating prevalence rates ranging from 20% in Australian Midwives [20] to 32–43% in Chinese nurses [11,19,24], 40–46% in Iranian nurses [4,25], 44–66% in Brazilian nurses [21,26], and 22–24% of American nurses who showed PTSD symptomology [27,28]. The level of stress among nurses can generally range from moderate to high [29,30] and the few prevalence rates that have been presented range from approximately 40–90% [31–34]. Predictive factors such as job satisfaction, high workloads, shift work, sleep disturbance, years of employment, and marital status [10,17–19,35] were commonly implicated with these mental disorders.

Hence, the current study aimed to

1. Assess the prevalence of depression, anxiety, and stress in a cohort of Australian nurses.
2. Determine demographic and work characteristics associated with each mental state.

2. Materials and Methods

2.1. Participants and Sampling

A cross-sectional study design was used to examine the prevalence and correlates of depression, anxiety, and stress symptoms in a cohort of Australian nurses. Data from 102 clinically active nurses were used in the current analysis. Prior to inclusion, all participants were screened for chronic disease/illness (including clinically diagnosed depression, anxiety, and other mental health issues), medication use, smoking habits (in excess of 10 cigarettes a day), and alcohol intake (in excess of 16 standard drinks a day) via an in-house designed lifestyle questionnaire. Participants were excluded if they answered yes to any of the screening questions above. All participants provided informed consent prior to the commencement of the study. At the commencement and conclusion of each session, the participant's blood pressure (BP) was measured three times with an automated blood pressure monitor (Omron IA1B, Kyoto, Japan), and then averaged to derive an average BP value to determine further inclusion into the study (requiring BP < 160/100 mmHg).

2.2. Data Collection/Measures

Demographic, lifestyle, and work-related data were collected using in-house designed questionnaires; developed to determine lifestyle risk factors/habits and determine inclusion/exclusion criteria for the study.

The 42-item Depression Anxiety Stress Scale (DASS) [36] was applied to assess symptom severity of each mental state. Together, each scale of the DASS assessed a comprehensive range of psychological distress symptoms to identifying psychological disturbances perceived by an individual ranging from situational anxiety, anhedonia, and dysphoria to levels of chronic non-specific arousal such as irritability and difficulty relaxing [36,37]. It can be noted that perceived job strain and control are commonly associated with self-reported mental health outcomes [38,39]. As the scale examines general mental health and is based on self-perception, it accounts for environmental and work-related factors that may influence how an individual is feeling.

2.3. Statistical Analysis

Data was initially subject to descriptive statistical analysis. Pearson's correlation analysis was conducted to assess associations between blood pressure and Depression, Anxiety, and Stress. Variables were then dichotomised to enable a good comparison of outcomes; participants with a cut-off score of ≥10 in depression, ≥8 in anxiety, and >15 in stress were considered as having these disorders as referenced by the DASS [36]. A forward-stepwise (conditional) binominal logistic regression was utilised to measure the strength of associations between variables and sought to identify significant predictors for the outcomes of interest to the study. The level of statistical significance was defined as $p < 0.05$. Statistical analysis was performed using SPSS Version 23.0 for the Windows platform (SPSS Inc.; Chicago, IL, USA).

3. Results

3.1. Demographics

Participants demographics are presented in Table 1. As seen in Table 1, a majority of the participants were females working as Assistants in Nursing (AIN's) and Registered nurses. A majority of the participants also worked in aged care and hospital environments, reflecting the large number of AIN's and registered nurses. Finally, most of the nurses assessed in the current study engaged in shiftwork.

Table 1. Demographics (n = 102).

Demographic/work factor	Mean ± SD or %
Age	30.91 ± 11.52
Gender (female)	79.41% (81F: 21M)
Position	
Assistant in Nursing	43.14% (44)
Enrolled nurse	15.69% (16)
Registered Nurse/Midwife	39.22% (40)
Other	1.96% (2)
Facility	
Aged care	33.33% (34)
Hospital	34.31% (35)
Multiple facilities	9.80% (10)
Other	5.88% (6)
Unspecified	16.67% (17)
Shift workers	78.43% (80)
Job satisfaction	
Yes	37.25% (38)
No	26.47% (27)
Unspecified	36.27 (37)

Mean DASS scores and prevalence for each mental state are displayed in Table 2. In the total sample, according to DASS scores, 32.4% of participants scored over the normal threshold for depression. Of those individuals, 21.57% fell into the mild/moderate categories while 4.9% showed sufficient scores for severe depression and 5.88% for extremely severe depression. However, though some individuals did not have scores over the normal threshold, 86.27% of the total cohort did report some level of depressive symptoms.

Similarly, 41.2% of participants scored over the normal threshold for anxiety. Of those individuals, 20.59% fell into the mild/moderate categories while 9.8% showed sufficient scores for severe anxiety and 10.78% for extremely severe anxiety. Though not all the scores were over the threshold, 91.18% of the total cohort did report some level of anxiety.

Finally, 41.2% of participants also scored over the normal threshold for stress. Of those individuals, 24.51% fell into the mild/moderate categories while 10.8% showed sufficient scores for severe stress and 5.88% for extremely severe stress. Once again, though some individuals did not score over the threshold, 95.10% of the total cohort did report some level of distress.

Table 2. Prevalence and Average scores for Depression, Anxiety, and Stress (n = 102).

	Normal Threshold	Cohort Mean ± SD	Interpretation	Prevalence (%)
Depression	<10	8.38 ± 8.81	Normal	32.4
Anxiety	<8	8.47 ± 7.86	Mild	41.2
Stress	<15	13.90 ± 9.94	Normal	41.2

As previously mentioned, blood pressure was assessed for inclusion criteria. Associations between blood pressure and depression, anxiety, and stress were non-significant, as seen in Table 3

Table 3. Correlations between blood pressure and depression, anxiety, and stress.

	Pre Systolic	Pre Diastolic	Pre Heart Rate	Post Systolic	Post Diastolic	Post Heart Rate
Depression	r = 0.03, p = 0.849	r = 0.10, p = 0.493	r = −0.14, p = 0.346	r = 0.05, p = 0.758	r = −0.10, p = 0.540	r = −0.15, p = 0.330
Anxiety	r = 0.03, p = 0.848	r = 0.07, p = 0.646	r =−0.07, p = 0.632	r = 0.10, p = 0.492	r = −0.07, p = 0.647	r = 0.01, p = 0.931
Stress	r = 0.01, p = 0.929	r = 0.09, p = 0.537	r = 0.01, p = 0.959	r = 0.09, p = 0.554	r = −0.05, p = 0.728	r = −0.004, p = 0.979

3.2. Binary Logistic Regression Models

The logistic regression model for depression was significant (p = 0.007), explaining 14.2% (Nagelkerke R2) of the variance in depression, and correctly classified 67.7% of cases. Job dissatisfaction significantly predicted depression (S.E. = 0.538, Exp(B) = 4.07, df = 1, p = 0.009) with individuals who reported not being satisfied being more likely to present with depression.

The logistic regression model for anxiety was non-significant. The association between the study variables showed no significance between anxiety and the following: age, gender, facility, shift work, shift type, shift length, job satisfaction, physical issues, and registration level.

The logistic regression model for stress was significant (p = 0.009), explaining 13.2% (Nagelkerke R2) of the variance in stress, and correctly classified 66.2% of cases. Job dissatisfaction significantly predicted stress (S.E. = 0.53, Exp(B) = 3.85, df = 1, p = 0.011) with individuals who reported not being satisfied also being more likely to present with symptoms of distress.

4. Discussion

We assessed the status of depression, anxiety and stress symptomology in a representative sample of Australian nurses. Our study demonstrated that depressive symptoms were common in nurses with a prevalence rate of over 30%, compared to only 4% of the general Australian population [16]. Thus, the results suggested that more than a quarter of the current sample complied with DASS cut-off criteria for depression (scores of 10 and above). Notably, multiple had presented with severe depressive symptoms. Depression prevalence among nurses in our study was also within the ranges reported in previous literature around the world with depression rates ranging from approximately 18–53% [10,18–21]. Likewise, the prevalence of anxiety symptoms was common among the current sample, with a prevalence rate of over 40% compared to 14% of the general Australian population [16]. Again, more than a quarter of the current sample complied with the DASS cut off criteria for anxiety (8 and above) and among these individuals, over 10% had presented with severe anxiety. The prevalence of anxiety among nurses in our study also fell within the ranges commonly reported in the literature (ranging between 20–60%) [4,11,19–21,24,26,29]. Finally, levels of distress were high with over 40% of the current nursing sample complying with the DASS cut-off criteria for stress (scores of 15 and above) and once again multiple individuals presented with severe levels of distress while our prevalence rate was similar to those of other countries [32,34].

As previously mentioned, rates of depression, anxiety, and stress in the current cohort were much higher than population norms. Ignoring the signs of anguish and depression presented by nursing professionals may not only increase the amount of physical and emotional stress on the individual but may also result in low-quality patient care and higher work burdens on establishments [40]. Literature suggests that poor mental health may lead to a decrease in cognitive performance such as an individual's ability to focus and process information, in turn, resulting in inadequate performance [41,42]. Such consequences in the workplace can include decreased alertness and reduced job performance, which could endanger human lives and increase the risk of adverse medical events [43,44].

Australian state spending on mental health services has increased over the past few years, now costing approximately $9 billion [45] and more notably, the cost and number of workers' compensation claims associated with stress and stress-related mental disorders are noticeably higher in medicine and healthcare compared to other occupations [46,47]. Individuals who suffer from mental health issues also tend to have more days out of role, taking approximately five days off work and having 11 days of reduced productivity annually; adding billions of dollars lost to absenteeism and lost productivity [48,49]. Although the number of nurses in Australia has increased over the last decade [50], nurse shortages remain an ongoing issue [51]. High turnover, absenteeism, and lost productivity within the health workforce could amplify shortages and easily leave facilities understaffed and unable to meet patient demands, placing patients at risk [3,52]. Thus, as the prevalence of mental health disorders increases within the profession so too will the economic, social, and individual impacts of these disorders.

The current findings suggested that demographic and occupational factors associated with an increased incidence of developing symptoms of depression, anxiety, and stress were limited as only one occupational factor was associated with poor mental health outcomes. While job dissatisfaction was associated with an increased risk of distress and depression, no factors were found to significantly increase the likelihood of developing anxiety. Further, blood pressure parameters were similarly not associated with depression, anxiety, or stress. However, previous literature has implicated various demographic and work-related predictors for the relatively high prevalence of negative mental states among nurses. Previous studies have found common predictors such as age, job satisfaction, sleep disturbance, years of employment, and marital status [10,17–19,53] to increase the likelihood of developing stress, anxiety and depression. Associations between highly stressful work and its impact on mental wellbeing necessitate the consideration of interventions which aim to improve working conditions and reduce the personal and occupational stress of nurses in an aid to reduce and/or prevent symptoms of depression, stress, and anxiety [43].

Limitations (such as a small representative sample and cross-sectional study design) do exist in the current study, and hence further research may benefit from longitudinal study designs to fully determine predictors of stress, depression, and anxiety in nurses. As the current data was collected as part of a larger study, limited information was collected and available for analysis. A more comprehensive assessment of demographic, personal, and work-related factors that may be considered predictors for negative mental states may also be beneficial.

5. Conclusions

Nursing is an important role in our health care system, and patient care is heavily reliant upon their ability to work optimally and deliver the best care possible [54]. It is becoming increasingly recognised that nurses are affected by symptoms of stress, depression, and anxiety [9]. The prevalence of nurses affected by negative mental states in the current study was high, and it is possible that poor mental health can be detrimental to both the individual and the industry [2,10]. Further research is needed to help care for the well-being of nurses and minimize poor mental health in the workplace. Additionally, the development of short and long-term support strategies and interventions aimed at improving the mental health needs of nursing professionals should be a priority to combat the physical and psychological exhaustion associated with these mental states.

The stress, depression, and anxiety experienced by nursing professionals may not be entirely preventable but realising its prevalence in the workplace is considerably important [55]. A healthy workforce is essential in ensuring that both personal wellbeing and quality patient outcomes are achieved [55].

Author Contributions: Investigation, S.M.; Supervision, S.L.; Data Curation, X.X.; Writing-Original Draft Preparation, S.M.; Writing-Review & Editing, T.L.

Acknowledgments: The authors would like to acknowledge the School of Life Sciences at the University of Technology Sydney, where this research was conducted and the participants for their time and interest.

References

1. Australian Institute of Health and Wellbeing. Nursing and Midwifery Workforce. 2015. Available online: https://www.aihw.gov.au/reports/workforce/nursing-and-midwifery-workforce-2015/contents/who-are-nurses-and-midwives (accessed on 15 May 2018).
2. Gong, Y.; Han, T.; Yin, X.; Yang, G.; Zhuang, R.; Chen, Y.; Lu, Z. Prevalence of depressive symptoms and work-related risk factors among nurses in public hospitals in southern China: A cross-sectional study. *Sci. Rep.* **2014**, *4*, 7109. [CrossRef] [PubMed]

3. DeLucia, P.R.; Ott, T.E.; Palmieri, P.A. Performance in Nursing. *Rev. Hum. Factors Ergon.* **2009**, *5*, 1–40. [CrossRef]
4. Ghods, A.A.; Sotodehasl, N.; Khalaf, M.E.; Mirmohamadkhani, M. Situational Anxiety among Nurses. *Middle East J. Rehabil. Health* **2017**, *4*. [CrossRef]
5. Pikó, B. Work-related stress among nurses: A challenge for health care institutions. *J. R. Soc. Promot. Health* **1999**, *119*, 156–162. [CrossRef]
6. Lim, J.; Bogossian, F.; Ahern, K. Stress and coping in Australian nurses: A systematic review. *Int. Nurs. Rev.* **2010**, *57*, 22–31. [CrossRef] [PubMed]
7. Letvak, S.; Ruhm, C.J.; McCoy, T. Depression in hospital-employed nurses. *Clin. Nurse Spec.* **2012**, *26*, 177–182. [CrossRef]
8. Stetz, M.C.; Thomas, M.L.; Russo, M.B.; Stetz, T.A.; Wildzunas, R.M.; McDonald, J.J.; Wiederhold, B.K.; Romano, J.A. Stress, mental health, and cognition: A brief review of relationships and countermeasures. *Aviat. Space Environ. Med.* **2007**, *78*, B252–B260. [PubMed]
9. Chiang, Y.-M.; Chang, Y. Stress, depression, and intention to leave among nurses in different medical units: Implications for healthcare management/nursing practice. *Health Policy* **2012**, *108*, 149–157. [CrossRef]
10. Welsh, D. Predictors of Depressive Symptoms in Female Medical-Surgical Hospital Nurses. *Issues Ment. Health Nurs.* **2009**, *30*, 320–326. [CrossRef]
11. Gao, Y.-Q.; Pan, B.-C.; Sun, W.; Wu, H.; Wang, J.-N.; Wang, L. Anxiety symptoms among Chinese nurses and the associated factors: A cross sectional study. *BMC Psychiatry* **2012**, *12*, 141. [CrossRef]
12. Dyrbye, L.N.; Thomas, M.R.; Shanafelt, T.D. Systematic Review of Depression, Anxiety, and Other Indicators of Psychological Distress Among U.S. and Canadian Medical Students. *Acad. Med.* **2006**, *81*, 354–373. [CrossRef] [PubMed]
13. Schneiderman, N.; Ironson, G.; Siegel, S.D. STRESS AND HEALTH: Psychological, Behavioral, and Biological Determinants. *Annu. Rev. Clin. Psychol.* **2005**, *1*, 607–628. [CrossRef] [PubMed]
14. Sinha, R. Chronic Stress, Drug Use, and Vulnerability to Addiction. *Ann. N. Y. Acad. Sci.* **2008**, *1141*, 105–130. [CrossRef] [PubMed]
15. Yau, Y.H.C.; Potenza, M.N. Stress and Eating Behaviors. *Minerva Endocrinol.* **2013**, *38*, 255–267. [PubMed]
16. Australian Bureau of Statistics (ABS) National Survey of Mental Health and Wellbeing: 2008 Summary of Results. Available online: http://www.abs.gov.au/ausstats/abs@.nsf/Latestproducts/4326.0Main%20Features32007 (accessed on 18 September 2018).
17. Tabrizi, K.N.; Kavari, S.H. P02-45—A study of depression prevalence in nurses and it's effective factors in shiraz namazi hospital. *Eur. Psychiatry* **2011**, *26*, 640. [CrossRef]
18. Ardekani, Z.Z.; Kakooei, H.; Ayattollahi, S.M.; Choobineh, A.; Seraji, G.N. Prevalence of mental disorders among shift work hospital nurses in Shiraz, Iran. *Pak. J. Biol. Sci.* **2008**, *11*, 1605–1609. [CrossRef] [PubMed]
19. Cheung, T.; Yip, P.S.F. Depression, Anxiety and Symptoms of Stress among Hong Kong Nurses: A Cross-sectional Study. *Int. J. Environ. Res. Public Health* **2015**, *12*, 11072–11100. [CrossRef] [PubMed]
20. Creedy, D.K.; Sidebotham, M.; Gamble, J.; Pallant, J.; Fenwick, J. Prevalence of burnout, depression, anxiety and stress in Australian midwives: A cross-sectional survey. *BMC Pregnancy Childbirth* **2017**, *17*, 13. [CrossRef]
21. Schmidt, D.R.C.; Dantas, R.A.S.; Marziale, M.H.P. Anxiety and depression among nursing professionals who work in surgical units. *Revista da Escola de Enfermagem da USP* **2011**, *45*, 487–493. [CrossRef]
22. Nourry, N.; Luc, A.; Lefebvre, F.; Sultan-Taïeb, H.; Béjean, S. Psychosocial and organizational work environment of nurse managers and self-reported depressive symptoms: Cross-sectional analysis from a cohort of nurse managers. *Int. J. Occup. Med. Environ. Health* **2014**, *27*, 252–269. [CrossRef] [PubMed]
23. Ohler, M.C.; Kerr, M.S.; Forbes, D.A. Depression in Nurses. *Can. J. Nurs. Res. Arch.* **2010**, *42*, 66–82.
24. Li, S.; Li, L.; Zhu, X.; Wang, Y.; Zhang, J.; Zhao, L.; Li, L.; Yang, Y. Comparison of characteristics of anxiety sensitivity across career stages and its relationship with nursing stress among female nurses in Hunan, China. *BMJ Open* **2016**, *6*, e010829. [CrossRef] [PubMed]
25. Nooryan, K.; Sasanpour, M.; Sharif, F.; Ghafarian Shirazi, H.R. Anxiety in Physicians and Nurses Working in Intensive Care Units in Yasuj's Hospitals/Iran. *Procedia Soc. Behav. Sci.* **2014**, *122*, 457–460. [CrossRef]
26. Veloso, L.U.P.; Laurindo, L.M.B. Prevalance of anxiety in nursing professionals of urgency medicine. *J. Nurs. UFPE* **2016**, *8*, 3969–3976. [CrossRef]

27. Mealer, M.L.; Shelton, A.; Berg, B.; Rothbaum, B.; Moss, M. Increased Prevalence of Post-traumatic Stress Disorder Symptoms in Critical Care Nurses. *Am. J. Respir. Crit. Care Med.* **2007**, *175*, 693–697. [CrossRef]
28. Mealer, M.; Burnham, E.L.; Goode, C.J.; Rothbaum, B.; Moss, M. The prevalence and impact of post traumatic stress disorder and burnout syndrome in nurses. *Depress. Anxiety* **2009**, *26*, 1118–1126. [CrossRef]
29. Opie, T.; Lenthall, S.; Wakerman, J.; Dollard, M.; Macleod, M.; Knight, S.; Rickard, G.; Dunn, S. Occupational stress in the Australian nursing workforce: A comparison between hospital-based nurses and nurses working in very remote communities. *Aust. J. Adv. Nurs.* **2011**, *28*, 36–43.
30. Subih, M.; Alamer, R.; Hadid, L.A.; Alsatari, M. Stressors Amongst Jordanian Nurses Working in Different Types of Hospitals and the Effect of Selected Demographic Factors: A Descriptive-Explorative Study. *Jordan Med. J.* **2012**, *45*, 331–340.
31. Al-Makhaita, H.M.; Sabra, A.A.; Hafez, A.S. Predictors of work-related stress among nurses working in primary and secondary health care levels in Dammam, Eastern Saudi Arabia. *J. Fam. Community Med.* **2014**, *21*, 79–84. [CrossRef]
32. Gheshlagh, R.G.; Parizad, N.; Dalvand, S.; Zarei, M.; Farajzadeh, M.; Karami, M.; Sayehmiri, K. The prevalence of job stress among nurses in Iran: A meta-analysis study. *Nurs. Midwifery Stud.* **2017**, *6*, 143–148. [CrossRef]
33. Khan, N.; Anwar, H.; Sayed, M. Prevalence of Stress Factors in Nurses in Leady Reading Hospital (LRH), Khyber Teaching Hospital (KTH) and Hayatabad Medical Complex (HMC) Hospitals, Peshawar, KPK. *Int. J. Innov. Res. Dev.* **2015**, *4*, 4.
34. Kibria, M.G. Prevalence of Stress and Coping Mechanism Among Staff Nurses of Intensive Care Unit in a Selected Hospital. *Int. J. Neurosurg.* **2018**, *2*, 8–12. [CrossRef]
35. Khodadadi, E.; Hosseinzadeh, M.; Azimzadeh, R.; Fooladi, M. The relation of depression, anxiety and stress with personal characteristics of nurses in hospitals of Tabriz, Iran. *Int. J. Med. Res. Health Sci.* **2016**, *5*, 140–148.
36. Lovibond, S.H.; Lovibond, P.F. *Manual for the Depression Anxiety Stress Scales*, 2nd ed.; Psychology Foundation: Sydney, Australia, 1995.
37. Crawford, J.; Henry, J. The Depression Anxiety Stress Scales (DASS): Normative data and latent structure in a large non-clinical sample. *Br. J. Clin. Psychol.* **2003**, *42*, 111–131. [CrossRef] [PubMed]
38. Karasek, R. Job demands, job decision latitude, and mental strain: Implications for job redesign. *Adm. Sci. Q.* **1979**, *24*, 285–308. [CrossRef]
39. De Jonge, J.; van Vegchel, N.; Shimazu, A.; Schaufeli, W.; Dormann, C. A longitudinal test of the demand-control model using specific job demands and specific job control. *Int. J. Behav. Med.* **2010**, *17*, 125–133. [CrossRef]
40. De Vargas, D.; Dias, A.P.V. Depression prevalence in Intensive Care Unit nursing workers: A study at hospitals in a northwestern city of São Paulo State. *Revista Latino-Americana de Enfermagem* **2011**, *19*, 1114–1121. [CrossRef]
41. Marazziti, D.; Consoli, G.; Picchetti, M.; Carlini, M.; Faravelli, L. Cognitive impairment in major depression. *Eur. J. Pharmacol.* **2010**, *626*, 83–86. [CrossRef]
42. Maharaj, S.; Lees, T.; Lal, S. Negative Mental States and Their Association to the Cognitive Function of Nurses. *J. Psychophysiol.* **2018**, 1–12. [CrossRef]
43. Johnson, J.; Hall, L.H.; Berzins, K.; Baker, J.; Melling, K.; Thompson, C. Mental healthcare staff well-being and burnout: A narrative review of trends, causes, implications, and recommendations for future interventions. *Int. J. Ment. Health Nurs.* **2018**, *27*, 20–32. [CrossRef]
44. Berland, A.; Natvig, G.K.; Gundersen, D. Patient safety and job-related stress: A focus group study. *Intensive Crit. Care Nurs.* **2008**, *24*, 90–97. [CrossRef] [PubMed]
45. Australian Institute of Health and Welfare. Mental Health Services in Australia, Expenditure on Mental Health-Related Services 2018. Available online: https://www.aihw.gov.au/reports/mental-health-services/mental-health-services-in-australia/report-contents/expenditure-on-mental-health-related-services (accessed on 15 May 2018).
46. Statistics Main Features—Doctors and Nurses. Available online: http://www.abs.gov.au/AUSSTATS/abs@.nsf/Lookup/4102.0Main+Features20April+2013 (accessed on 15 May 2018).

47. Australian Safety and Compensation Council. *Work-Related Mental Disorders in Australia—Report*; Australian Safety and Compensation Council, Australian Government: Canberra, Australia, 2006.
48. Safe Work Australia. *Incidence of Accepted Workers' Compensation Claims for Mental Stress in Australia*; Safe Work Australia: Canberra, Australia, 2013.
49. Slade, T.; Johnston, A.; Teesson, M.; Whiteford, H.; Burgess, P.; Pirkis, J.; Saw, S. *The Mental Health of Australians 2: Report on the 2007 National Survey of Mental Health and Wellbeing*; Department of Health and Ageing: Canberra, Australia, 2009.
50. Beyond Blue—Insure Workforce Report 2011. Available online: https://www.beyondblue.org.au/docs/default-source/policy-submissions/bw0088-policy-submission---insecure-work-in-australia.pdf?sfvrsn=ab4fa9e9_2 (accessed on 15 May 2018).
51. APH Nurse Shortages and the Impact on Health Services. 2004. Available online: https://www.aph.gov.au/Parliamentary_Business/Committees/Senate/Community_Affairs/Completed_inquiries/2002-04/nursing/report/c02 (accessed on 15 May 2018).
52. Tuckett, A.; Winters-Chang, P.; Bogossian, F.; Wood, M. "Why nurses are leaving the profession. Lack of support from managers": What nurses from an e-cohort study said. *Int. J. Nurs. Pract.* **2015**, *21*, 359–366. [CrossRef] [PubMed]
53. Ruggiero, J.S. Health, work variables, and job satisfaction among nurses. *J. Nurs. Adm.* **2005**, *35*, 254–263. [CrossRef] [PubMed]
54. Gatchel, R. The importance of the profession of nursing in health care: Current and future issues. *J. Appl. Biobehav. Res.* **2018**, *23*, e12127. [CrossRef]
55. Brandford, A.A.; Reed, D.B. Depression in Registered Nurses: A State of the Science. *Workplace Health Saf.* **2016**, *64*, 488–511. [CrossRef]

12

A Cognitive Behavioural Intervention Programme to Improve Psychological Well-Being

Birgitta Ojala [1,2,*], Clas-Håkan Nygård [1], Heini Huhtala [1], Philip Bohle [3] and Seppo T. Nikkari [2,4]

1 Faculty of Social Science, Health Unit, University of Tampere, 33014 Tampere, Finland; Clas-Hakan.Nygard@staff.uta.fi (C.-H.N.); Heini.Huhtala@staff.uta.fi (H.H.)
2 Tullinkulma Occupational Health Unit, 33100 Tampere, Finland; Seppo.Nikkari@staff.uta.fi
3 Tasmanian School of Business and Economics, University of Tasmania, Private Bag 84 Hobart, Tasmania 7001, Australia; philip.bohle@sydney.edu.au
4 Faculty of Medicine and Health Technology, Tampere University, 33100 Tampere, Finland
* Correspondence: ojala.birgitta@gmail.com;

Abstract: Psychosocial risk factors have increased in today's work environment, and they threaten work ability. Good workplace atmosphere, psychosocial support, the ability to cope with stress, and skills and knowledge are all connected to more successful coping. Faster changes in the work environment and an increased workload can lead to a chain of fatigue and illness. The aim of this study was to evaluate a cognitive behavioural intervention as an early rehabilitation strategy to improve employees' well-being, in intervention group N446 and in control group N116. The well-being measures used were the Bergen Burnout Inventory (BBI 15), Utrecht Work Engagement Scale (UWES), and depression and stress screening questions. Data were obtained by a self-report survey at baseline and at a nine-month follow-up. Differences were analysed within and between groups. The results suggest that cognitive behavioural intervention as an early rehabilitation programme will increase employees' well-being measured by BBI 15, UWES, and depression and stress screening questions. In the intervention group, the total BBI 15 score ($p < 0.01$) and each of the three subdimensions of burnout (exhaustion, cynicism, and sense of inadequacy) decreased at follow-up. Mental health issues are the commonest reasons for sick leave and early retirement. We need ways to prevent these issues.

Keywords: stress; occupational health; intervention; burnout; well-being

---

1. Introduction

Work is changing, and so are work-related occupational hazards [1]. Work-related psychosocial factors are considered a new type of occupational hazard. They include work characteristics and demands, overload and mental stress, workers' opportunities to influence work tasks and procedures, their use of knowledge and skills, and difficulty and hurry at work [1,2].

These factors increasingly influence workers' capacity to cope at work. A prolonged discrepancy between employees' capacities and work demands may produce burnout, which consists of three main symptoms: Exhaustion, cynicism, and reduced professional efficiency. Burnout is typically associated with absenteeism, sick leave, job turnover or physical health issues [3–5]. Approximately 5% of the Finnish population suffer from depression annually, and there is a reciprocal relationship between burnout and depression symptoms [6,7].

Participatory interventions that focus on the individual as well as on the organisational level have been shown to be effective in treating burnout [8]. Successful intervention programmes against burnout can be enhanced with refresher courses [9]. It is also important to recognise different burnout patterns and to focus activities effectively [10–12].

Employee engagement can be built at work through meaningful experiences and by enabling workers to understand why they are doing the work. In the health sector, people usually describe their work as meaningful and valuable. Everybody ascribes meanings to their work—for example, to the nature of the work role, and to the relationships that they build with others—and these have implications for their experiences of work. Employees are usually fully engaged in contexts where a source of meaningfulness is present. Agreeable identities with clear roles, important work relationships, challenging work, supportive leadership, and the pursuit of rewards all increase engagement. Employees' engagement can thus be improved by supervisors, leaders, human resources staff, and other co-workers. Under these conditions, workers do their best, are loyal to their employer, and are willing to be flexible if the work so requires [13]. It has been shown that the quality of nurses' work improves with such engagement [14].

Job strain may precipitate clinical depression among employees, according to a review of six studies with a total of 27,461 participants and 914 incident cases of clinical depression [5]. In some organisations, best practices for managing workplace stress have included context-specific interventions, combined organisational and individual interventions, a participative approach, and a change in culture [15]. When office employees were allocated to social and physical environmental intervention groups, social–environmental intervention showed an improvement in task performance, whereas physical environmental intervention showed an improvement in absorption [15]. Workplace-based, high-intensity psychological interventions may improve work disability outcomes for workers with common mental health conditions [16,17]. However, in a meta-analysis of effects of occupational stress management intervention programmes, cognitive behavioural therapy (CBT) interventions consistently produce larger effects than other types of intervention [18].

The CBT model of intervention encourages individuals to act by themselves to achieve their own goals by supporting them to take actions towards those goals [18]. CBT has been found to be effective in improving work-related stress, depression, anxiety, chronic pain, chronic fatigue syndrome, and insomnia. It has also been found to increase work engagement within a working population [19].

Burnout reflects a negative relationship of hostility and alienation between the person and his/her job, the positive opposite of which is engagement, a relationship of reconciliation, and acceptance [20]. We conducted a prospective study to evaluate the effects of a CBT intervention to improve employees' well-being, as measured by outcome of questionnaires on psychosocial variables from positive and negative directions.

2. Material and Methods

2.1. Participants

In 2011–2014, our outpatient intervention study recruited a total of 779 municipal employees. Participants were volunteers who met the inclusion criteria for the study: Being employed in the public sector and working as permanent or long-term temporary staff with at least one year of service. The study was a nine-month follow-up designed to study the causal impact of the intervention on an intervention group, with a control group that did not take part in the intervention. Of the 779 total participants, 594 took part in the intervention group and 185 in the control group. Control group members had the opportunity to take part in the intervention after they had answered follow-up questionnaires before the intervention started. The intervention sessions lasted for four months, with one session every two weeks; five months after that came the follow-up tests and group meetings.

The intervention was conducted during paid working hours, and participants were required to commit to the entire programme.

Of the 779 participants, 80% were women and 20% were men. The mean age of subjects intervention group and the control group in age, gender, body mass index, marital status or years of work experience (Table 1). However, there was a difference in education: The intervention group had less vocational training than the control group. The subjects were recruited from different vocational areas for the intervention programme. The largest participation of women came from health services (37.3%), and of men from construction and transport (70.4%) (Table 2).

Table 1. Background characteristics of study population.

	N	Intervention	*N*	Control	*p*
Age (years)	578	49.2 (7.8)	173	48.1	0.205
Gender, female (%)	463	80.1	138	79.8	1
Married (%)	578	56.6	173	61.5	1
Years of professional experience	547	19.2 (10.1)	165	18.2 (10.6)	0.702
Education					
No vocational training (%)	38	7.1	9	5.3	
Vocational school (%)	344	64.3	108	63.9	
University of applied science (%)	55	10.3	25	14.8	0.61
University degree (%)	98	18.3	27	16	
Total	535	100	169	100	

Table 2. Main occupations of study population.

	Intervention				Control			
	Female *N*	%	Male *N*	%	Female *N*	%	Male *N*	%
Health service	173	37.3	0	0	53	38.4	0	0
Construction and transport	0	0	81	70.4	0	0	22	62.9
Education and day care	69	14.9	9	7.8	22	15.9	4	11.4
Other services	68	14.7	0	0	18	13.1	0	0
Food services	66	14.3	0	0	21	15.2	0	0
Office work	48	10.4	7	6.1	18	13.1	0	0
Management specialist	39	8.4	18	15.7	6	4.3	9	25.7
Total	463	100	115	100	138	100	35	100

In the intervention group, 446 (75.1%) completed the questionnaires at both baseline and follow-up. There were missing responses in 148 cases. In 28 of these, there was natural movement, such as changes of workplace, absence, changes of job, and death. Nineteen cases did not want to take part in the study, and 101 answered incompletely at the baseline or follow-up. In the control group, 116 (62.7%) answered at baseline and follow-up, there was natural movement with six participants, and 63 answered incompletely at baseline or follow-up (Figure 1).

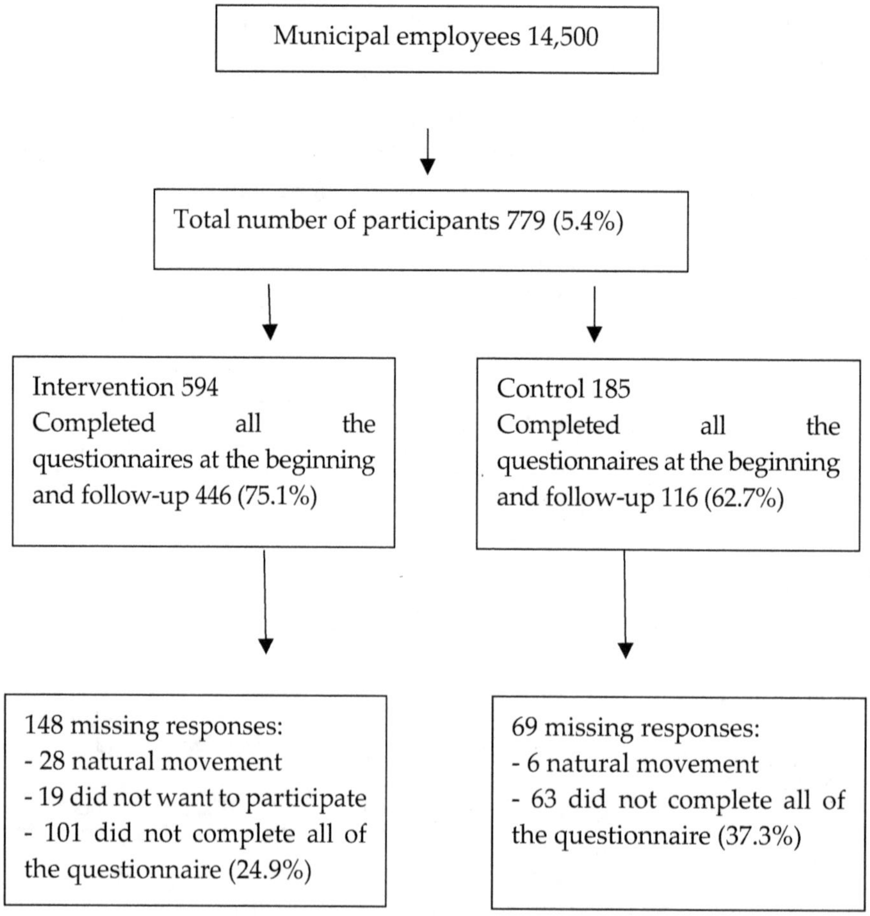

Figure 1. Participants in this study.

2.2. *Intervention*

An interdisciplinary, goal-oriented multi-professional team (a doctor, an occupational physiotherapist, an occupational psychologist, and a nurse) facilitated each intervention subgroup. The total intervention group was broken down into smaller subgroups for the purposes of the intervention. Goals were set with the participants, who each defined their own goals to improve their work ability. The subgroups met regularly for four months (one day every two weeks). After a further five months, there was the follow-up, which consisted of a three-hour subgroup meeting.

The intervention consisted of different educational components—for example, related to physical training, it was important that all participants understood their own physical test results and how to improve their aerobic condition, muscle strength, balance, and coordination. Physical training included identifying several aspects of one's physical condition and conducting practices based on those aspects, such as aerobic training focused on one's pulse level, or training for strength, balance, and coordination. During group reflection, all participants shared their experiences for last two-week period, providing feedback on what have they done to achieve their goals. Work well-being is in direct connection to the work and coping at work. Participants analysed their everyday work-related problems and found ways to understand changes at work and change-related phenomena and they learned new problem-solving skills and skills to talk with their supervisors at work about their work and develop work relationships in everyday life. Work-related problem-solving skills were practised by analysing the elements of one's work. Skills to talk and develop work relationships in everyday life were practised by starting recommended conversations in the workplace with one's supervisor concerning one's work and its daily challenges. Participants had experience on how to set short- and long-term individual goals and what kind of changes are realistic in their life situation.

On each intervention day, there were discussions of the issues affecting participants' work ability. Every meeting started with individual reflections on the previous two weeks, including things that had been successful, as well as challenging situations. Groups were directed to try to find solutions to challenging situations, rather than to concentrate on problems; to analyse their own work with tools that would help them to see changes in their working lives from a new perspective; to start conversations with their supervisors according to their own interests; and to plan their own paths towards their goals. Peer support was available during the group conversations, which were described as very meaningful by the participants. The group discussions were well received by the participants.

It was considered important that learning should be transferred to everyday health-related activities as soon as possible, to facilitate long-term effects. The rhythm of sessions supported this self-reliance: The sessions were every two weeks, and between sessions, everybody followed their own schedule. This process made it possible to implement practices around all the relevant issues in everyday life. This would be less easy in institutional rehabilitation, where participants usually spend longer periods away from ordinary life situations.

2.3. Study

The study was a nine-month trial to estimate the causal impact of the intervention on an intervention group, with a no-treatment control group that did not take part in the intervention. Only data from participants who had responded to all questions during the intervention and follow-up were included in the data analysis. Invitations to participate in the intervention and control groups were sent out to these employees through their workplace management.

Since this intervention was undertaken at an early, pre-clinical stage, there was no need for a medical certificate to take part. The main purpose was to offer an opportunity for intervention to those who needed some support to maintain their own work ability. This approach ensured that the intervention was offered at a time the participants believed was appropriate for them.

Participants were selected for the intervention by occupational health service professionals who had knowledge of the participants' medical histories, together with the participants' employers, who were aware of their work demands and workloads. Selection for intervention was thus undertaken collaboratively between occupational health service professionals and the employer. The employer, however, made the final decision as to whether the person could take paid leave from work on the outpatient intervention days. Employers paid the costs of the implementation, and employees took part during paid work hours. Social security paid compensation for the wage costs.

Widely used questionnaires with established reliability and validity were used. Questionnaires were completed at the beginning of the intervention and during follow-up. All questionnaires were administered to the intervention and control groups at the same time: Before the intervention and after nine months, just before the monitoring day.

The study was approved by the ethics committees of the Pirkanmaa Hospital District and the University of Tampere (No: R11068). Written informed consent was obtained from all study participants.

2.4. Measurement

The measurement tools used in this study were the Bergen Burnout Inventory (BBI) and the Utrecht Work Engagement Scale (UWES). All measurements were taken at baseline during the information session (autumn 2011); the intervention group completed the measurements at the follow-up test meeting, and the same measurements were taken for the control group at the same time (autumn 2014). The intervention and control subgroups who answered the questionnaires were from the same work units. Each question, including personal information, such as name and social security number, was numbered. The questionnaires were saved in folders, and the folders were archived according to healthcare requirements. The data were stored in a password-protected Excel file, with personal information removed, for statistical tests.

BBI 15 was used to measure burnout. It includes three sub-dimensions: Exhaustion (five items), cynicism (five items), and sense of inadequacy (five items). The internal validity of this test has been previously described [20,21]. The percentiles for age and gender are presented in the manual: Zero to 74 indicates no burnout, 75 to 84 indicates slight burnout, 85 to 94 indicates moderate burnout, and 95 to 100 indicates serious burnout. In this study, we considered only the total sum of BBI 15 and its subdimensions. The BBI 15 measurement can be used in research and occupational health contexts, because BBI 15 has high item–scale reliabilities and good concurrent validity among managers in Finland and Estonia [3,22].

UWES 9 was used to define three dimensions of work engagement: Vigour (three items), dedication (three items), and absorption (three items) [3]. Persons with high vigour scores report high energy, are willing to invest high effort in their work, and display mental resilience while working; persons with high scores on dedication are inspired by their work, see their work as important, and feel pride in their work; persons with high scores on absorption report giving full attention to their work, and the majority find it difficult to detach from work. The UWES assesses a mental state of accomplishment, which is the opposite to burnout [3,22]. Intercorrelations between the three UWES scales exceed 0.65, and the internal consistency of Cronbach's α is equal to the critical value of 0.70 [23,24]. UWES 9 was developed by Schaufeli and Bakker in the Netherlands [24,25].

Two questions were used to screen for depression: (1) "During the last month, have you often been worried, dismal, depressed or hopeless? Answer yes or no"; (2) "During the last month, have you often been worried about experiencing a lack of interest or unwillingness to accomplish things? Answer yes or no". One or more affirmative answers indicated probable depression [26]. The stress screening question consisted of a single item: "Stress refers to a situation in which a person feels tense, restless, nervous or anxious, or where it is difficult to sleep because of issues constantly on your mind/due to worry. Are you currently experiencing this kind of stress?" The question was answered on a scale from one (not at all) to five (very much) [27].

2.5. Data Collection

The primary measurement tools used in this study were quantitative, like the Bergen Burnout Inventory (BBI15) and the Utrecht Work Engagement Scale (UWES). The intervention and control groups who answered these questionnaires were from the same work unit and they had the same criteria for taking part to the intervention. At the time of the first measurements filling, there was not any group division. We tried to randomise these groups, but we did not totally succeed because of working conditions. All measurements were taken at baseline in the information session of the intervention for both groups; the intervention group completed the measurements at the follow-up test meeting, and the same measurements were posted for the control group at the same time. The questionnaires were distributed to study participants in autumn 2011 and autumn 2014. The participants could fill in the questionnaires during their working hours.

2.6. Statistical Analyses

Differences between the groups at baseline were tested using the Mann–Whitney U test or chi-square test for categorical variables. Within-group comparisons between baseline and nine-month follow-up scores were performed using the Wilcoxon signed-ranks test. The main effects and interactions for the scores of the intervention and control groups at baseline and follow-up were tested using repeated measures analysis of variance. p Values of less than 0.05 were considered statistically significant. The data analysis was performed with SPSS 23.0 software (IBM Corporation, Armonk, NY, USA).

3. Results

The results contain only those answers where all items had been filled in at the beginning and end of the study. Baseline, follow-up, and the changes between baseline values and follow-up for the intervention and control groups are shown in Table 3 for the BBI 15 and UWES.

Table 3. Intervention and control groups at baseline and follow-up on total Bergen Burnout Inventory (BBI) 15 and Utrecht Work Engagement Scale (UWES) and all items, and changes in BBI 15 and UWES, related factors.

BBI 15		Baseline		Follow-Up				
	Intervention Group *N* = 425, Control Group *N* = 109	**Mean**	**SD**	**Mean**	**SD**	**Change from Baseline**	***p*-Value**	**Difference in Changes between Groups**
Total BBI 15	Intervention Control	36.9 37.6	11.8 12.2	33.9 37.5	12.3 14.4	−3 0.1	<0.001 0.912	0.023
Exhaustion (5 items)	Intervention Control	13.2 12.9	4.8 4.6	12.1 13.1	5.2 5.3	−1.1 0.2	<0.001 0.477	<0.001
Cynicism (5 items)	Intervention Control	10.6 11.2	4 4.2	10 11	4 5.1	−0.6 0.2	<0.001 0.622	0.927
Sense of inadequacy (5 items)	Intervention Control	13.1 13.6	4.8 4.9	11.8 13.4	4.9 5.5	−1.3 0.2	<0.001 0.68	0.016
UWES 9		**Baseline**		**Follow-Up**				
	Intervention Group *N* = 446, Control Group *N* = 116	**Mean**	**SD**	**Mean**	**SD**	**Change from Baseline**	***p*-Value**	**Difference in Changes between Groups**
Total UWES 9	Intervention Control	4.3 4.2	1.1 1	4.5 4.4	1.1 1.1	0.2 0.2	<0.001 0.142	0.711
Vigour (3 items)	Intervention Control	4.3 4.2	1 1	4.5 4.4	1 1	0.2 0.2	<0.001 0.154	0.555
Dedication (3 items)	Intervention Control	4.4 4.4	1.1 1.1	4.6 4.5	1.1 1.1	0.2 0.1	<0.001 0.054	0.919
Absorption (3 items)	Intervention Control	4.1 4.1	1.1 1	4.3 4.3	1.1 1.1	0.2 0.2	<0.001 0.232	0.659

Notes: Within-group changes in intervention and control groups after nine months (2) were compared with baseline (1). Difference in changes between groups measured by analysis of variance. Table shows only answers where all items were filled in at the beginning and end of the study.

Total BBI 15 values for the intervention group were 36.9 (standard deviation (SD) 11.8) at baseline and 33.9 (SD 12.3) at follow-up. The change from baseline was −3.0 ($p < 0.001$). Values for the control group were 37.6 (SD 12.2) at baseline and 37.5 (SD 14.4) at follow-up. The change from baseline was 0.1 ($p = 0.912$). The difference in changes between groups was statistically significant ($p = 0.023$).

In the intervention group, the total BBI 15 score ($p < 0.01$) and each of the three subdimensions of burnout (exhaustion, cynicism, and sense of inadequacy) decreased at follow-up. There was no corresponding decrease in BBI 15 scores for the control group. The difference in changes between groups in BBI 15 sub-scores was statistically significant for exhaustion ($p < 0.001$), but not for cynicism ($p = 0.927$) or sense of inadequacy ($p = 0.016$).

Total UWES 9 values for the intervention group were 4.3 (SD 1.1) at baseline and 4.5 (SD 1.1) at follow-up ($p < 0.001$). Values for the control group were 4.2 (SD 1.0) at baseline and 4.4 (SD 1.1) at follow-up ($p = 0.142$). There was no difference in changes (0.2) between the groups ($p = 0.711$), although the change in p-value was significant in the intervention group ($N = 446$) compared with the control group ($N = 116$). The total UWES 9 score and all three of its dimensions of work engagement improved in the intervention group ($p < 0.001$).

There was also a similar improvement in total UWES scores and two of its dimensions (vigour and absorption) compared with the control group (0.2), change in dedication in the intervention group was also 0.2, and in the control group, 0.1. It is possible that the questionnaire itself acted as intervention and led to some positive change. However, there were no statistically significant differences in the changes in any UWES scores from baseline to follow-up between the groups, because the change from baseline was very similar in both groups (Table 3).

The composite score for the two depression screening items decreased significantly from baseline to follow-up for the intervention group ($N = 451$), in which 6.4% of scores increased, 13.3% decreased, and 80.3% were at the same level as baseline ($p = 0.001$). There was no significant change for the control group ($N = 115$), in which 12.2% of scores increased, 7.8% decreased, and 80% were at the same level as baseline ($p = 0.405$).

The composite score for the one stress screening question compared with the baseline showed significant differences in the follow-up of the intervention group ($N = 445$): 39% increased, 15.5% decreased, and 45.5% were at the same level as baseline ($p < 0.001$). In the control group ($N = 117$), 24% increased, 26% decreased, and 50% were at the same level as baseline ($p = 0.596$).

4. Discussion

The principal finding of this study is a statistically significant improvement in several measures of psychosocial well-being (BBI 15, UWES, stress, depression) for participants who completed the cognitive behavioural intervention programme. No corresponding changes were identified in the control group. There was a significantly greater change in BBI 15 from baseline for the intervention group than for the control group. The UWES questionnaires seemed to produce nearly the same improvement in both the intervention and control groups, although the improvement in the control group was not statistically significant because of the group size. Factors associated with social processes at work seem to be crucial to burnout as measured by BBI 15. Burnout is connected to job demands, a lack of job resources, and health problems. When intervention leads to positive changes in participants' physical condition or work environment, participants have been shown to be able to modify their self-perceptions, resulting in psychological and behavioural changes, such as increased self-approval, self-mercy, and recognition of their inner needs and limits [28–30].

It seems that the effects of our cognitive behavioural intervention to improve employees' well-being was able to meet some challenges in the improvement of attitudes as measured by BBI 15. The UWES 9, used to define three dimensions of work engagement, showed significant improvement in the intervention group, for whom goals were set in collaboration with the participants, and every participant defined their own goals to improve their work ability. An earlier study also suggested that focusing on work engagement might benefit the individual. Employees who seem to perform better have elevated levels of energy and identification with their work [29].

All three UWES dimensions were at average levels at the beginning and follow-up, although absorption increased to an elevated level in both the intervention and control groups. It may be that the questionnaire acted as an intervention for both groups, regardless of other interventions [30,31].

The composite of two depression screening items showed significant improvement at follow-up for the intervention group. This result contrasts somewhat with earlier evidence that the use of screening for depression is associated with only a modest increase in its recognition. If used alone, screening questionnaires for depression appear to have little or no impact on the management of depression [25]. However, our intervention was performed after initial screening and appeared to influence depressive thoughts positively. The stress screening consisted of a single question, and stress was lower after the intervention. This result is in line with previous findings that cognitive behavioural stress management interventions are more effective than other intervention types [32].

The practical point of intervention is to be aware of the different profiles among employees regarding adjustments in the work and non-work demands they face. It is important to create interventions to support work cultures for diverse ways of working, because there is no single optimal way to manage boundaries between work and non-work. Person-oriented interventions that are tailored to support different profiles are needed [33].

Limitations of the Study

One limitation is that the participants represent a relatively small population in Finland. The intervention and control groups were selected partly according to the participants' own interests.

The overall workload of every employee in the workplace was considered during the selection process by the employer. This selection may have produced differences between the groups at baseline, and selection for the intervention might be one driver of some changes in the scores. Supervisors played a key role in allocating participants to groups.

A randomised control group could not be used for the intervention because of workplace constraints. Issues that needed to be considered included the timetable of the entire process, holidays, individuals' work situations, and the need to achieve a sufficient number of participants in the intervention group—there were not the same numbers of participants in the control group. However, the control group was from the same work unit as the intervention group, and participants were chosen as randomly as possible from that environment.

Question-based research may suffer from bias if the participants feel satisfied with the service and therefore respond positively when they answer the second time. Two dimensions of the UWES 9 results also improved in the control group, and statistically, the same change was significant in the larger intervention group, but not in the smaller control group; the change between the groups showed no statistical difference. This kind of long-lasting service includes many changing variables, which makes it difficult to define the causes of the results. A third measurement point would have enabled broader statistical analysis.

In this study, we had a respectable amount of data to ensure its adequacy for possible dropouts. Dropout is a prevalent complication in the analysis of data from follow-up studies, but in this study, there were no differences between those who responded compared with those who did not in terms of age, gender, years of work or work unit.

As part of our results suggest that the cognitive behavioural intervention was effective in increasing employees' well-being, we currently have no measures to show its financial benefits to the employer. One recent systematic review has found that it is difficult to draw conclusions about the cost-effectiveness of intervention outcomes, because of the shifting quality of the studies [33].

5. Conclusions

This study suggests that a cognitive behavioural intervention achieved significant improvements in several measures of mental health. The results imply that this kind of intervention is needed to give early support on mental health issues for the working-age population. Early rehabilitation allows participants to play an active role while they still have the resources to make changes in their own lives. Overall, the results of this study permit the conclusion that this kind of service does support working ability in today's municipal sector. It is important to act preventively while participants have the resources to play an active role. Peer support also has remarkable value for finding solutions in different life situations.

Author Contributions: All authors were involved in the development of the study design. B.O. was responsible for the data collection and for writing the manuscript. S.T.N., C.-H.N. and P.B. participated in the general coordination of the study and corrected draft versions of the manuscript. H.H. provided statistical consultation.

Acknowledgments: We wish to thank all employees who participated in this study, and the personnel department of the City of Tampere. We thank Eeva Saarela and Tullinkulma Occupational Health Unit for their cooperation, for conducting the interventions, and for data management.

References

1. Sparks, K.; Faragher, B.; Cooper, C.L. Well-being and occupational health in the 21st century workplace. *J. Occup. Organ. Psychol.* **2001**, *1*, 489–509. [CrossRef]

2. Kuoppala, J.; Kekoni, J. At the sources of one's well-being: Early rehabilitation for employees with symptoms of distress. *Occup. Environ. Med.* **2013**, *55*, 817–823. [CrossRef] [PubMed]
3. Salmela-Aro, K.; Rantanen, J.; Hyvönen, K.; Tilleman, K.; Feldt, T. Bergen Burnout Inventory: Reliability and validity among Finnish and Estonian managers. *Int. Arch. Occup. Environ. Health* **2011**, *84*, 635–645. [CrossRef]
4. Schaufeli, W.B.; Leiter, M.P.; Maslach, C. Burnout: 35 years of research and practice. *Career Dev. Int.* **2009**, *14*, 204–220. [CrossRef]
5. Madsen, I.E.H.; Nyberg, S.T.; Magnusson Hanson, L.L.; Ferrie, J.E.; Ahola, K.; Alfredsson, L.; Batty, G.D.; Bjorner, J.B.; Borritz, M.; Burr, H.; et al. Job strain as a risk factor for clinical depression: Systematic review and meta-analysis with additional individual participant data. *Psychol. Med.* **2017**, *47*, 1342–1356. [CrossRef]
6. Ahola, K.; Toppinen-Tanner, S.; Huuhtanen, P.; Koskinen, A.; Väänänen, A. Occupational burnout and chronic work disability: An eight-year cohort study on pensioning among Finnish forest industry workers. *J. Affect. Disord.* **2009**, *115*, 150–159. [CrossRef] [PubMed]
7. Ahola, K.; Väänänen, A.; Koskinen, A.; Kouvonen, A.; Shirom, A. Burnout as a predictor of all-cause mortality among industrial employees: A 10-year prospective register-linkage study. *J. Psychosom. Res.* **2010**, *69*, 51–57. [CrossRef]
8. Siukola, A.; Virtanen, P.J.; Luukkaala, T.H.; Nygård, C.-H. Perceived working conditions and sickness absence: A four-year follow-up in the food industry. *Saf. Health Work* **2011**, *2*, 313–320. [CrossRef] [PubMed]
9. Awa, W.L.; Plaumann, M.; Walter, U. Burnout prevention: A review of intervention programs. *Patient Educ. Couns.* **2010**, *78*, 184–190. [CrossRef] [PubMed]
10. Hätinen, M.; Kinnunen, U.; Pekkonen, M.; Kalimo, R. Comparing two burnout interventions: Perceived job control mediates decreases in burnout. *Int. J. Stress Manag.* **2007**, *14*, 227–248. [CrossRef]
11. Kuoppala, J.; Lamminpaa, A.; Husman, P. Work health promotion, job well-being, and sickness absences: A systematic review and meta-analysis. *J. Occup. Environ. Med.* **2008**, *50*, 1216–1227. [CrossRef] [PubMed]
12. Hätinen, M.; Kinnunen, U.; Pekkonen, M.; Aro, A. Burnout patterns in rehabilitation: Short-term changes in job conditions, personal resources, and health. *J. Occup. Health Psychol.* **2004**, *9*, 220–237. [CrossRef]
13. Kahn, W.A.; Fellows, S. Employee engagement and meaningful work. In *Purpose and Meaning in the Workplace*; Dik, B.J., Byrne, Z.S., Steger, M.F., Eds.; American Psychological Association: Washington, DC, USA, 2013; pp. 105–126.
14. García-Sierra, R.; Fernández-Castro, J.; Martínez-Zaragoza, F. Work engagement in nursing: An integrative review of the literature. *J. Nurs. Manag.* **2016**, *24*, E101–E111. [CrossRef]
15. Coffeng, J.; Hendriksen, I.; Duijts, S.; Twisk, J.; van Mechelen, W.; Boot, C. Effectiveness of a combined social and physical environmental intervention on presenteeism, absenteeism, work performance, and work engagement in office employees. *J. Occup. Environ. Med.* **2014**, *56*, 258–265. [CrossRef]
16. Pomaki, G.; Franche, R.; Murray, E.; Khushrushahi, N.; Lampinen, T.M. Workplace-based work disability prevention interventions for workers with common mental health conditions: A review of the literature. *J. Occup. Rehabil.* **2012**, *22*, 182–195. [CrossRef]
17. Ruotsalainen, J.; Serra, C.; Marine, A.; Verbeek, J. Systematic review of interventions for reducing occupational stress in health care workers. *Scand. J. Work Environ. Health* **2008**, *34*, 169–178. [CrossRef]
18. Richardson, K.M.; Rothstein, H.R. Effects of occupational stress management intervention programs: A meta-analysis. *J. Occup. Health Psychol.* **2008**, *13*, 69–93. [CrossRef]
19. Imamura, K.; Kawakami, N.; Furukawa, T.A.; Matsuyama, Y.; Shimazu, A.; Umanodan, R.; Kawakami, S.; Kasai, K. Does Internet-based cognitive behavioral therapy (iCBT) prevent major depressive episode for workers? A 12-month follow-up of a randomized controlled trial. *Psychol. Med.* **2015**, *45*, 1907–1917. [CrossRef]
20. Naatanen, P.; Aro, A.; Matthiesen, S.B.; Salmela-Aro, K. *Bergen Burnout Indicator 15*; Edita: Helsinki, Finland, 2003.
21. Schaufeli, W.B.; Bakker, A.B. *Test Manual for the Utrecht Work Engagement Scale*; Utrecht University Occupational Health Psychology Unit: Utrecht, The Netherlands, 2003; Available online: http://www.schaufeli.com (accessed on 12 October 2018).
22. Schaufeli, W.; Martínez, I.; Pinto, A.; Salanova, M.; Bakker, A. Burnout and engagement in university students: A crossnational study. *J. Cross Cult. Psychol.* **2002**, *33*, 464–481. [CrossRef]

23. Bakker, A.B.; Leiter, M.P. *Work Engagement: A Handbook of Essential Theory and Research*, 1st ed.; Imprint Psychology Press: London, UK, 2010.
24. Bakker, A.B.; Albrecht, S.L.; Leiter, M.P. Key questions regarding work engagement. *Eur. J. Work Organ. Psychol.* **2011**, *20*, 4–28. [CrossRef]
25. Shuck, B.; Zigarmi, D.; Owen, J. Psychological needs, engagement, and work intentions. *Eur. J. Train. Dev.* **2015**, *39*, 2–21. [CrossRef]
26. Arroll, B.; Khin, N.; Kerse, N. Screening for depression in primary care with two verbally asked questions: Cross sectional study. *BMJ* **2003**, *327*, 1144–1146. [CrossRef]
27. Elo, A.; Leppänen, A.; Jahkola, A. Validity of a single-item measure of stress symptoms. *Scand. J. Work Environ. Health* **2003**, *29*, 444–451. [CrossRef] [PubMed]
28. Gilbody, S.; Richards, D.; Brealey, S.; Hewitt, C. Screening for depression in medical settings with the patient health questionnaire (PHQ): A diagnostic meta-analysis. *J. Gen. Intern. Med.* **2007**, *22*, 1596–1602. [CrossRef] [PubMed]
29. Schaufeli, W.B.; Bakker, A.B.; Salanova, M. The measurement of work engagement with a short questionnaire: A cross-national study. *Educ. Psychol. Meas.* **2006**, *66*, 701–716. [CrossRef]
30. Schaufeli, W.B.; Bakker, A.B.; Van Rhenen, W. How changes in job demands and resources predict burnout, work engagement, and sickness absenteeism. *J. Organ. Behav.* **2009**, *30*, 893–917. [CrossRef]
31. Schaufeli, W.B.; Salanova, M.; Gonzalez-Roma, V.; Bakker, A.B. The measurement of burnout and engagement: A confirmatory factor analytic approach. *J. Happiness Stud.* **2002**, *3*, 71–92. [CrossRef]
32. Van der Klink, J.; Blonk, R.; Schene, A.; van Dijk, F. The benefits of interventions for work-related stress. *Am. J. Public Health* **2001**, *91*, 270–276.
33. Kinnunen, U.; Rantanen, J.; de Bloom, J.; Mauno, S.; Feldt, T.; Korpela, K. The role of work-nonwork boundary management in work stress recovery. *Int. J. Stress Manag.* **2016**, *23*, 99–123. [CrossRef]

13

Developing Wellbeing Through a Randomised Controlled Trial of a Martial Arts Based Intervention: An Alternative to the Anti-Bullying Approach

Brian Moore *, Stuart Woodcock and Dean Dudley

Department of Educational Studies, Faculty of Human Sciences, Macquarie University, North Ryde, NSW 2109, Australia; stuart.woodcock@mq.edu.au (S.W.); dean.dudley@mq.edu.au (D.D.)

* Correspondence: brian.william.moore@det.nsw.edu.au

Abstract: Anti-bullying policies and interventions are the main approach addressing bullying behaviours in Australian schools. However, the evidence supporting these approaches is inconsistent and its theoretical underpinning may be problematic. The current study examined the effects of a martial arts based psycho-social intervention on participants' ratings of resilience and self-efficacy, delivered as a randomised controlled trial to 283 secondary school students. Results found a consistent pattern for strengths-based wellbeing outcomes. All measures relating to resilience and self-efficacy improved for the intervention group, whereas results declined for the control group. These findings suggest that a martial arts based psycho-social intervention may be an efficacious method of improving wellbeing outcomes including resilience and self-efficacy. The study proposes utilising alternatives to the anti-bullying approach and that interventions should be aimed towards helping individuals develop strengths and cope more effectively, which has specific relevance to bullying and more generalised importance to positive mental health.

Keywords: bullying; martial arts; mental health; resilience; self-efficacy; wellbeing

---

1. Introduction

Bullying is a complex and controversial subject that receives frequent media and academic attention. However, there is no standard definition of bullying [1–3], and definitions inclusive of all bullying behaviours are difficult to establish [4]. Bullying behaviours can occur directly and indirectly; and include verbal, physical, and/or relational characteristics. Research suggests bullying can be defined as: (a) a type of aggression [5], (b) systematic and repeated [6], and (c) based upon an imbalance of power [7,8].

Anti-bullying policies and interventions are the main approach addressing bullying behaviours in Australian schools [9]. However, the evidence supporting these approaches is indeterminate (for example: [1,10,11]) and their theoretical underpinnings are problematic [4,5].

Examining Australian state and territory educational policies and related documents suggests there is a relatively consistent approach to bullying policy across Australia. While education is primarily a state and territory responsibility in Australia, there has been a collaborative approach to addressing bullying across Australian education jurisdictions. For example, the Bullying. No way! website [9] is a collaborative product of the Australian Government's (AG) Department of Education, the state and territory government education departments, the National Catholic Education Commission, and the Independent Schools Council of Australia. This consistency is also due to school-based anti-bullying interventions being the main strategy addressing bullying behaviours [12]. Table 1 lists key policies across Australia, and Table 2 provides details of the characteristics of anti-bullying programs across Australian education jurisdictions.

Table 1. Australian educational bullying policy and associated documents.

Education Jurisdiction	Bullying Policy Accessible Online	Policy Document Title
ACT (Territory)	Yes	Safe and supportive schools policy [13]
AG (Federal)	No [a]	Disability Discrimination Act 1992 [14] Human Rights and Equal Opportunity Commission (HREOC) Act 1986 [15] Racial Discrimination Act 1975 [16] Racial Hatred Act 1995 [17] Sex Discrimination Act 1984 [18]
NSW (State)	Yes	Bullying of students—Prevention and response policy [19]
NT (Territory)	Limited	Health and wellbeing of students: Bullying, cyberbullying and cybersafety [20]
QLD (State)	Yes	Preventing bullying and violence [21]
SA (State)	Limited	Keeping children safe from bullying [22]
TAS (State)	No	n/a
VIC (State)	Yes	School Policy—Bullying [23]
WA (State)	Yes	Guidelines for preventing and managing bullying in schools [24]

Note. ACT: Australian Capital Territory, AG: Australian Government, NSW: New South Wales, NT: Northern Territory, QLD: Queensland, SA: South Australia, TAS: Tasmania, VIC: Victoria, WA: Western Australia. [a] While there is no specific Federal policy regarding school bullying the listed Federal legislation is relevant to this area.

As indicated by Table 2, Australian anti-bullying policies have relatively consistent characteristics. Policies typically define bullying as: (a) involving the misuse of power in a relationship, (b) ongoing and repeated behaviour, and (c) involving behaviours intended to cause harm [9]. It is important to consider differences between the former (research oriented) and latter (policy oriented) definitions of bullying. First, the latter definition omits the notion that bullying is a form of aggression [5]. Second, while the issue of power is noted in the latter definition, the meaning of this is moderated by including the term misuse. Third, the latter definition includes a focus on intent and harm causation. While this issue is not excluded from the former definition, its use in the latter frames the way bullying is conceptualised in terms of victims and perpetrators of bullying.

In response to these definitions, anti-bullying interventions typically fall into several categories. These include behavioural rule-based, non-punitive, social-emotional learning, and student intervention approaches. Policies typically mandate schools have official bullying or anti-bullying plans but suggest a flexible approach to implementation. Consequently, while policy and associated documents suggest a variety of strategies, it is difficult to know what anti-bullying actions are enacted at the school level.

Table 2. Characteristics of Australian anti-bullying programs based on policy and associated documents.

Education Jurisdiction	Defines Bullying	Mandates Bullying Plan	Whole School	Preventative Strategies	Awareness Raising	Staff Training	Engage Carers	Behaviour Sanctions	Non-Punitive	Social-Emotional	Bystander Intervention
ACT (Territory)	√	√	√	√	√	√	√	√	√	√	x
AG (Federal)	√	n/a	√	√	√	√	√	√	√	√	√
NSW (State)	√	√	√	√	√	√	√	√	√	√	√
NT (Territory)	√	x	x	x	x	x	x	x	x	x	x
QLD (State)	√	√	√	√	√	√	√	x	√	√	√
SA (State)	√	√	√	√	x	√	√	x	x	x	x
TAS (State)	n/a	n/a	n/a	n/a	n/a	n/a	n/a	n/a	n/a	n/a	n/a
VIC (State)	√	√	√	√	√	√	√	x	√	√	√
WA (State)	√	√	√	√	√	√	√	x	√	√	x

Note. ACT: Australian Capital Territory, AG: Australian Government, NSW: New South Wales, NT: Northern Territory, QLD: Queensland, SA: South Australia, TAS: Tasmania, VIC: Victoria, WA: Western Australia, √ = yes, x = not stated, n/a = not applicable.

1.1. *The Failure of Anti-Bullying Policy*

Anti-bullying literature frequently claims substantial empirical support to address bullying [1,25]. However, these claims should be viewed with caution. Case in point, a meta-analysis published by the Australian Government's Attorney General's Department reported that "with several exceptions . . . the outcomes from the evaluations reviewed were . . . positive in reducing overall bullying behaviour" [1] (p. 2). Despite Rigby's [1] assertion that research shows bullying behaviours among school children can be "significantly reduced" (p. 1), this is not wholly supported by the evidence presented in the meta-analysis. Notably, of the 13 studies reviewed by the meta-analysis three studies reported no change and six studies cited increased bullying behaviour post-intervention.

Evidence provided by other meta-analyses vary considerably in the level of support they provide for the efficacy of anti-bullying approaches. Ttofi and Farrington [11], reported that anti-bullying programs reduced bullying behaviours by an average of 20–23 per cent; and Jiménez-Barbero, Ruiz-Hernández, Llor-Zaragoza, Pérez-García, and Llor-Esteban [26] reported that anti-bullying programs resulted in significant reductions in the frequency of bullying behaviours. By contrast, Merrell, Gueldner, Ross and Isava [10] reported mixed results regarding anti-bullying programs changing rates of bullying; and Smith, Schneider, Smith and Ananiadau [27] reported that only a small number of programs produced positive outcomes regarding bullying and victimisation. Despite claims of substantial empirical support, the evidence to date is largely inconclusive.

The published meta-analyses raise another issue regarding anti-bullying policy and interventions to-date. It appears that the construct has become so broad that included studies contain almost any program that mentions bullying as a potential outcome variable. This leads to complicated methodologies and instruments being applied and it is therefore unsurprising that research to-date has not established what elements of anti-bullying strategies are crucial for reducing bullying behaviours [1]. Nonetheless, Farrington and Ttofi's [12] meta-analysis suggested that several anti-bullying strategies appear to be associated with decreased bullying. The most important of these being disciplinary methods including using explicit consequences regarding bullying, followed by parent training and meetings, and the duration and intensity of bullying programs.

1.2. *An Evolutionary Perspective of Bullying*

Bullying is a complex phenomenon that resists simple solutions [9]. Consequently, it is important to consider the narrative underpinning the anti-bullying approach to understand why the evidence regarding anti-bullying programs is inconclusive. As noted, anti-bullying policies typically omit the notion that bullying is a form of aggression [5] from their definitions. Aggression can be conceptualised as an exercise of power and relational power imbalances are critical to understanding bullying behaviours [28]. While anti-bullying literature proposed that bullying involves the abuse and exploitation of power [3,8], an evolutionary psychology perspective explores the use of power and rationalises why power imbalances exist.

Evolutionary psychology proposes that behaviours exist because they are adaptive [28]. Consequently, it is important to consider the adaptive nature of bullying, which appears to be a ubiquitous human behaviour [3,4]. Social dominance theory proposed that bullying can be used as a strategy to establish and maintain social dominance which facilitates access to valued resources, and can be understood in terms of the costs and benefits associated with using aggression [5]. It appears that many of the strategies used by the anti-bullying approach attempt to shift the relational balance of power without accounting for an evolutionary understanding of bullying behaviour. This occurs across behavioural, non-punitive, and student intervention anti-bullying strategies.

Bystander intervention has been identified as a "core tenant" of anti-bullying programs [29] (pp. 31–32), and involves shifting bystanders to become "active defenders of bullied students" [25] (p. 8). This approach can be interpreted as attempting to change the relational balance of power and may be a conceptually optimistic strategy. Research regarding the bystander effect was developed due to the observation that bystanders are unlikely to help others [30]. Latane and Darley [30] suggested that there are many factors that inhibit helping and make bystander intervention less likely including bystanders noticing that something is happening, interpreting the event and deciding something is wrong, assuming personal responsibility for helping, and deciding how to help.

1.3. Resilience and Bullying

Resilience is a complex construct [31] that is often defined as the attainment of positive outcomes despite significant adversity, risk, or stress [32,33]. This is evident in the varying operational definitions of resilience which include hardiness, optimism, competence, self-esteem, social-skills, achievement, and absence of pathology in the face of adversity [34]. Resilience can be conceptualised as a multi-level construct that includes: (a) protective processes, (b) the interaction of protection and risks, and (c) conceptual tools used in predictive models [35]. Examining resilience in terms of protective factors offers a viable means of measuring the construct [36] and recent research has suggested specific resilience factors may have greater efficacy in developing resilience based approaches to bullying [37].

Generally, the research examining the relationship between resilience and bullying is limited. Positively, students who reported higher levels of resilience were found to be less likely to engage in bullying behaviours or be victims of bullying [38]. Resilience towards bullying behaviours appeared to improve when individuals could disclose their experiences to a peer or family member [39] which is supported by research finding family factors, such as warm relationships and positive home environments were associated with greater resilience to bullying [40]. Resilience programs that improved social skills also appeared to decrease bullying behaviours [41]. Greater resilience and self-efficacy to bullying was reported as correlating with students completing an adventure based anti-bullying initiative [42], however the study reported weak correlations (ranging from $r = 0.25$ to $r = 0.26$) to support its claims.

A recent study by Moore and Woodcock [28] examining the mental health impacts of bullying considered resilience from a factorial perspective and conceptualised resilience as incorporating a sense of mastery, relatedness to others, and emotional reactivity. The study found higher levels of mastery and relatedness were a protective factor regarding depression, lower levels of emotional reactivity were a protective factor regarding depression and anxiety, and that higher levels of emotional reactivity were associated with an increased likelihood of bullying and being a victim of bullying behaviours. In a follow-up study, Moore and Woodcock [37] examined the resilience sub-scales underpinning these factors and found a pattern of effect sizes that suggested the sub-scale factors optimism, trust, tolerance, sensitivity and impairment may be more important for developing efficacious interventions that promote resilience to the effects of bullying.

1.4. Martial Arts Based Therapeutic Intervention and Developing Wellbeing

Martial arts are an ancient human behaviour which are often associated with promoting psychological benefits such as increased well-being, self-esteem and confidence [43]. The term martial arts are often used to describe many of the combat arts that developed in Eastern cultures [44] and martial arts participation exhibited substantial growth during the 20th century [45]. Perceptions of the martial arts are mixed [46]. The views range from martial arts promoting psychological benefits [43] to the assumption that martial arts training results in negative socialization processes such as increased aggression and hostility [46]. The focus of existing research has examined the physical aspects of martial arts training, such as health benefits and injuries resulting from martial arts practice [44]. Few studies have examined whether martial arts training can address mental health problems or promote mental health and wellbeing.

In a recent meta-analysis Moore, Dudley and Woodcock [47] reported that martial arts training had a positive effect on mental health outcomes. The analysis found that martial arts training had a small effect size regarding increasing wellbeing, and medium effect size regarding reducing internalising mental health issues, such as anxiety and depression. Several studies have reported martial arts training promoted characteristics associated with wellbeing. For example, a study examining a six-month taekwondo program reported increased self-esteem following the intervention [48]; while another found that participants reported higher self-concept compared to a comparison group after studying taekwondo for eight weeks [49]. Similarly, several studies reported that martial arts training reduced the symptoms associated with anxiety and depression. For example, karate students have been reported as being less prone to depression compared to reported norms for male college students [50]; and training in tai-chi reduced anxiety and depression compared to a non-treatment condition [51]. However, studies examining the psychological effects of martial arts training exhibit significant methodological problems that limit the generalisability of findings [46,52]. These include theoretical problems such as conceptual and definitional issues; and research design problems including a reliance on cross-sectional designs, small sample sizes, self-selection effects, limited use of follow-up measures, and not accounting for gender differences.

1.5. *Bullying and a Martial Arts Based Psycho-Social Intervention*

This study proposes an evolutionary perspective of bullying and considers the term bullying as a synonym for power imbalances in relationships. If it is assumed that bullying behaviours have an adaptive function, it may be optimistic to believe that bullying behaviours can be systemically modified.

An alternative approach could involve more generalised interventions promoting mental health through developing strengths, wellbeing and the ability to cope. Martial arts training can be conceptualised as a sports-based mental health intervention, where sport provides "the hook" [53] (p. 124) with which to deliver psycho-social interventions. Given its emphasis on respect, self-regulation and health promotion, martial arts training may be efficacious alternative to the anti-bullying approach. However, the efficacy of martial arts based interventions has received little research attention [54]. This study examined a martial arts based intervention using a randomised controlled trial design, and considered whether this type of sports-based psycho-social approach has the potential to improve participants' ratings of resilience and self-efficacy.

1.6. *Theoretical Framework*

The theoretical framework of this study is based on the bipartite martial arts model. Research examining the effects of martial arts training on mental health outcomes has typically used a bipartite model [55] which distinguishes between traditional and modern martial arts practice. This model assumes that the martial arts can be classified according to various criteria. The distinction between traditional and modern martial arts is based upon whether mediation, patterns practice and ethical and philosophical teachings are included (traditional martial arts) or excluded (modern martial arts) [56]. Traditional martial arts emphasize the non-aggressive aspects of martial arts, whereas modern martial arts typically emphasize competition and aggression [57]. The study is based on a traditional martial arts perspective.

1.7. *Research Questions*

Based on the literature review including identified gaps, methodological issues, and theoretical orientation; the following questions are proposed for investigation:

1. How does participation in a 10-week martial arts based intervention affect mental health factors, including resilience and self-efficacy?; and,
2. What is the relationship of mental health factors, including resilience and self-efficacy:
    a) before a 10-week martial based intervention (pre-intervention)?
    b) immediately after a 10-week martial based intervention (post-intervention)? and,
    c) three months after a 10-week martial based intervention (follow-up)?

2. Materials and Methods

2.1. Research Design

The study was a 10-week secondary school-based intervention that has been evaluated using a randomised controlled trial. Ethics approval for the study was obtained from an Australian University Human Research Ethics Committee. The study was registered with the Australian and New Zealand Clinical Trials Registry (ACTRN12618001405202). Additionally, the study protocol was also reviewed externally by school psychologists employed by the NSW Department of Education.

The researchers conducted pre-intervention (baseline) assessments at participating schools after the initial recruitment process. Following pre-intervention assessments and randomisation, the intervention group received the intervention program after which post-intervention assessment was conducted. At the time of writing this article results from the planned 12-week post-intervention (follow-up) assessment were not available. The control group received the same intervention program after the first post-intervention assessment. The design, conduct and reporting of this study adhered to the Consolidation Standards of Reporting Trials (CONSORT) guidelines for a randomised controlled trial [58]. Participants and caregivers provided written informed consent.

2.2. Participants

Two hundred and eighty-three ($N = 283$) students from five secondary schools in NSW, Australia were recruited to participate in the study. Participants had an age range of 12 to 14 years ($M = 12.76$, $SD = 0.68$) and were recruited from grade 7 ($n = 192$) and grade 8 ($n = 91$) at participating schools. One hundred and forty-three females and 136 males participated in the program. Four participants did not identify their biological sex. The socio-economic status of participants was reported as high ($n = 70$), high average ($n = 85$), low average ($n = 49$), and low ($n = 78$). The cultural background of the sample was predominantly reported as Australian ($n = 251$). Other reported cultural backgrounds included Aboriginal ($n = 2$), African ($n = 1$), Arabic ($n = 1$), Asian ($n = 14$), European ($n = 3$), and Pacific ($n = 8$). Two hundred and forty-one ($N = 241$) participants completed the post-intervention assessment. Of the 42 drop-outs from the study 20 participants chose to discontinue participation, 13 participants changed schools, and nine participants did not complete the assessment for unknown reasons.

Power calculations were conducted to determine the sample size required to detect changes in resilience and self-efficacy outcomes resulting from martial arts training. Statistical power calculations assumed baseline-post-test expected effect size gains of $d = 0.3$, and were based on 90% power with alpha levels set at $p < 0.05$. The minimum completion sample size was calculated as $N = 234$. As participant drop-out rates of 20% are common in randomised controlled trials [59] the maximum proposed sample size was $N = 293$.

2.3. Intervention Program

The intervention was delivered in a face-to-face group format onsite at participating schools. The intervention dose was 10×50 min sessions, once per week for 10 weeks. Each intervention session included:

(a) Psycho-education—based on facilitator guided group discussion. Topics included respect, goal-setting, self-concept and self-esteem, courage, resilience, bullying and peer pressure, self-care and caring for others, values, and, optimism and hope;
(b) Warm up activities—basic exercises including jogging, star jumps, push ups, and sit ups;
(c) Stretching activities—a variety of stretching activities were used during the program including hamstring stretch, triceps stretch, figure four stretch, butterfly stretch, lunging hip flexor stretch, knee to chest stretch, and standing quad stretch; and,
(d) Technical martial arts practice—including stances, blocks, punching, and kicking.

Additionally, the following activities were alternated during the program:

(e) Patterns practice—a pattern is a choreographed sequence of movements consisting of combinations of blocks, punches and kicks, performed as though defending against imaginary opponents;
(f) Sparring—an activity based on the tai-chi sticking hands exercise was included as an alternative to traditional martial arts sparring; and,
(g) Meditation—based on breath focusing exercise.

It should be noted that aggressive physical contact was not part of the intervention program. The intervention was delivered by a (1) registered psychologist with minimum 6 years of experience, and (2) 2nd Dan/level black-belt taekwondo instructor with minimum 5 years of experience.

2.4. Instruments

Evaluation of the intervention program involved a variety of standardised psychometric instruments to report on mental health related outcomes. Instruments included the Strengths and Difficulties Questionnaire (SDQ) [60], Child and Youth Resilience Measure (CYRM-28) [61], and the Self-Efficacy Questionnaire for Children (SEQ-C) [62].

The SDQ is a 25-item instrument that measures various aspects of children's and adolescents' behaviour. The scale provided a total problems scale and five subscales including an emotional scale, conduct scale, hyperactivity-inattention scale, peer problems scale, and a prosocial behaviour scale. The English language self-report version of the scale was used which has a good internal consistency (0.76) [63] and good convergent validity. Items are scored on a 3-point Likert scale with 0 = not true, 1 = somewhat true, and 2 = certainly true. An example of SDQ items include: (1) I have one good friend or more, and (2) I am kind to younger children.

The CYRM-28 is a 28-item instrument that measures various aspects of children's and adolescents' resilience. The scale provided a total resilience scale and three subscales including an individual capacities and resources scale, relationship with primary caregiver scale, and contextual factors scale. The self-report version of the scale was used which has good internal consistency (.66 to .81) [64] and good construct validity. Items are scored on a 5-point Likert scale with 0 = not at all, 1 = a little, 2 = somewhat, 3 = quite a bit, and 4 = a lot. An example of CYRM-28 items include: (1) I have people I look up to, and (2) I feel supported by my friends.

The SEQ-C is a 24-item instrument that measures various aspects of children's and adolescents' self-efficacy. The scale provided a total self-efficacy scale and three subscales including an academic self-efficacy scale, a social self-efficacy scale, and an emotional self-efficacy scale. The SEQ-C scales have good internal consistency (>0.70) [65]. Items are scored on a 5-point Likert scale with 0 = not at all, 1 = a little, 2 = somewhat, 3 = quite a bit, and 4 = very well. An example of SEQ-C items include: (1) How well can you become friends with other children? and (2) How well can you control your feeling?.

2.5. Data Collection

The sampling plan utilised a randomised controlled sample to generate data for the study. All eligible government or catholic secondary schools in an urban area of New South Wales, Australia (n = 140) were sent an initial email with an invitation to participate in the study. Schools that responded to the initial email were pooled and received a follow up call in random order from the project researchers to discuss their participation. The first five schools that demonstrated interest were then recruited into the study.

All students enrolled in grades 7 and 8 (target age range 12–14 years) at participating schools were invited to participate in the study. Participant and caregiver information and consent forms were provided to students. Two follow-up letters were subsequently sent at two week intervals. Students who responded to the invitation were pooled and randomly allocated into the study, or not included in the study. Concurrent martial arts training were exclusion criteria for participation in the study, however previous experience of martial arts training was not an exclusion criterion.

Data was collected at pre-intervention (baseline), post-intervention, and 12-week post-intervention (follow-up). Randomisation into intervention and control group occurred after pre-intervention assessments. A simple computer algorithm was used to randomly allocate participants into intervention or control groups. The researchers were blinded to this randomisation of intervention and control group allocations.

During data collection participants were withdrawn from regular classes in small groups (pre-intervention), or the groups in which they completed the program (post-intervention). This enabled the researchers to explain, monitor and provide assistance while participants completed the survey. Participants were reminded that the survey was confidential and that they could discontinue the survey at any point. Instructions given to participants included: (a) an explanation of rating scales, and (b) how to make corrections if necessary. Surveys were then given to participants. Upon completion participants placed the survey into a locked box to ensure confidentiality.

2.6. Data Analysis

Statistical analysis of the psychometric test data was conducted using Statistical Package for the Social Sciences version 25 (IBM SPSS Statistics, Chicago, IL, USA) and alpha levels were set at $p < 0.05$.

The collected psychometric test data was consolidated into subscale variables using factor analysis and the internal consistency of each variable was examined to determine reliability. This was completed for pre-intervention and post-intervention measures. Table 3 reports pre-intervention and post-intervention internal consistency for the SDQ, CYRM-28 and SEQ-C. During factor analysis the SDQ converged in four factors (the conduct subscale and attention subscale converged in one factor which was renamed behaviour problems). For the emotional problems subscale item 6 did not converge across pre-intervention and post-intervention factor analysis and was discarded from the study. Internal consistency for the emotional problems scale was good. For the behaviour problems subscale items 12 and 22 did not converge across pre-intervention and post-intervention factor analysis and were discarded from the study. Internal consistency for the behaviour problems scale was good. For the peer problems subscale items 12, 14 and 19 did not converge across pre-intervention and post-intervention factor analysis and were discarded from the study. Internal consistency for the peer problems scale was poor and the subscale was discarded from the study. All items converged for the prosocial behaviour subscale across pre-intervention and post-intervention factor analysis, however internal consistency for the prosocial behaviour scale was poor and the scale was discarded from the study. The internal consistency for the SDQ total problems scale was good across pre-intervention and post-intervention factor analysis.

Table 3. Internal consistency for SDQ, CYRM-28 and SEQ-C across pre-intervention and post-intervention measures.

Measure	Scale	Pre-Intervention α	Post-Intervention α
SDQ	Emotional problems	0.72	0.73
	Behaviour problems	0.81	0.81
	Peer problems	0.18	0.12
	Prosocial behaviour	0.50	0.45
	Total problems	0.72	0.76
CYRM-28	Individual capacities and resources	0.85	0.89
	Relationship with primary carer	0.80	0.81
	Contextual factors	0.73	0.74
	Total resilience	0.89	0.91
SEQ-C	Academic self-efficacy	0.83	0.84
	Social self-efficacy	0.78	0.82
	Emotional self-efficacy	0.81	0.85
	Total self-efficacy	0.89	0.91

During factor analysis the CYRM-28 converged in three factors. For the individual capacities and resources subscale all factors converged across pre-intervention and post-intervention factor analysis, and internal consistency for the scale was good. For the relationship with primary caregiver subscale all factors converged across pre-intervention and post-intervention factor analysis, and internal consistency for the scale was good. For the contextual factors subscale all factors converged across pre-intervention and post-intervention factor analysis, and internal consistency for the scale was good. The internal consistency for the CYRM-28 total resilience scale was good across pre-intervention and post-intervention factor analysis.

During factor analysis the SEQ-C converged in three factors. For the academic self-efficacy subscale all factors converged across pre-intervention and post-intervention factor analysis, and internal consistency for the scale was good. For the social self-efficacy subscale all factors converged across pre-intervention and post-intervention factor analysis, and internal consistency for the scale was good. For the emotional self-efficacy subscale item 8 did not converge across pre-intervention and post-intervention factor analysis and was discarded from the study. Internal consistency for the emotional self-efficacy scale was good. The internal consistency for the SEQ-C total self-efficacy scale was good across pre-intervention and post-intervention factor analysis.

Items to be included in the scale variables were added and computed to create composite scores for pre-intervention and post-intervention data. Multivariate analysis of variance (MANOVA), analysis of variance (ANOVA) and Chi-square analyses were used to examine test data. Interpretation of effect sizes reflected Cohen's suggested small, medium, and large effect sizes, where η_p^2 sizes are equal to 0.10, 0.25, and 0.40 respectively [66].

3. Results

3.1. Behaviour and Emotion Problems

The hypothesis that martial arts training would decrease total problems and related sub-factors was not supported. Using Pillai's trace, martial arts training had no significant effect on participants' emotional problems, $V = 0.004$, $F(2, 238) = 0.52$, $p = 0.59$, $\eta_p^2 = 0.004$; behavioural problems, $V = 0.014$, $F(2, 237) = 1.65$, $p = 0.19$, $\eta_p^2 = 0.014$; or total problems, $V = 0.006$, $F(2, 237) = 0.75$, $p = 0.47$, $\eta_p^2 = 0.006$. Means and standard deviations are summarized in Table 4.

Table 4. Means and standard deviations for SDQ strengths and difficulties scales by experimental condition.

Scale	Condition	Baseline		Post-Test	
		Mean	SD	Mean	SD
Emotional difficulties	Intervention	0.69	0.51	0.66	0.47
	Control	0.74	0.51	0.73	0.51
Behavioural difficulties	Intervention	0.77	0.42	0.77	0.45
	Control	0.78	0.48	0.68	0.43
Total difficulties	Intervention	0.82	0.23	0.81	0.24
	Control	0.81	0.24	0.78	0.25

3.2. Resilience

The intervention improved levels of the overall resilience and resilience sub-factors. Means and standard deviations are summarized in Table 5.

Individual capacities and resources: Using Pillai's trace, there was a significant effect of the experimental condition on participants' individual capacities and resources, $V = 0.10$, $F(2, 238) = 13.35$, $p < 0.001$, $\eta_p^2 = 0.10$. Separate univariate ANOVAs revealed no significant difference between the intervention and control condition pre-intervention, $F(1, 239) = 1.64$, $p = 0.20$, $\eta_p^2 = 0.007$; however there was a significant difference between the intervention and control condition post-intervention, $F(1, 239) = 18.87$, $p < 0.001$, $\eta_p^2 = 0.07$.

Relationship with primary caregiver: There was a significant effect of the experimental condition on participants' relationship with primary caregiver, $V = 0.09$, $F(2, 238) = 11.59$, $p < 0.001$, $\eta_p^2 = 0.09$. Separate univariate ANOVAs revealed no significant difference between the intervention and control condition pre-intervention, $F(1, 239) = 1.06$, $p = 0.30$, $\eta_p^2 = 0.004$; however there was a significant difference between the intervention and control condition post-intervention, $F(1, 239) = 23.04$, $p < 0.001$, $\eta_p^2 = 0.09$.

Contextual factors: There was a significant effect of the experimental condition on participants' contextual factors, $V = 0.09$, $F(2, 238) = 11.94$, $p < 0.001$, $\eta_p^2 = 0.09$. Separate univariate ANOVAs revealed no significant difference between the intervention and control condition pre-intervention, $F(1, 239) = 1.54$, $p = 0.22$, $\eta_p^2 = 0.006$; however there was a significant difference between the intervention and control condition post-intervention, $F(1, 239) = 22.10$, $p < 0.001$, $\eta_p^2 = 0.09$.

Total resilience: There was a significant effect of the experimental condition on participants' total resilience score, $V = 0.14$, $F(2, 238) = 18.58$, $p < 0.001$, $\eta_p^2 = 0.14$. Separate univariate ANOVAs revealed no significant difference between the intervention and control condition pre-intervention, $F(1, 239) = 0.00$, $p = 0.98$, $\eta_p^2 = 0.000$; however there was a significant difference between the intervention and control condition post-intervention $F(1, 239) = 32.80$, $p < 0.001$, $\eta_p^2 = 0.12$.

Table 5. Means and standard deviations for CYRM-28 resilience scales by experimental condition.

Scale	Condition	Baseline		Post-Test	
		Mean	SD	Mean	SD
Individual capacities and resources	Intervention	2.96	0.60	3.10	0.53
	Control	3.06	0.59	2.75	0.69
Relationship with primary carer	Intervention	3.14	0.68	3.17	0.65
	Control	3.05	0.74	2.73	0.79
Contextual factors	Intervention	2.51	0.76	2.62	0.72
	Control	2.38	0.77	2.18	0.71
Total resilience	Intervention	2.90	0.51	3.01	0.45
	Control	2.90	0.56	2.62	0.61

3.3. *Self-Efficacy*

In terms of self-efficacy, the intervention improved levels of the overall self-efficacy and self-efficacy sub-factors. Means and standard deviations are summarized in Table 6.

Table 6. Means and standard deviations for SEQ-C self-efficacy scales by experimental condition.

Scale	Condition	Baseline		Post-Test	
		Mean	SD	Mean	SD
Academic self-efficacy	Intervention	2.56	0.71	2.77	0.64
	Control	2.48	0.73	2.41	0.69
Social self-efficacy	Intervention	2.57	0.74	2.84	0.62
	Control	2.78	0.57	2.60	0.67
Emotional self-efficacy	Intervention	2.23	0.80	2.63	0.70
	Control	2.34	0.73	2.25	0.79
Total self-efficacy	Intervention	2.45	0.60	2.75	0.52
	Control	2.54	0.52	2.42	0.59

Academic self-efficacy: Using Pillai's trace, there was a significant effect of the experimental condition on participants' academic self-efficacy, $V = 0.07$, $F(2, 238) = 9.19$, $p < 0.001$, $\eta_p^2 = 0.07$.

Separate univariate ANOVAs revealed no significant difference between the intervention and control condition pre-intervention, $F(1, 239) = 0.67$, $p = 0.41$, $\eta_p^2 = 0.003$; however there was a significant difference between the intervention and control condition post-intervention $F(1, 239) = 17.98$, $p < 0.001$, $\eta_p^2 = 0.07$.

Social self-efficacy: There was a significant effect of the experimental condition on participants' social self-efficacy, $V = 0.09$, $F(2, 238) = 12.14$, $p < 0.001$, $\eta_p^2 = 0.09$. Separate univariate ANOVAs revealed a significant difference between the intervention and control condition pre-intervention, $F(1, 239) = 6.24$, $p < 0.05$, $\eta_p^2 = 0.03$; and there was a significant difference between the intervention and control condition post-intervention, $F(1, 239) = 8.58$, $p < 0.01$, $\eta_p^2 = 0.04$.

Emotional self-efficacy: There was a significant effect of the experimental condition on participants' emotional self-efficacy, $V = 0.09$, $F(2, 238) = 11.64$, $p < 0.001$, $\eta_p^2 = 0.09$. Separate univariate ANOVAs revealed no significant difference between the intervention and control condition pre-intervention, $F(1, 239) = 1.24$, $p = 0.27$, $\eta_p^2 = 0.005$; however there was a significant difference between the intervention and control condition post-intervention, $F(1, 239) = 15.95$, $p < 0.001$, $\eta_p^2 = 0.06$.

Total self-efficacy: There was a significant effect of the experimental condition on participants' total self-efficacy, $V = 0.11$, $F(2, 238) = 14.94$, $p < 0.001$, $\eta_p^2 = 0.11$. Separate univariate ANOVAs revealed no significant difference between the intervention and control condition pre-intervention, $F(1, 239) = 1.48$, $p = 0.23$, $\eta_p^2 = 0.006$; however there was a significant difference between the intervention and control condition post-intervention, $F(1, 239) = 21.16$, $p < 0.001$, $\eta_p^2 = 0.08$.

3.4. Post-Program Martial Arts Participation

The intervention condition was asked whether they would like to continue practising martial arts after completing the program. Of the 125 participants who completed the intervention condition, 94 (75.2%) reported they would like to continue the program or participate in another martial art based program after the intervention. Chi square analysis of covariates found no significant differences for age, $\chi^2 = 2.86$, $p > 0.05$; grade, $\chi^2 = 0.14$, $p > 0.05$; biological sex, $\chi^2 = 5.25$, $p > 0.05$; cultural background $\chi^2 = 4.85$, $p > 0.05$; or socio-economic status $\chi^2 = 7.83$, $p > 0.05$.

4. Discussion

The results of the current study found a consistent pattern for wellbeing outcomes. All primary and secondary measures relating to resilience and self-efficacy improved for the intervention group and declined for the control group at statistically significant levels, which supports previous research [48,49]. The results provide valid and reliable evidence that psycho-social interventions based on a traditional martial arts model can be considered as an efficacious method of improving strengths and wellbeing outcomes. Interventions using this approach should promote an individual's ability to cope with the effects of bullying.

For resilience, the intervention had the greatest effect on total resilience which observed the largest effect size in the study. This is an important result given that students who report higher levels of resilience are less likely to become victims of bullying [38]. The resilience sub-factors relationship with primary caregivers and contextual factors exhibited the same effect size which was slightly smaller than for total resilience; and the resilience sub-factor individual capacities and resources exhibited the smallest resilience effect size resulting from the intervention program. The result regarding improved relationships with primary caregivers is particularly important given previous resilience research found that family factors including warm relationships and positive home environments are associated with greater resilience to bullying [40], and that resilience to bullying behaviours was improved when individuals could disclose their experiences to a family member [39]. The result that participants' resilience improved for the intervention group and declined for the control group suggests the intervention may improve participants' resilience to bullying.

A similar pattern was evident for self-efficacy insofar as the intervention had the greatest effect for total self-efficacy when compared to the self-efficacy sub-scales. Academic and emotional self-efficacy exhibited a similar effect size, which was slightly smaller than for total self-efficacy; while social self-efficacy exhibited the smallest self-efficacy effect size resulting from the intervention program. As the victims of bullying report lower self-efficacy compared to non-victims [37] the result that all self-efficacy scales improved for the intervention group and declined for the control group suggests the intervention may improve participants' ability to cope with bullying.

While the study exhibited increased resilience and self-efficacy for the intervention group and decreases for the control group, comparison of effect sizes suggests that the intervention had a greater effect on resilience outcomes. To this end, it is notable that the intervention program had a greater effect regarding total resilience and two of the resilience subscales (relationship with primary caregivers and contextual factors); than for total self-efficacy. It is also interesting that the relationship with primary caregivers resilience sub-scale exhibited a larger effect size compared to the social self-efficacy sub-scale, as they are intuitively related scales. Further, it is important to note that while the specific wellbeing scales considered in the current study differ from previous research, the current results support previous findings which reported martial arts training improved wellbeing factors such as self-esteem [48] and self-concept [49].

Although the effect sizes for resilience and self-efficacy were in the small range, this is nonetheless an important result. First, the meta-analyses conducted by Moore, Dudley and Woodcock [47] found that martial arts training resulted in improvements to factors associated with wellbeing, but that observed effect sizes were small. Results from the current study are consistent with this. Second, as noted there is a clear pattern regarding all resilience and self-efficacy scales increasing for the intervention group and decreasing for the control group. Third, the study recruited a randomised sample from a normal population and the intervention program was a 10-week group program. Consequently, the intervention's resilience and self-efficacy results should be viewed as promising.

However, results from the current study do not support previous research findings [50,51] and a meta-analysis [47] suggesting that martial arts training had a significant impact on internalising mental health issues. The current study found no significant internalising mental health differences between the intervention and control groups post-intervention, which is intriguing in view of previous research and positive finding from the current study regarding wellbeing outcomes.

It is encouraging that a large majority of the intervention group reported they would elect to continue martial arts participation post-program. Co-variate analysis was similarly encouraging, finding no differences for age, grade, biological sex, cultural background or socio-economic status regarding participants choosing to continue practicing martial arts. While the issue of self-selection effects cannot be entirely discounted, the result suggests the intervention program successfully engaged participants and may be applicable for a variety of different groups.

4.1. *Explanation of Intervention Effects*

The positive wellbeing outcomes found by the study are important, however explaining the casual factors associated with these effects is difficult. Resilience is a complex construct, and there are many elements in the intervention program incorporated from resilience literature that could result in improving resilience outcomes. These include empathic modelling, changing negative scripts, accepting participants for who they are and establishing realistic goals, encouraging participants to learn from mistakes, developing a social conscience, and encouraging problem solving and self-discipline [67]. Additionally, other social psychological constructs may have utility in explaining the intervention effects. For example, participants in the intervention program may have benefited from the development of an in-group identity [68] and the development of group superordinate goals [69]. From the current results the authors do not propose to isolate which factors may have been more important for developing greater resilience, however the above may be a useful conceptualisation towards this. These factors may also have utility in explaining participants' improved self-efficacy resulting from the intervention program.

The lack of observed effect post-intervention regarding internalising mental health issues may be explained by a variety of factors including scale issues, sample issues, as well as consideration of the null hypothesis. Scale issues may have impacted the study's capacity to measure participants' reports of internalising mental health issues. The SDQ exhibited problems regarding factor analysis and poor internal reliability, which resulted in several elements of the scale being discarded from the study. Consequently, it would be interesting to examine the effects of martial arts training regarding internalising mental health using an alternate measure. Sample bias may also have contributed to the study not detecting changes regarding internalising mental health. Given that the sample was randomly recruited from a normal population, the current study may not have had the same capacity to detect changes to participants' internalising mental health issues compared to previous research that recruited from targeted pathological samples. For example, Trulson's [48] study recruited from a sample of males diagnosed with behaviour disorders. Finally, it is important to consider the null hypothesis. It is possible that martial arts based training does not have a significant effect on internalising mental health outcomes. However, the authors propose that the noted scale and sample issues require further investigation before making conclusions regarding the null hypothesis.

4.2. Limitations

Several issues may limit the results of the current study. First, while the study has addressed many of limitations evident in prior research, the current study did not obtain third party corroboration of self-report measures. Inclusion of third party report measures should be considered in future research. Longer term effects of martial art training on mental health outcomes are unclear, given that follow-up data was not available at the time of writing this article. Finally, the issue of psycho-education versus martial arts training may be a confound in the current study. Psycho-education and martial arts training were presented as part of a single intervention program, hence it is not possible to separate their effects. However, it is arguable that combined psycho-education and martial arts training is consistent with the practice of many traditional martial arts, hence this issue may only have superficial significance.

4.3. Implications Regarding Interventions to Reduce Bullying

The current study's results have multiple implications to policy, practice and future research regarding bullying. Bullying behaviours are difficult to address, and the results attributed to the anti-bullying approach are inconsistent. Despite this, the anti-bullying approach maintains a dominant position informing educational policy regarding bullying. Arguably, the theoretical underpinning informing educational policy should be modified to account for other explanations of bullying behaviour, such as evolutionary perspectives on power and bullying. This should lead to questions regarding whether the aims of the anti-bullying approach (namely: no bullying) are achievable. The current study proposes an alternate approach to educational policy and suggests that instead of focusing resources towards eliminating bullying behaviours, policy should focus on promoting mental health through developing wellbeing. Results from the current study suggest that martial arts based psycho-social interventions have the potential to improve participants' strengths, wellbeing and ability to cope; which is important to consider in terms of educational policy regarding bullying.

The study has significant implications to practice regarding bullying behaviour. The institutional failure of the anti-bullying approach is potentially damaging to individuals. It is important to consider the impact and message understood by students when they continue to experience bullying behaviours despite the explicit anti-bullying policies and strategies used by schools. Further, because schools combine a wide variety of anti-bullying strategies flexibly, it is difficult to know what anti-bullying actions occur at the school level, and concerns should exist regarding whether the specific combinations used by schools are empirically supported. Given the inconsistent results attributed to the anti-bullying approach, alternate practices regarding bullying behaviour should be considered. Specifically, the current results have implications for practice by suggesting that intervention programs that develop strengths, including resilience and self-efficacy, have the potential to improve participants' sense of wellbeing and ability to cope with bullying.

The current study employed a robust design and rigorous evaluation, and suggests a promising approach to addressing bullying behaviours through improving wellbeing and mental health. The current results have a variety of implications for future research including sample considerations, methodological variations and developing a teacher professional learning program based on the study. Future research should examine the intervention program's effects on different population samples. Consideration should be given to implementing the intervention as a universal program with primary school students (ages 10–11); targeting specific populations such as participants diagnosed with (a) mental health issues such as anxiety and depression, (b) Autism Spectrum Disorder, (c) intellectual disability, and (d) behavioural disorders such as Oppositional Defiance Disorder, and participants who have experienced violent incidents including domestic and sexual violence; and extending the study to international settings to examine the intervention's efficacy in different cultural milieus. Future research should incorporate methodological changes including utilising third party measures to corroborate self-report measures, using alternate measures of mental health pathology such as the Kessler 10 Psychological Distress Scale [70], including a qualitative approach to supplement quantitative information, and varying the longitudinal parameters of the study by extending the follow-up period and lengthening the intervention program (e.g., 3/6/12 month interventions). Finally, future research should develop a professional learning program for teachers to facilitate similar programs which could be embedded within a physical education curriculum or welfare/pastoral care curriculum. Such a program would require piloting and ongoing measurement to ensure program efficacy.

5. Conclusions

Despite inconsistent evidence, the anti-bullying approach dominates educational policy and practice regarding bullying behaviours. While bullying is a complex phenomenon, the inconsistent evidence regarding the anti-bullying approach may be explained by problems with its theoretical underpinning. The authors propose the primary aim regarding bullying behaviours should change from attempted reduction of the behaviour, to improving individual ability to cope with the effects of bullying. The current study offers a strengths-based method of achieving this which is consistent with previous research. The results suggest that psycho-social interventions based on a traditional martial arts model can successfully promote wellbeing characteristics such as resilience and self-efficacy. Interventions that promote these strengths can help individuals develop better mental health and should be a focus of efforts to address the effects of bullying.

Author Contributions: B.M. conceptualized the article. Methodology was developed by all authors. B.M. conducted the investigation. Formal analysis was conducted by B.M., and all authors provided feedback and approved the final analysis. The paper was written by B.M., and all the authors provided feedback on the draft manuscript and approved the final version.

References

1. Rigby, K. *A Meta-Evaluation of Methods and Approaches to Reducing Bullying in Pre-Schools and Early Primary School in Australia*; Commonwealth Attorney-General's Department: Canberra, Australia, 2002.
2. Rigby, K. An overview of approaches to managing bullying and victim problems. In *Bullying Solutions: Evidence Based Approaches to Bullying in Australian Schools*; McGrath, H., Noble, T., Eds.; Pearson: Sydney, Australia, 2006; pp. 161–173.
3. Rigby, K. *Children and Bullying: How Parents and Educators Can Reduce Bullying at Schools*; Blackwell: Victoria, Australia, 2008.
4. Lines, D. *The Bullies: Understanding Bullies and Bullying*; Jessica Kingsley: London, UK, 2008.

5. Pellegrini, A. Bullying during the middle school years. In *Bullying: Implications for the Classroom*; Saunders, C., Pyne, G., Eds.; Elsevier Academic Press: New York, NY, USA, 2004.
6. Olweus, D. *Bullying at School*; Blackwell: Oxford, UK, 1993.
7. Bouman, T.; van der Meulen, M.; Goossens, F.; Olthaf, T.; Vermande, M.; Aleva, E. Peer and self-reports of victimization and bullying: Their differential association with internalizing problems and social adjustment. *J. Sch. Psychol.* **2012**, *50*, 759–774. [CrossRef]
8. Smith, P.; Sharp, S. *School Bullying: Insights and Perspectives*; Routledge: London, UK, 1994.
9. Australian Education Authorities. Bullying. No Way! Available online: https://bullyingnoway.gov.au (accessed on 15 December 2018).
10. Merrell, K.; Gueldner, B.; Ross, S.; Isava, D. How effective are school bullying intervention programs? A meta-analysis of intervention research. *Sch. Psychol. Q.* **2008**, *23*, 26–42. [CrossRef]
11. Ttofi, M.; Farrington, D. Effectiveness of school-based programs to reduce bullying: A systematic and meta-analytic review. *J. Exp. Criminol.* **2011**, *7*, 27–56. [CrossRef]
12. Farrington, P.; Ttofi, M. School-Based Programs to Reduce Bullying and Victimization. Campbell Collaboration, 2009. Available online: https://www.ncjrs.gov/pdffiles1/nij/grants/229377.pdf (accessed on 28 December 2018).
13. ACT Education Directorate. Safe and Supportive Schools Policy. Available online: https://www.education.act.gov.au/publications_and_policies/School-and-Corporate-Policies/wellbeing/safety/safe-and-supportive-schools-policy (accessed on 15 December 2018).
14. Australian Government. Disability Discrimination Act 1992. Available online: https://www.legislation.gov.au/Details/C2018C00125 (accessed on 15 December 2018).
15. Australian Government. Human Rights and Equal Opportunity Commission (HREOC) Act 1986. Available online: https://www.legislation.gov.au/Details/C2017C00143 (accessed on 15 December 2018).
16. Australian Government. Racial Discrimination Act 1975. Available online: https://www.legislation.gov.au/Details/C2014C00014 (accessed on 15 December 2018).
17. Australian Government. Racial Hatred Act 1995. Available online: https://www.legislation.gov.au/Details/C2004A04951 (accessed on 15 December 2018).
18. Australian Government. Sex Discrimination Act 1984. Available online: https://www.legislation.gov.au/Details/C2014C00002 (accessed on 15 December 2018).
19. NSW Department of Education. Bullying of Students—Prevention and Response Policy. Available online: https://education.nsw.gov.au/policy-library/policies/bullying-of-students-prevention-and-response-policy (accessed on 15 December 2018).
20. NT Department of Education. Health and Wellbeing of Students: Bullying, Cyberbullying and Cybersafety. Available online: https://nt.gov.au/learning/primary-and-secondary-students/health-and-wellbeing-of-students/bullying-cyberbullying-and-cybersafety (accessed on 15 December 2018).
21. QLD Department of Education. Preventing Bullying and Violence. Available online: http://behaviour.education.qld.gov.au/bullying-and-violence/Pages/default.aspx (accessed on 15 December 2018).
22. SA Department for Education. Keeping Children Safe from Bullying. Available online: https://www.education.sa.gov.au/supporting-students/health-e-safety-and-wellbeing/keeping-children-safe-bullying (accessed on 15 December 2018).
23. VIC Department of Education and Training. School Policy—Bullying. Available online: https://www.education.vic.gov.au/school/principals/spag/safety/Pages/bullying.aspx (accessed on 15 December 2018).
24. WA Department of Education. Guidelines for Preventing and Managing Bullying in Schools. Available online: http://det.wa.edu.au/studentsupport/behaviourandwellbeing/detcms/school-support-programs/behaviour-and-wellbeing/safe-and-supportive-schools/guidelines-for-preventing-and-managing-bullying-in-schools.en?title=Guidelines+for+preventing+and+managing+bullying (accessed on 15 December 2018).
25. Centre for Education Statistics and Evaluation. Anti-Bullying Interventions in Schools—What Works? NSW Department of Education, 2017. Available online: https://www.cese.nsw.gov.au/images/stories/PDF/anti_bullying_in_schools_what_works_AA.pdf (accessed on 28 December 2018).
26. Jiménez-Barbero, J.; Ruiz-Hernández, J.; Llor-Zaragoza, L.; Pérez-García, M.; Llor-Esteban, B. Effectiveness of anti-bullying school programs: A meta-analysis. *Child. Youth Serv. Rev.* **2016**, *61*, 165–175. [CrossRef]

27. Smith, J.; Schneider, B.; Smith, P.; Ananiadau, K. The effectiveness of whole-school antibullying programs: A synthesis of evaluation research. *Sch. Psychol. Rev.* **2004**, *33*, 547–560.
28. Moore, B.; Woodcock, S. Bullying and resilience: Towards an alternative to the anti-bullying approach. *Educ. Psychol. Pract.* **2017**, *33*, 65–80. [CrossRef]
29. Ansary, N.; Elias, M.; Greene, M.; Green, S. Guidance for schools selecting antibullying approaches: Translating evidence-based strategies to contemporary implementation realities. *Educ. Res.* **2015**, *44*, 27–36. [CrossRef]
30. Latane, B.; Darley, J. *The Unresponsive Bystander: Why Doesn't He Help?* Appleton Century Crofts: New York, NY, USA, 1970.
31. Kaplan, H. Understanding the concept of resilience. In *Handbook of Resilience in Children*; Goldstein, S., Brooks, R., Eds.; Springer: New York, NY, USA, 2006; pp. 39–48.
32. Goldstein, S.; Brooks, R. Why study resilience? In *Handbook of Resilience in Children*; Goldstein, S., Brooks, R., Eds.; Springer: New York, NY, USA, 2006; pp. 3–16.
33. Naglieri, J.; LeBuffe, P. Measuring resilience in children. In *Handbook of Resilience in Children*; Goldstein, S., Brooks, R., Eds.; Springer: New York, NY, USA, 2006; pp. 107–123.
34. Prince-Embury, S. *Resilience Scales for Children and Adolescents: A Profile of Personal Strengths*; Pearson: Minneapolis, MN, USA, 2007.
35. Elias, M.; Parker, S.; Rosenblatt, J. Building educational opportunity. In *Handbook of Resilience in Children*; Goldstein, S., Brooks, R., Eds.; Springer: New York, NY, USA, 2006; pp. 315–336.
36. Fuller, A. A resilience based approach to helping the victims of bullying and their families. In *Bullying Solutions: Evidence Based Approaches to Bullying in Australian Schools*; McGrath, H., Noble, T., Eds.; Pearson: Sydney, Australia, 2006; pp. 161–173.
37. Moore, B.; Woodcock, S. Resilience, bullying, and mental health: Factors associated with improved outcomes. *Psychol. Sch.* **2017**, *54*, 689–702. [CrossRef]
38. Donnon, T. Understanding how resiliency development influences adolescent bullying and victimization. *Can. J. Sch. Psychol.* **2010**, *25*, 101–113. [CrossRef]
39. Rivers, I.; Cowie, H. Bullying and homophobia in UK schools: A perspective on factors affecting resilience and recovery. *J. Gay Lesbian Issues Educ.* **2006**, *3*, 11–43. [CrossRef]
40. Bowes, L.; Maughan, B.; Caspi, A.; Moffitt, T.; Arseneault, L. Families promote emotional and behavioural resilience to bullying: Evidence of an environmental effect. *J. Child Psychol. Psychiatry* **2010**, *51*, 809–814. [CrossRef] [PubMed]
41. Lisboa, C.; Killer, S. Coping with peer bullying and resilience promotion: Data from Brazilian at-risk children. *Int. J. Psychol.* **2008**, *43*, 711.
42. Beightol, J.; Jevertson, J.; Gray, S.; Carter, S.; Gass, M. The effect of an experiential, adventure-based 'anti-bullying initiative' on levels of resilience: A mixed methods study. *J. Exp. Educ.* **2009**, *31*, 420–424. [CrossRef]
43. Daniels, K.; Thornton, E. An analysis of the relationship between hostility. *J. Sport Sci.* **1990**, *8*, 95–101. [CrossRef] [PubMed]
44. Burke, D.; Al-Adawi, S.; Lee, Y.; Audette, J. Martial Arts as sport and therapy and training in the martial arts. *J. Sport Med. Phys. Fit.* **2007**, *47*, 96–102.
45. Cox, J. Traditional Asian martial arts training: A review. *Quest* **1993**, *45*, 366–388. [CrossRef]
46. Vertonghen, J.; Theeboom, M. The socio-psychological outcomes of martial arts practice among youth: A review. *J. Sport Sci. Med.* **2010**, *9*, 528–537.
47. Moore, B.; Dudley, D.; Woodcock, S. The effect of martial arts training on mental health outcomes: A systematic review and meta-analysis. *BMC Public Health* **2018**, under review.
48. Trulson, M. Martial arts training: A "novel" cure for juvenile delinquency. *Hum. Relat.* **1986**, *39*, 1131–1140. [CrossRef]
49. Finkenberg, M. Effect of participation in Taekwondo on college women's self-concept. *Percept. Mot. Skill* **1990**, *71*, 891–894. [CrossRef]
50. McGowan, R.; Jordan, C. Mood states and physical activity. *Louis Assoc. Health Phys. Educ. Rec. Dan J.* **1988**, *15*, 32.

51. Li, F.; Fisher, K.; Harmer, P.; Irbe, D.; Tearse, R.; Weimer, C. Tai Chi and self rated quality of sleep and daytime sleepiness in older adults: A randomised controlled trial. *J. Am. Geriatr. Soc.* **2004**, *52*, 892–900. [CrossRef] [PubMed]
52. Tsang, T.; Kohn, M.; Chow, C.; Singh, M. Health benefits of Kung Fu: A systematic review. *J. Sport Sci.* **2008**, *26*, 1249–1267. [CrossRef] [PubMed]
53. Hartmann, D. Theorizing sport as social intervention: A view from the grassroots. *Quest* **2003**, *55*, 118–140. [CrossRef]
54. Macarie, I.; Roberts, R. Martial arts and mental health. *Contemp. Psychother.* **2010**, *2*, 1–4.
55. Donohue, J.; Taylor, K. The classification of the fighting arts. *J. Asian Martial Art* **1994**, *3*, 10–37.
56. Nosanchuk, T.; MacNeil, C. Examination of the effects of traditional and modern martial arts training on aggressiveness. *Aggress. Behav.* **1989**, *15*, 153–159. [CrossRef]
57. Twemlow, S.; Biggs, B.; Nelson, T.; Venberg, E.; Fonagy, P.; Twemlow, S. Effects of participation in a martial arts based antibullying program in elementary schools. *Psychol. Sch.* **2008**, *45*, 947–959. [CrossRef]
58. Moher, D.; Liberati, A.; Tetzlaff, J.; Altman, D. PRISMA Group Preferred reporting items for systematic reviews and meta-analyses: The PRISMA statement. *PLoS Med.* **2009**, *6*. [CrossRef]
59. Wood, A.; White, I.; Thompson, S. Are missing outcome data adequately handled? A review of published randomized controlled trials in major medical journals. *Clin. Trials* **2004**, *1*, 368–376. [CrossRef]
60. Goodman, R. Strengths and Difficulties Questionnaire. Available online: http://www.sdqinfo.com (accessed on 14 December 2018).
61. Ungar, M.; Liebenberg, L. Assessing Resilience across Cultures Using Mixed-Methods: Construction of the Child and Youth Resilience Measure-28. *J. Mixed-Methods Res.* **2011**, *5*, 126–149. [CrossRef]
62. Muris, P. A Brief Questionnaire for Measuring Self-Efficacy in Youths. *J. Psychopathol. Behav. Assess.* **2001**, *23*, 145–149. [CrossRef]
63. Muris, P.; Meesters, C.; Eijkelenboom, A.; Vincken, M. The self-report version of the Strengths and Difficulties Questionnaire: Its psychometric properties in 8- to 13-year-old non-clinical children. *Br. J. Clin. Psychol.* **2004**, *43*, 437–448. [CrossRef] [PubMed]
64. Sanders, J.; Munford, R.; Thimasarn-Anwar, T.; Liebenberg, L. Validation of the Child and Youth Resilience Measure (CYRM-28) on a Sample of At-Risk New Zealand Youth. *Res. Soc. Work Pract.* **2017**, *27*, 827–840. [CrossRef]
65. Minter, A.; Pritzker, S. Measuring Adolescent Social and Academic Self-Efficacy: Cross-Ethnic Validity of the SEQ-C. *Res. Soc. Work Pract.* **2015**, *27*, 818–826. [CrossRef]
66. Richardson, J. Eta squared and partial eta squared as measures of effect size in educational research. *Educ. Res. Rev.* **2011**, *6*, 135–147. [CrossRef]
67. Brooks, R. The power of parenting. In *Handbook of Resilience in Children*; Goldstein, S., Brooks, R., Eds.; Springer: New York, NY, USA, 2006; pp. 297–313.
68. Kurzban, R.; Leary, M. Evolutionary origin of stigmatization: The functions of social exclusion. *Psychol. Bull.* **2001**, *127*, 187–208. [CrossRef]
69. Sherif, M.; Harvey, L.; White, B.; Hood, W.; Sherif, C. *The Robbers Cave Experiment: Intergroup Conflict and Cooperation*; Wesleyan University Press: Middletown, CT, USA, 1961.
70. Kessler, R.; Barker, P.; Colpe, L.; Epstein, J.; Gfroerer, J.; Hiripi, E.; Howes, M.J.; Normand, S.L.T.; Manderscheid, R.W.; Walters, E.E.; et al. Screening for serious mental illness in the general population. *Arch. Gen. Psychiatry* **2003**, *60*, 184–189. [CrossRef]

14

Microbiome—The Missing Link in the Gut-Brain Axis: Focus on its Role in Gastrointestinal and Mental Health

Karolina Skonieczna-Żydecka [1], Wojciech Marlicz [2,*], Agata Misera [3], Anastasios Koulaouzidis [4] and Igor Łoniewski [1]

1 Department of Biochemistry and Human Nutrition, Pomeranian Medical University in Szczecin, 71-460 Szczecin, Poland; karzyd@pum.edu.pl (K.S.-Z.); igorloniewski@sanum.com.pl (I.L.)
2 Department of Gastroenterology, Pomeranian Medical University, 71-252 Szczecin, Poland
3 Department of Child and Adolescent Psychiatry, Charité Universitätsmedizin, 13353 Berlin, Germany; agata.misera@charite.de
4 Endoscopy Unit, The Royal Infirmary of Edinburgh, EH16 4SA Edinburgh, UK; akoulaouzidis@hotmail.com
* Correspondence: marlicz@hotmail.com;

Abstract: The central nervous system (CNS) and the human gastrointestinal (GI) tract communicate through the gut-brain axis (GBA). Such communication is bi-directional and involves neuronal, endocrine, and immunological mechanisms. There is mounting data that gut microbiota is the source of a number of neuroactive and immunocompetent substances, which shape the structure and function of brain regions involved in the control of emotions, cognition, and physical activity. Most GI diseases are associated with altered transmission within the GBA that are influenced by both genetic and environmental factors. Current treatment protocols for GI and non-GI disorders may positively or adversely affect the composition of intestinal microbiota with a diverse impact on therapeutic outcome(s). Alterations of gut microbiota have been associated with mood and depressive disorders. Moreover, mental health is frequently affected in GI and non-GI diseases. Deregulation of the GBA may constitute a grip point for the development of diagnostic tools and personalized microbiota-based therapy. For example, next generation sequencing (NGS) offers detailed analysis of microbiome footprints in patients with mental and GI disorders. Elucidating the role of stem cell–host microbiome cross talks in tissues in GBA disorders might lead to the development of next generation diagnostics and therapeutics. Psychobiotics are a new class of beneficial bacteria with documented efficacy for the treatment of GBA disorders. Novel therapies interfering with small molecules involved in adult stem cell trafficking are on the horizon.

Keywords: gut brain axis; microbiota; functional gastrointestinal disorders; inflammatory bowel disease (IBD); adult stem cells

---

1. Introduction

Recently, a new United Nation's (UN) Commission goals on global mental health and sustainable development has been published [1]. This Commission is in line with other UN General Assembly and High-Level Meeting report and explores the issues of mental health from those with mental disorders to whole populations [2]. Accordingly, good mental health is viewed as fundamental to individual's well-being and overall health. In addition, efforts are being focused on systemic and global changes in order to align mental health across all medical specialties [3,4]. In the context of the previously mentioned documents, the relationship between gut microbiota and mental health seems to be very interesting.

Intestinal microbiota represent one of the richest ecosystems in nature. Professor Rob Knight of the University of California, San Diego [5] reported that more than half of all cells in the human body are microorganisms, which are mainly bacteria as well as fungi and viruses. Until recently, the general belief was that intestinal microbes were mainly involved in digestive processes. With the advent of new molecular techniques and bioinformatics, in-depth research has unraveled the role of intestinal microbiota in a number of physiological processes [6,7]. The topic of global microbial diversity is so crucial and important to human health and wellbeing that scientists from Rutgers University-New Brunswick—In a recent issue of *Science*—Called for the creation of a global microbiota vault to protect humanity's long-term health [8].

The role of the gut microbiome on human health is very diverse and implicated in the pathophysiology of various diseases. Its role in metabolism and obesity development has been clearly documented [9]. More recently, gut microbes have been implicated in the pathogenesis of cancer and microbial contribution in cancer treatment [10]. The pathogenesis and natural history of chronic GI, non-communicable diseases e.g., non-alcoholic steatohepatitis (NASH) [11], functional gastrointestinal disorders (FGIDs) [12], and non-GI disorders e.g., cardiovascular disease (CVD) [13] have been linked to GI tract microbes. The alterations of gut microbiota have been associated with neurodegenerative diseases as well as mood disturbance and depression [14–16]. In fact, mental health alterations are frequently observed in many GI diseases [17–20].

2. Paradigm Changer—Rome IV Criteria and FGIDs

For years, FGIDs were viewed as purely functional disorders with no scientific confirmation of a clear pathogenetic mechanism. According to Rome IV criteria, the phenotype of FGIDs results from an altered transmission of nerve and biochemical signals within the gut-brain-microbiota axis with mechanisms controlled by both genetic and environmental factors [21]. Additionally, few studies conducted in patients suffering from functional dyspepsia (FD) and irritable bowel syndrome (IBS) found alterations in small bowel microbiota. Zhong et al. [22] showed that *Actinomyces*, *Atopobium*, *Leptotrichia*, *Prevotella*, and *Veilonella* counts differ between FD and control patients. The finding was preceded by an observation that, in FD patients, gut barrier integrity is impaired and expressed as lowered transepithelial resistance, diminished expression of proteins of tight junctions, and, lastly, elevated levels of mast cells, eosinophils, and interstitial lymphocytes [23]. Giamarellos-Bourboulis reported a significant reduction in the diversity of small-bowel microbiota and the number of species [24]. Furthermore, Martinez et al. reported that the proportion of dilated junctions and intercellular distance between enterocytes in their apical part was elevated [25]. They also found that higher tryptase mRNA expression leads to overactive bowel movements and looser stool as per Bristol stool scale. Importantly, the degranulation of mast cells was found to positively affect the firing of visceral-nociceptive sensory neurons in IBS [26]. According to the new ROME IV criteria, the following factors contribute to the pathogenesis of FGIDs: (i) motility disturbance, (ii) visceral hypersensitivity, (iii) altered mucosal and immune function, (iv) altered gut microbiota, and (v) altered central nervous system (CNS). All of them are also associated with the concept of the microbiota-gut-brain axis.

The overlap of FGIDs and CNS disorders has been discussed in a few studies. It has been demonstrated that approximately one third of IBS patients suffer from depression [27]. More recently, Batmaz et al. [28] reviewed patients referred either directly to psychiatric clinics or from gastroenterology wards to psychiatrists and concluded that these patients were complaining of both GI and psychiatric symptoms. Furthermore, patients of the latter group complained more frequently of constipation, abdominal pain, and bloating and were more frequently diagnosed with psychotic disorders in comparison to those directly referred to psychiatric clinics. It is estimated that psychiatric symptoms occur in at least 36.5% of FGIDs patients [17]. Stasi et al. found that the highest prevalence of mental or spectrum disorders is in patients with functional constipation (60%) as compared to patients diagnosed with FD (52.4%) and/or functional bloating (47.6%). The most prevalent psychiatric disorder observed in FGIDs were the general anxiety disorder and panic diagnosis [17]. Furthermore,

Wilder-smith et al. [29] identified both GI and CNS symptom profiles secondary to fructose or lactose ingestion.

3. The Emerging Role of the Microbiota-Gut-Brain Axis

Studies in animal models have shown that microbiota play an essential role in shaping the structure and function of the CNS [30]. Using sophisticated strategies for manipulating the microbiome, researchers observed the consequences of these changes one the brain and behavior. For example, it has been found out that the thickness of the myelin sheath, the length of dendrites, and the density of dendritic spines are controlled by microbiota [31,32]. A recent study by Lu et al. [33] conducted in humanized germ-free mice demonstrated that slow-growing mice presented skewed neuron and oligodendrocyte development as well as evident signs of neuro-inflammation. Social competences and repetitive behaviors are, at least in part, a reflection of the composition of intestinal bacteria [34]. These dependencies result directly from the existence of a physical and functional connection between the human digestive tract and the CNS. This concept called the gut-brain axis (GBA) with the participation of neural and biochemical mechanisms can be exploited for the development of new therapies for mental health disorders.

The CNS utilizes neural and endocrine pathways to cooperate with the gut. The sympathetic part of the autonomic nervous system and the hypothalamus-pituitary-adrenal axis (HPA) co-modulate the secretion, motility, and blood flow affecting intestinal permeability and influencing various GI disorders [35]. Gut neural signals are passed through the enteric nervous system (ENS) and the vagus nerve [36]. Biochemical information is carried out by cytokines, chemokines, neurotransmitters, and micro-vesicles [37] as well as directly by-products of gut microbiota metabolic activity, i.e., short chain fatty acids (SCFAs). Eventually, once in the circulation, these molecules influence HPA and GBA [38]. An elevated stress response may impair the psychosomatic well-being [39]. With pioneering work, Sudo et al. [40] demonstrated that gut microbiota is essential to proper stress hormones release and the restoration of intestinal ecosystem may reverse abnormal stress response. More recently, in vivo experimentation has demonstrated that stress mediators and their receptors' expression are reduced in pathogen-free animals [41].

4. How the Gut/Brain Talks to the Brain/Gut

Intestinal microbiota as an integral part of the intestinal barrier controls the transport of antigens through the peri-cellular route to the *lamina propria* where the gut associated lymphoid tissue (GALT) is located [42]. The composition of intestinal microbiota can, therefore, influence intestinal barrier permeability, which guarantees the flow of molecules through the peri-cellular route to blood vessels. Gut microbes permanently train GALT to create immunity against commensal bacteria and food antigens but also to provide defense against pathogenic microorganisms [43]. During dysbiosis, due to GALT activation, effector cells and inflammatory mediators disrupt gut barrier integrity and result in elevated intestinal permeability [44]. The interaction of the intestinal barrier elements, thus, provides a physiologic and selective ability to absorb and secrete specific substances while inhibiting the translocation of microorganisms and the penetration of toxins and other harmful antigens [45,46].

The effects of increased intestinal permeability may manifest locally—In the GI tract—As well as extra-intestinally. For example, the concentration of zonulin—A protein that activates the intracellular signaling pathway leading to tight junctions [47] modulation and a marker of intestinal permeability increases in people with inflammatory and autoimmune diseases [48]. Of importance, the gut barrier resembles in structure and function the blood brain barrier (BBB) [49]. Both barriers are composed of epithelial and endothelial cells laced with lymphatic vessels, macrophages, and cellular tight junctions. It has already been suggested that both IBS and pseudomembranous colitis [50,51] are consequences of microbiota and intestinal barrier dysfunctions and these entities frequently coexist with depression [52,53].

5. Microbiota-Gut-Brain Axis and Susceptibility to Neuropsychiatric and Gastrointestinal Disease and Response to Therapy

The structure of intestinal microbiota is strongly influenced by diet and environmental stressors such as drugs. It seems that these factors dominate over the impact of genotype on the gut flora composition [54]. Consequently, it has been recognized that it may be the optimal marker of susceptibility to express certain clinical phenotypes and, thus, the response to pharmacotherapy [55]. Since the concept of bidirectional signaling between the gut and the brain started to evolve, scientists have made attempts to discover microbial fingerprints in neurology and psychiatry. Emerging research suggested that gut-brain axis dysfunction may be involved in the etiology of depression and anxiety, schizophrenia, addiction, and neurodevelopmental and neurodegenerative diseases as well as age-related cognitive decline [14,56–59]. Major microbiota-related alterations in particular neuropsychiatric conditions are summarized in Table 1.

Table 1. Microbiota and its metabolites alterations in various psychiatric conditions.

The Disease	Microbiota-Related Fingerprint	Reference
Depression	↑ *Bacteroidetes, Proteobacteria, Actinobacteria, Enterobacteriaceae, Alistipes,* propionic, isobutyric, and isovaleric acids ↓ *Faecalibacterium, Bifidobacterium, Lactobacillus;* serotonin, noradrenalin, SCFAs, kynurenic acid, kynurenine	[60–63]
Schizophrenia	↑ *Corinobacteriaceae, Prevotella, Succinivibrio, Collinsella, Megasphaera, Klebsiella, Methanobrevibacter, Clostridium* ↓ *Blautia, Coprococcus, Roseburia,*	[64,65]
Bipolar disorder	↑ *Bacteroides, Actinobacteria, Coriobacteria* ↓ *Faecalibacterium, Roseburia, Alistipes,*	[66,67]
Parkinson's disease	↑ *Bacteroides, Roseburia* ↓ *Blautia, Coprococcus, Dorea, Oscillospira, Akkermansia*	[68]
Autism Spectrum Disorder	↑ *Streptococcus, Clostridiales, Comamonadaceae, Akkermansia, Rhosococcus, Oscillospira, Desulvibrio, Burkholderia, Collinsella, Corynebacterium, Dorea, and Lactobacillus;* acetic and propionic acid, p-cresol, Glutamate, ↓ *Firmicutes, Faecalibacterium, Ruminococcus, Proteobacteria, Fuscobacteria, Verrumicrobia, Bifidobacterium, Neisseria, Alistipes, Bilophila, Dialister, Parabacteroides,* and *Veillonella,* butyric acid, tryptophan, kynurenic acid,	[69–73]
Attention-Deficit Hyperactivity Disorder	↑ *Actinobacteria (Bifidobacterium* genus) ↓ *Firmicutes (Clostridiales* order)	[74]
Alzheimer's disease	↑ *Blautia, Phascolarctobacterium, Gemella, E.coli, Shigella, Ps. aueruginosa* ↓ *Ruminococcaceae, Turicibacteraceae, Peptostreptococcaceae, Clostridiaceae, Mogibacteriaceae,* and the genera *SMB53* (family, *Clostridiaceae) Dialister, Clostridium, Turicibacter,* and cc115 (family *Erysipelotrichaceae)*	[75,76]
Multiple sclerosis	↑ *Akkermansia muciniphila, Acinetobacter calcoaceticus* ↓ *Parabacteroides distasonis*	[77]
Anorexia nervosa	↑ *Methanobrevibacter smithii*	[78]

Nevertheless, uninterrupted stress regulation is pivotal to mental health and altered stress response has been implicated in the origin of psychiatric diseases [58]. Numerous studies conducted in animals and humans have demonstrated that both acute and chronic stress interfere with intestinal barrier integrity and induce adverse alterations in intestinal microbiota composition. This has been confirmed in models of early-life [79] stress and prenatal stress [80]. Yarandi et al. [81] showed that water and ion in the gut might be reduced and elevated, respectively, under stressful conditions. This, in turn, impairs the physical protection of the gut barrier against both pathogenic microorganisms and nociceptive molecules. Furthermore, HPA activation, in particular corticotropin-releasing factor (CRF), showed a causative role in gut integrity disruption [82]. Elevated intestinal permeability was also found to be linked to stress-induced hypersensitivity of the rectum in animals, which were studied by means of partial restraint stress [83]. Winter et al. merged microbiome data from both animals and humans and selected bacterial genera that were either over-represented or appeared in a reduced number following stressor exposure. The first group included: *Desulfovibrio, Eggerthella, Holdemania, Turicibacter, Clostridium, Blautia, Anaerofilum* and *Roseburia* whereas those found in reduced numbers were: *Prevotella, Bacteroides, Mucispirillum, Dialister, Allobaculum, Faecalibacterium, Oscillospira, Ruminococcus, Dorea, Coprococcus,* and *Pseudobytyrivibrio* [84].

Emerging New Concepts in the Development of Neurodegenerative and GI Disease—Gut Microbes, Innate Immunity, and Bone Marrow Stem Cells as Partners in Crime

Mood and psychiatric disorders as well as numerous GI disorders are related to chronic inflammation [85]. For example, post-infectious IBS alters GI tract motility and behavior [86]. A similar effect appears in patients with FD [87]. Behavioral alterations predominate in chronic GI inflammatory disorders [88]. Chronic inflammation of the ENS can easily affect the CNS. However, knowledge on mechanisms behind this phenomenon is still scarce. For decades, inflammation in the brain, which were recently implicated in the pathogenesis of psychiatric diseases, has been considered "sterile." However, recent reports reveal the presence of the gut-vascular barrier (GVB), which, in structure and function, resembles the blood brain barier (BBB) and their communication is mediated via blood and bone marrow systems [89]. GVB controls the dissemination of bacteria from the gut into the bloodstream and the *Salmonella typhimirum* infection has been shown to decrease the Wnt/β catenin-inducible gene Axin2 (a marker of stem cell renewal) in the gut endothelium.

Importantly, the Wnt/β catenin signaling pathway is universally involved in trafficking (mobilization and proliferation) of stem cells deposited in adult tissues [90] including those located in GI tract [91]. Wnt/β catenin system has also been involved in the developmental control of BBB formation [92]. It has been demonstrated that various types of bone marrow-derived stem cells are mobilized into peripheral blood in patients and experimental animals in response to tissue/organ injury [93]. Examples include myocardial infarction [94], stroke [95], deep skin burns [96], and gut inflammation [97]. It has been previously shown that circulating peripheral bone marrow mononuclear cells (PBMNCs) were enriched with cells expressing mRNA of leucine-rich repeat-containing G-protein coupled receptor 5 (lgr-5), Achaete-scute complex homolog 2 (Ascl-2), Doublecortin Like Kinase 1 (Dclk-1), Male-specific lethal 1 homolog (MSL1), and B lymphoma Mo-MLV insertion region 1 homolog (BML-1). These markers are involved in the development of early intestinal lineage [97]. These circulating in PB cells could potentially be involved in reparatory mechanisms of peripheral tissues including the brain [98].

In fact, the release of very small embryonic-like stem cells (VSELs) and more differentiated neural stem cells (NSCs) from bone marrow into the peripheral blood in response to brain injury in rodents [99] and humans [95] has been well documented. Recent research indicates the involvement of other factors such as small bioactive lipids that may direct mobilization and trafficking of stem cells to injured organs [100]. Notably, release of sphingiosine-1-phosphate (S1P) correlates with the activation of the complement cascade and formation of the C5b-C9 membrane attack complex (MAC). Activation of proteolytic and fibrynolitis complement cascades. The release of cleavage fragments (e.g., C5a and desArgC5a fragments) could enhance the mobilization of stem cells from their niche in the bone marrow [101]. Moreover, these stem cells can be attracted from the bone marrow and from the intestinal epithelium in response to tumor or injured tissue derived plasma chemo-atractants such as stromal derived factor-1 (SDF-1), vascular endothelial growth factor (VEGF), zonulin, hepatocyte growth factor (HGF) or shphingosine-1-phosphate (S1P), ceramides, and extracellular nucleotides [102,103]. On the other hand, stem cells may secrete their own growth factors, cytokines, or even membrane-derived micro-vesicles that accelerate the regeneration process [104]. The previously mentioned factors have been frequently implicated in the pathogenesis of gastrointestinal and psychiatric disorders [89,105].

We envision that stem cells together with the GI microbiome are mutually involved in the pathogenesis of disorders of GBA by employing different mechanisms (e.g., autocrine, paracrine, or hormonal effects, immunomodulatory effects, replacement of damaged cells, cytotoxic effects, and neurotoxic effects) in distant tissues and organs. Further studies are needed to assess more accurately the mechanisms of cell-host-microbe interactions (Figure 1). Knowledge around these mechanisms already allows the design of novel treatments targeting GBA. For example, structural analog of S1P —Fingolimod and Ozanimod, functional antagonists of S1P receptors have already been applied in the treatment of relapsing forms of multiple sclerosis [106] as well as ulcerative colitis [107]. Similarly, supplementation with multi-species probiotics (Ecologic® Barrier, Amsterdam, The Netherlands) in a 12-week, placebo-controlled, randomized clinical study, which favorably modified both functional and biochemical markers (e.g., VEGF) of vascular dysfunction in obese postmenopausal women [108].

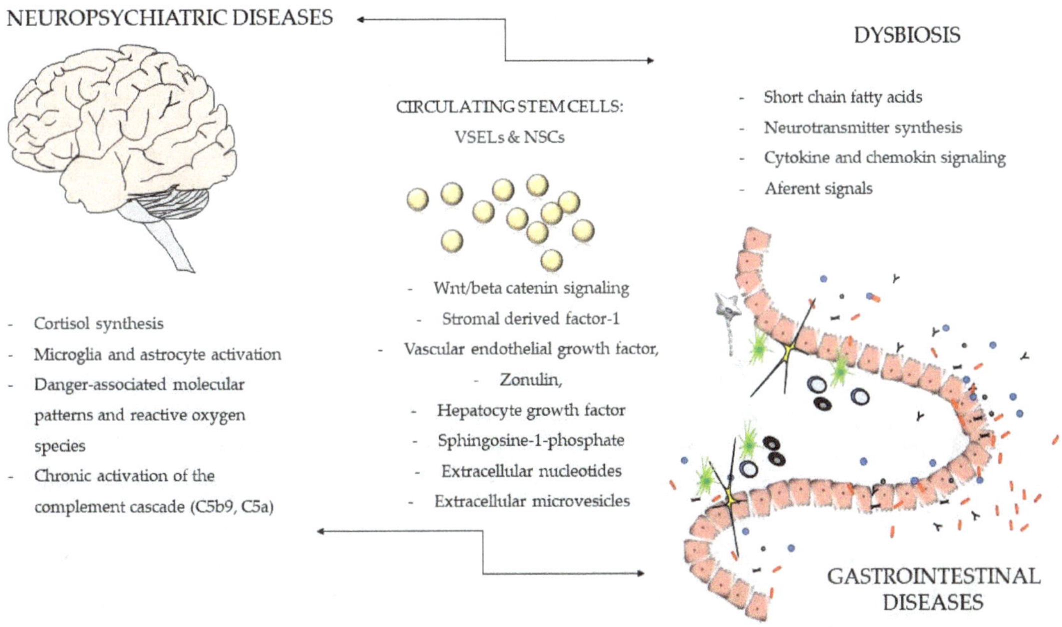

Figure 1. The bidirectional signaling within the GBA with the involvement of sterile inflammation of the brain and actions of microbiota and circulating adult stem cells. For details, see the text.

Emerging scientific data show that rapid changes in diet and lifestyle significantly contribute to the weakening of old evolutionary cell door-keeping mechanisms (e.g., Wnt/β catenin system) in the gut and the brain. The notion that even minor and subclinical stimuli to the gut mucosal and vascular barrier (e.g., infection) can result in significant, though delayed, consequences that may seriously affect the health of an individual is attractive [109], it still requires further detailed studies.

6. Drug-Microbiome Interactions—Still Neglected Problem in Clinical Medicine

Although microbiota alterations play—At least in part—A role in the etiology of neuropsychiatric diseases. Paradoxically, the treatment of these conditions may adversely affect the composition of intestinal microbiota. In fact, multiple drugs were found to be involved in dysbiosis origin [110–112]. Recently, Maier [113] reported that approximately one-fourth of about 10,000 non-antibiotic drugs were found to be able to reduce the in vitro growth of particular bacteria strain. Among these, the psychiatric drugs were predominant. In fact, certain pharmaceuticals utilized in neurology and psychiatry, which are predominantly antidepressants and antipsychotics, were historically characterized for being antibacterial agents. Evidence gathered mostly from animal studies but also in humans suggests that second-generation antipsychotics (SGA), which are mainly olanzapine and risperidone, change the composition of intestinal bacteria toward bacterial species promoting obesity. As demonstrated by several authors, the administration of these psychotropic drugs may increase the *Firmicutes/Bacteroidetes* ratio [114–118] previously found to be a microbiota profile of the obese [119].

The majority of studies aimed to look for the link between antipsychotic-induced metabolic malfunctions and microbiota dysbiosis were in vivo models. In rats treated with olanzapine (OLZ) and mice fed with a high fat diet and administered with OLZ, the microbiome diversity was found to be reduced [115,118]. When treated with another neuroleptic agent, namely risperidone (RIS), fewer operational taxonomy units (OTUs) were found in female mice [117]. Davey et al. demonstrated gender-dependent elevation of *Firmicutes* abundance and a decrease of *Bacteroidetes* [115,116]. Antipsychotic-driven dysbiosis in rodents resulted in decreased counts of beneficial *Actinobacteria* and *Proteobacteria* [115]. The OLZ regimen introduced higher abundance of *Erysipelotrichia* and *Gammaproteobacteria* and lower abundance of *Bacteroidia*. Lastly, OLZ suppressed the growth of anaerobic bacteria [117] and *Escherichia coli* NC101 [118].

In parallel, very few studies in humans explored the alterations of the gut microbiome following SGA treatment. Skewed intestinal microbiota following the psychotropic pharmacotherapy in humans expressed as elevated phylogenetic diversity and evaluated by means of PcoA of unweighted UniFrac distances [120] and reduced Simpson diversity in females [121] have been reported. Chronic use of RIS in children elevated the levels of *Clostridium*, *Lactobacillus*, *Ralstonia*, and *Eubacterium*. This occurred only in patients with a significant gain in BMI [120]. Flowers et al. conducted gut microbiota analyses in adult patients diagnosed with bipolar disorder and demonstrated that psychotropic treatment increased concentration of family *Lachnospiraceae* in the whole cohort of patients treated with SGA and a group of obese subjects. In addition, lowered counts of *Akkermansia* genera were noticed in the whole cohort of patients receiving treatment [121]. Yuan et al. lowered the levels of *Clostridium coccoides* Kaneuchi and *Lactobacillus* spp. and elevated the numbers of *Escherichia coli* Castellani and Chalmers in adult schizophrenia patients since six weeks of RIS treatment, which demonstrated that these variations may have induced body weight gain and increased fasting plasma glucose, homeostasis model assessment of insulin resistance (HOMA-IR), and low density lipoprotein (LDL) cholesterol concentration [122]. As far as metabolic disturbances are concerned, studies by Bahr et al. [120] and Flowers et al. [121] microbiota alteration during psychotropic treatment may correlate with weight gain.

We previously demonstrated that SGA-induced dysbiosis may potentially result in body weight and metabolic disturbances with low-level inflammation and decreased energy expenditure involved in the mechanism. However, since the majority of studies were conducted in rodent models with a high number of unclear risk of bias assessments, these findings need to be considered cautiously and may not be fully replicated in humans [123]. More studies regarding the involvement of psychiatric medications on gut microbiota composition in humans are warranted and, ccurrently, our research team undertook this effort.

The first antidepressant—Iproniazid—Via producing isonicotinoyl radicals may interrupt the bacterial cell cycle and inhibit their growth [124,125]. Tricyclic antidepressants were found to possess anti-plasmid activity and inhibit the growth of *Escherichia coli* Castellani and Chalmers, *Yersinia enterocolitica* Schleifstein & Coleman [126] and *Giardia lamblia* Kofoid & Christiansen [127] by means of decreasing the activity of DNA gyrase [128]. Tricyclic antidepressants are active relative to Plasmodium falciparum [129] and *Leishmania* spp. [130]. Selective serotonin re-uptake inhibitors may inhibit the growth of *Staphylococcus*, *Enterococcus* [131–133], *Citrobacter* spp, *Pseudomonas aeruginosa* Migula, *Klebsiella pneumoniae* Trevisan, *Morganella morganii* Brenner et al., *Clostridium perfringens* Hauduroy et al., and *Clostridium difficile* Prevot [131,134]. Efflux pump inhibition may be involved in these properties [135]. Ketamine may control the growth of *Staphylococcus aureus* Rosenbach, *Staphylococcus epidermidis* Evans, *Entercoccus faecalis* Schleifer and Kilpper-Bälz, *Streptococcus pyogenes* Rosenbach, *Pseudomonas aeruginosa* Migula and *Candida albicans* (C.P.Robin) Berkhout [134,136].

7. Modulation of Microbiota-Gut-Brain Axis as a Promising Tool to Manage Gastrointestinal and Mental Health

Mood disorders and depression are associated frequently with other GI conditions such as liver disease, inflammatory bowel disease (IBD), food intolerance, enteropathies (e.g., celiac disease), and cancer. Recently, Felice and O'Mahony [137] explained the origin of the high coincidence between stress-related psychiatric conditions and GI symptoms. Dysbiotic gut microbiota via synthesizing neuroactive metabolites are able to counteract secretion, motility, and blood flow within the GI tract and, additionally, transfer neural signals through vagus nerve and spinal cord routes. Therefore, the modulation of microbiota-gut-brain pathways opens up new avenues for the management of chronic diseases both of psychiatric and organic origin [12,138–143].

The new treatment avenues could be addressed through the modulation of the microbiota-gut-brain axis by means of prebiotic and probiotic administration. The World Gastroenterology Organization (WGO) recently issued a Global Guideline on Prebiotics and Probiotics use by healthcare professionals [144]. Among probiotics, those are recommended in the management of disorders of gut-brain interaction commonly known as FGIDs: *Lactobacillus plantarum* Bergey et al. 299V, *Bifidobacterium infantis* Reuter 35624, *Bifidobacterium animalis* Scardovi and Trovatelli DN-173 010, and *Saccharomyces boullardii* Henri Boulard CNCM I-745.

Psychobiotics—New Kid on the Block

Psychobiotics are a new class of probiotics which, when ingested, confer mental health benefits through interactions with the microbiota-gut-brain axis [145]. This term should also include prebiotics, which favorably influence the growth of beneficial gut bacteria [146]. Some of the properties of probiotics are prevalent among different strains, e.g., improvement of the intestinal epithelium renewal while the others are strain-specific, e.g., modulation of the CNS function [147]. Misra et al. noted that psychobiotic strains may be involved in the neuroactive substances synthesis, activate directly neural pathways, modulate neurotrophic factors, protect microbiota against stress, and others [148].

The action of psychobiotics was confirmed in mechanistic studies. For example, Ait-Belgnaoui et al. [149] demonstrated that psychobiotics may significantly reduce stress-induced neuronal activation in three brain regions i.e., hypothalamus, amygdala, and hippocampus, and promote the development of dendrites in the cingulate cortex-center of neurogenesis. Another study confirmed that psychobiotics decreased visceral hypersensitivity intensity and such an action correlated with the concentration of stress hormones (noradrenaline, adrenaline, corticosterone) and was possibly regulated by glucocorticoid receptors [150]. In vivo studies also reported that ingestion of psychobiotics improved GI function through the modulation of GBA in animals experiencing maternal separation [151] and *Citrobacter rodentium* infection [152].

Lately, the importance of psychobiotic use in humans has been acknowledged. Diop et al. was the first to demonstrate that probiotic supplementation reduces symptoms of GI disorders caused by stress in healthy people [153]. Messaoudi et al. showed that psychobiotic strains impact positively psychological stress exponents and reduce urinary free cortisol concentration [154]. Steenbergen et al. [155] demonstrated that, after 4 weeks of probiotic supplementation, a statistically significant improvement of aggression and rumination compared to placebo was found. Allen et al. [156] tested the psychobiotic strain to find that it may improve memory and reduce stress while Kato-Katoka [157] who analyzed a group of students during the exam session reported that the incidence of abdominal pain and cold as vegetative stress symptoms was significantly lowered in the group of students receiving probiotics compared to the placebo group. A recent study by Lv et al. [158] summarized that psychobiotics improve the function of the GI tract in patients with schizophrenia.

In addition, meta-analyses have shown that probiotic intervention may positively affect the mood in healthy persons as well as depressive patients [159]. McKean et al. [160] found that probiotic consumption may diminish the symptoms of depression, anxiety, and stress. Surprisingly, the latest meta-analysis concluded that such an intervention may significantly improve the mood of patients with mild to moderate depression but not the mood of healthy individuals [161]. Consequently, psychobiotics and neurobiotics, which are capable of GBA and HPA modulation, could be advocated in the management of patients endangered with iatrogenic complications associated with pharmacotherapy and polypharmacy. However, more studies—Especially of the highest evidence level—Are necessary to elucidate the psychobiotic potential to improve GBA function.

The use of these new probiotic compounds could be of great use in the daily management of stress and depression in FGIDs patients but also with other GI and extra-intestinal complaints associated with mental or mood alterations [162,163]. The data supporting their use are already strong and new studies that shall create even more evidence to medical societies as well as governmental agencies to help them evaluate the microbiota-gut-brain axis therapeutics in the management of stress in contemporary medicine [164,165]. Table 2 includes examples of psychobiotic strains and their clinical applications [144,148,166]. Since a few probiotic strains were found to be effective to counteract mood disorders and FGIDs, there is still limited data in individuals with ASD, Parkinson's disease, and Alzheimer's disease. There is an urgent need for a great investment in clinical trials in these entities [167–171].

Table 2. Probiotics strains with documented efficacy in gut-brain axis disorders [144,148,166,172].

Condition	Strain
Anxiety and depression	*Lactobacillus fermentum* NS8 and NS9, *Lactobacillus casei* Shirota, *Lactobacillus gasseri* OLL2809, *Lactobacillus rhamnosus* JB-1, *Lactobacillus helveticus* Rosell -52, *Lactobacillus acidophilus* W37, *Lactobacillus brevis* W63, *Lactococcus lactis* W19 and W58, *Bifidobacterium longum* Rosell-175, *Bifidobacterium longum* NCC3001, *Bifidobacterium longum* 1714, *Bifidobacterium bifidum* W23, *Bifidobacterium lactis* W52, *Lactobacillus plantarum* 299v
Stress	*Lactobacillus casei* Shirota, *Lactobacillus helveticus* Rosell -52, *Lactobacillus plantarum* PS128, *Bifidobacterium longum* Rosell-175, *Lactobacillus gasseri* CP230 *
FGIDs	*Lactobacillus plantarum 299v* (DSM 9843), *Escherichia coli* DSM17252, *Bifidobacterium animalis* DN-173, *Saccharomyces boulardii* CNCM I-745 *Bifidobacterium infantis* 35624, *Lactobacillus rhamnosus* NCIMB 30174, *Lactobacillus plantarum* NCIMB 30173, *Lactobacillus acidophilus* NCIMB 30175, *Enterococcus faecium* NCIMB 30176

* Para-psychobiotic-heat inactivated strain.

8. Conclusions

Our review suggests some involvements of GBA deregulation in the origin of disorders of the brain and gut. We hypothesize that stem cell-host microbiome cross talk is potentially involved in GBA disorders. Consequently, molecules mediating GBA signaling may constitute a grip point for the development of diagnostic tools and personalized microbiota-based therapies. In addition, novel treatment protocols based on new compounds interfering with gut derived metabolites as well as small molecules and bioactive lipids playing roles in adult stem cell trafficking are awaiting further developments.

Author Contributions: Conceptualization, K.S.-Ż., W.M., I.Ł. Investigation, all. Writing—Original Draft Preparation, K.S.-Ż. Writing—Review, editing, final approval, all. Supervision, W.M. and I.Ł.

References

1. World Health Organization. Mental Health Included in the UN Sustainable Development Goals. Available online: http://www.who.int/mental_health/SDGs/en/ (accessed on 25 November 2018).
2. World Health Organization. Third United Nations High-level Meeting on NCDs. Available online: http://www.who.int/ncds/governance/third-un-meeting/en/ (accessed on 25 November 2018).
3. Chandra, P.S.; Chand, P. Towards a new era for mental health. *Lancet* **2018**. [CrossRef]
4. Patel, V.; Saxena, S.; Lund, C.; Thornicroft, G.; Baingana, F.; Bolton, P.; Chisholm, D.; Collins, P.Y.; Cooper, J.L.; Eaton, J.; et al. The Lancet Commission on global mental health and sustainable development. *Lancet* **2018**. [CrossRef]
5. Gallagher, J. More than Half Your Body is not Human. Available online: https://www.bbc.com/news/health-43674270 (accessed on 6 December 2018).
6. Lynch, S.V.; Pedersen, O. The Human Intestinal Microbiome in Health and Disease. *N. Engl. J. Med.* **2016**, *375*, 2369–2379. [CrossRef] [PubMed]
7. Bloomfield, S.F.; Rook, G.A.; Scott, E.A.; Shanahan, F.; Stanwell-Smith, R.; Turner, P. Time to abandon the hygiene hypothesis: New perspectives on allergic disease, the human microbiome, infectious disease prevention and the role of targeted hygiene. *Perspect. Public Health* **2016**, *136*, 213–224. [CrossRef] [PubMed]
8. Bello, M.G.D.; Knight, R.; Gilbert, J.A.; Blaser, M.J. Preserving microbial diversity. *Science* **2018**, *362*, 33–34. [CrossRef] [PubMed]
9. Bretin, A.; Gewirtz, A.T.; Chassaing, B. Microbiota and metabolism: What's new in 2018? *Am. J. Physiol. Endocrinol. Metab.* **2018**, *315*, 1–6. [CrossRef] [PubMed]
10. Rea, D.; Coppola, G.; Palma, G.; Barbieri, A.; Luciano, A.; Del Prete, P.; Rossetti, S.; Berretta, M.; Facchini, G.; Perdonà, S.; et al. Microbiota effects on cancer: From risks to therapies. *Oncotarget* **2018**, *9*, 17915–17927. [CrossRef] [PubMed]
11. Chu, H.; Williams, B.; Schnabl, B. Gut microbiota, fatty liver disease, and hepatocellular carcinoma. *Liver Res.* **2018**, *2*, 43–51. [CrossRef] [PubMed]
12. Marlicz, W.; Yung, D.E.; Skonieczna-Żydecka, K.; Loniewski, I.; van Hemert, S.; Loniewska, B.; Koulaouzidis, A. From clinical uncertainties to precision medicine: The emerging role of the gut barrier and microbiome in small bowel functional diseases. *Expert Rev. Gastroenterol. Hepatol.* **2017**, *11*, 961–978. [CrossRef]
13. Sanduzzi Zamparelli, M.; Compare, D.; Coccoli, P.; Rocco, A.; Nardone, O.M.; Marrone, G.; Gasbarrini, A.; Grieco, A.; Nardone, G.; Miele, L. The metabolic role of gut microbiota in the development of nonalcoholic fatty liver disease and cardiovascular disease. *Int. J. Mol. Sci.* **2016**, *17*, 1225. [CrossRef]
14. Skonieczna-Żydecka, K.; Łoniewski, I.; Maciejewska, D.; Marlicz, W. Mikrobiota jelitowa iskładniki pokarmowe jako determinanty funkcji układu nerwowego. Część I. Mikrobiota przewodu pokarmowego. *Aktualności Neurologiczne* **2017**, *17*, 181–188. (In Polish) [CrossRef]
15. Cenit, M.C.; Sanz, Y.; Codoñer-Franch, P. Influence of gut microbiota on neuropsychiatric disorders. *World J. Gastroenterol.* **2017**, *23*, 5486–5498. [CrossRef] [PubMed]
16. Marizzoni, M.; Provasi, S.; Cattaneo, A.; Frisoni, G.B. Microbiota and neurodegenerative diseases. *Curr. Opin. Neurol.* **2017**, *30*, 630–638. [CrossRef] [PubMed]
17. Stasi, C.; Nisita, C.; Cortopassi, S.; Corretti, G.; Gambaccini, D.; De Bortoli, N.; Fani, B.; Simonetti, N.; Ricchiuti, A.; Dell'Osso, L.; et al. Subthreshold psychiatric psychopathology in functional gastrointestinal disorders: Can it be the bridge between gastroenterology and psychiatry? *Gastroenterol. Res. Pract.* **2017**, *2017*. [CrossRef]
18. Bernstein, C.N.; Hitchon, C.A.; Walld, R.; Bolton, J.M.; Sareen, J.; Walker, J.R.; Graff, L.A.; Patten, S.B.; Singer, A.; Lix, L.M.; et al. Increased burden of psychiatric disorders in inflammatory bowel disease. *Inflamm. Bowel Dis.* **2018**. [CrossRef]
19. Chan, W.; Shim, H.H.; Lim, M.S.; Sawadjaan, F.L.B.; Isaac, S.P.; Chuah, S.W.; Leong, R.; Kong, C. Symptoms of anxiety and depression are independently associated with inflammatory bowel disease-related disability. *Dig. Liver Dis.* **2017**, *49*, 1314–1319. [CrossRef]
20. Frolkis, A.D.; Vallerand, I.A.; Shaheen, A.-A.; Lowerison, M.W.; Swain, M.G.; Barnabe, C.; Patten, S.B.; Kaplan, G.G. Depression increases the risk of inflammatory bowel disease, which may be mitigated by the use of antidepressants in the treatment of depression. *Gut* **2018**. [CrossRef]

21. Drossman, D.A.; Hasler, W.L. Rome IV-functional GI disorders: Disorders of gut-brain interaction. *Gastroenterology* **2016**, *150*, 1257–1261. [CrossRef]
22. Zhong, L.; Shanahan, E.R.; Raj, A.; Koloski, N.A.; Fletcher, L.; Morrison, M.; Walker, M.M.; Talley, N.J.; Holtmann, G. Dyspepsia and the microbiome: Time to focus on the small intestine. *Gut* **2017**, *66*, 1168–1169. [CrossRef]
23. Vanheel, H.; Vicario, M.; Vanuytsel, T.; Van Oudenhove, L.; Martinez, C.; Keita, Å.V.; Pardon, N.; Santos, J.; Söderholm, J.D.; Tack, J.; et al. Impaired duodenal mucosal integrity and low-grade inflammation in functional dyspepsia. *Gut* **2014**, *63*, 262–271. [CrossRef]
24. Giamarellos-Bourboulis, E.; Tang, J.; Pyleris, E.; Pistiki, A.; Barbatzas, C.; Brown, J.; Lee, C.C.; Harkins, T.T.; Kim, G.; Weitsman, S.; et al. Molecular assessment of differences in the duodenal microbiome in subjects with irritable bowel syndrome. *Scand. J. Gastroenterol.* **2015**, *50*, 1076–1087. [CrossRef]
25. Martínez, C.; Lobo, B.; Pigrau, M.; Ramos, L.; González-Castro, A.M.; Alonso, C.; Guilarte, M.; Guilá, M.; de Torres, I.; Azpiroz, F.; et al. Diarrhoea-predominant irritable bowel syndrome: An organic disorder with structural abnormalities in the jejunal epithelial barrier. *Gut* **2013**, *62*, 1160–1168. [CrossRef]
26. Barbara, G.; Wang, B.; Stanghellini, V.; de Giorgio, R.; Cremon, C.; Di Nardo, G.; Trevisani, M.; Campi, B.; Geppetti, P.; Tonini, M.; et al. Mast cell-dependent excitation of visceral-nociceptive sensory neurons in irritable bowel syndrome. *Gastroenterology* **2007**, *132*, 26–37. [CrossRef]
27. Shah, E.; Rezaie, A.; Riddle, M.; Pimentel, M. Psychological disorders in gastrointestinal disease: Epiphenomenon, cause or consequence? *Ann. Gastroenterol.* **2014**, *27*, 224–230.
28. Gastrointestinal Symptoms in Psychiatry: Comparison of Direct Applications and Referrals. Available online: http://www.dusunenadamdergisi.org/ing/fArticledetails.aspx?MkID=1125 (accessed on 19 November 2018).
29. Wilder-Smith, C.H.; Olesen, S.S.; Materna, A.; Drewes, A.M. Fermentable sugar ingestion, gas production, and gastrointestinal and central nervous system symptoms in patients with functional disorders. *Gastroenterology* **2018**, *155*, 1034–1044. [CrossRef]
30. Codagnone, M.G.; Spichak, S.; O'Mahony, S.M.; O'Leary, O.F.; Clarke, G.; Stanton, C.; Dinan, T.G.; Cryan, J.F. Programming bugs: Microbiota and the developmental origins of brain health and disease. *Biol. Psychiatry* **2018**. [CrossRef]
31. Luczynski, P.; Whelan, S.O.; O'Sullivan, C.; Clarke, G.; Shanahan, F.; Dinan, T.G.; Cryan, J.F. Adult microbiota-deficient mice have distinct dendritic morphological changes: Differential effects in the amygdala and hippocampus. *Eur. J. Neurosci.* **2016**, *44*, 2654–2666. [CrossRef]
32. Hoban, A.E.; Stilling, R.M.; Ryan, F.J.; Shanahan, F.; Dinan, T.G.; Claesson, M.J.; Clarke, G.; Cryan, J.F. Regulation of prefrontal cortex myelination by the microbiota. *Transl. Psychiatry* **2016**, *6*, 774. [CrossRef]
33. Lu, J.; Lu, L.; Yu, Y.; Cluette-Brown, J.; Martin, C.R.; Claud, E.C. Effects of intestinal microbiota on brain development in humanized gnotobiotic mice. *Sci. Rep.* **2018**, *8*, 5443. [CrossRef]
34. Desbonnet, L.; Clarke, G.; Shanahan, F.; Dinan, T.G.; Cryan, J.F. Microbiota is essential for social development in the mouse. *Mol. Psychiatry* **2014**, *19*, 146–148. [CrossRef]
35. Marlicz, W.; Poniewierska-Baran, A.; Rzeszotek, S.; Bartoszewski, R.; Skonieczna-Żydecka, K.; Starzyńska, T.; Ratajczak, M.Z. A novel potential role of pituitary gonadotropins in the pathogenesis of human colorectal cancer. *PLoS ONE* **2018**, *13*, e0189337. [CrossRef]
36. Kaelberer, M.M.; Buchanan, K.L.; Klein, M.E.; Barth, B.B.; Montoya, M.M.; Shen, X.; Bohórquez, D.V. A gut-brain neural circuit for nutrient sensory transduction. *Science* **2018**, *361*. [CrossRef]
37. Paolicelli, R.C.; Bergamini, G.; Rajendran, L. Cell-to-cell communication by extracellular vesicles: Focus on microglia. *Neuroscience* **2018**. [CrossRef]
38. Kavvadia, M.; Santis, G.L.D.; Cascapera, S.; Lorenzo, A.D. Psychobiotics as integrative therapy for neuropsychiatric disorders with special emphasis on the microbiota-gut-brain axis. *Biomed. Prev.* **2017**, *2*, 8. [CrossRef]
39. Riboni, F.V.; Belzung, C. Stress and psychiatric disorders: From categorical to dimensional approaches. *Curr. Opin. Behav. Sci.* **2017**, *14*, 72–77. [CrossRef]
40. Sudo, N.; Chida, Y.; Aiba, Y.; Sonoda, J.; Oyama, N.; Yu, X.-N.; Kubo, C.; Koga, Y. Postnatal microbial colonization programs the hypothalamic-pituitary-adrenal system for stress response in mice. *J. Physiol. (Lond.)* **2004**, *558*, 263–275. [CrossRef]

41. Crumeyrolle-Arias, M.; Jaglin, M.; Bruneau, A.; Vancassel, S.; Cardona, A.; Daugé, V.; Naudon, L.; Rabot, S. Absence of the gut microbiota enhances anxiety-like behavior and neuroendocrine response to acute stress in rats. *Psychoneuroendocrinology* **2014**, *42*, 207–217. [CrossRef]
42. König, J.; Wells, J.; Cani, P.D.; García-Ródenas, C.L.; MacDonald, T.; Mercenier, A.; Whyte, J.; Troost, F.; Brummer, R.-J. Human intestinal barrier function in health and disease. *Clin. Transl. Gastroenterol.* **2016**, *7*, 196. [CrossRef]
43. Fond, G.; Boukouaci, W.; Chevalier, G.; Regnault, A.; Eberl, G.; Hamdani, N.; Dickerson, F.; Macgregor, A.; Boyer, L.; Dargel, A.; et al. The "psychomicrobiotic": Targeting microbiota in major psychiatric disorders: A systematic review. *Pathol. Biol.* **2015**, *63*, 35–42. [CrossRef]
44. Spadoni, I.; Zagato, E.; Bertocchi, A.; Paolinelli, R.; Hot, E.; Di Sabatino, A.; Caprioli, F.; Bottiglieri, L.; Oldani, A.; Viale, G.; et al. A gut-vascular barrier controls the systemic dissemination of bacteria. *Science* **2015**, *350*, 830–834. [CrossRef]
45. Brown, E.M.; Sadarangani, M.; Finlay, B.B. The role of the immune system in governing host-microbe interactions in the intestine. *Nat. Immunol.* **2013**, *14*, 660–667. [CrossRef]
46. Groschwitz, K.R.; Hogan, S.P. Intestinal barrier function: Molecular regulation and disease pathogenesis. *J. Allergy Clin. Immunol.* **2009**, *124*, 3–20. [CrossRef]
47. Tripathi, A.; Lammers, K.M.; Goldblum, S.; Shea-Donohue, T.; Netzel-Arnett, S.; Buzza, M.S.; Antalis, T.M.; Vogel, S.N.; Zhao, A.; Yang, S.; et al. Identification of human zonulin, a physiological modulator of tight junctions, as prehaptoglobin-2. *Proc. Natl. Acad. Sci. USA* **2009**, *106*, 16799–16804. [CrossRef]
48. Fasano, A. Zonulin and its regulation of intestinal barrier function: The biological door to inflammation, autoimmunity, and cancer. *Physiol. Rev.* **2011**, *91*, 151–175. [CrossRef]
49. Sharon, G.; Sampson, T.R.; Geschwind, D.H.; Mazmanian, S.K. The central nervous system and the gut microbiome. *Cell.* **2016**, *167*, 915–932. [CrossRef]
50. Al-Asmakh, M.; Anuar, F.; Zadjali, F.; Rafter, J.; Pettersson, S. Gut microbial communities modulating brain development and function. *Gut Microbes* **2012**, *3*, 366–373. [CrossRef]
51. Daneman, R.; Rescigno, M. The gut immune barrier and the blood-brain barrier: Are they so different? *Immunity* **2009**, *31*, 722–735. [CrossRef]
52. Mayer, E.A.; Craske, M.; Naliboff, B.D. Depression, anxiety, and the gastrointestinal system. *J. Clin. Psychiatry* **2001**, *62* (Suppl. 8), 28–37.
53. Carding, S.; Verbeke, K.; Vipond, D.T.; Corfe, B.M.; Owen, L.J. Dysbiosis of the gut microbiota in disease. *Microb. Ecol. Health Dis.* **2015**, *26*, 26191. [CrossRef]
54. Rothschild, D.; Weissbrod, O.; Barkan, E.; Kurilshikov, A.; Korem, T.; Zeevi, D.; Costea, P.I.; Godneva, A.; Kalka, I.N.; Bar, N.; et al. Environment dominates over host genetics in shaping human gut microbiota. *Nature* **2018**, *555*, 210–215. [CrossRef]
55. Foster, J.A.; Neufeld, K.-A.M. Gut-brain axis: How the microbiome influences anxiety and depression. *Trends Neurosci.* **2013**, *36*, 305–312. [CrossRef]
56. Sherwin, E.; Dinan, T.G.; Cryan, J.F. Recent developments in understanding the role of the gut microbiota in brain health and disease. *Ann. N. Y. Acad. Sci.* **2018**, *1420*, 5–25. [CrossRef]
57. Rogers, G.B.; Keating, D.J.; Young, R.L.; Wong, M.-L.; Licinio, J.; Wesselingh, S. From gut dysbiosis to altered brain function and mental illness: Mechanisms and pathways. *Mol. Psychiatry* **2016**, *21*, 738–748. [CrossRef]
58. Bastiaanssen, T.F.S.; Cowan, C.S.M.; Claesson, M.J.; Dinan, T.G.; Cryan, J.F. Making sense of ... the microbiome in psychiatry. *Int. J. Neuropsychopharmacol.* **2018**. [CrossRef]
59. Grochowska, M.; Wojnar, M.; Radkowski, M. The gut microbiota in neuropsychiatric disorders. *Acta Neurobiol. Exp.* **2018**, *78*, 69–81. [CrossRef]
60. Aizawa, E.; Tsuji, H.; Asahara, T.; Takahashi, T.; Teraishi, T.; Yoshida, S.; Ota, M.; Koga, N.; Hattori, K.; Kunugi, H. Possible association of Bifidobacterium and Lactobacillus in the gut microbiota of patients with major depressive disorder. *J. Affect. Disord.* **2016**, *202*, 254–257. [CrossRef]
61. Jiang, H.; Ling, Z.; Zhang, Y.; Mao, H.; Ma, Z.; Yin, Y.; Wang, W.; Tang, W.; Tan, Z.; Shi, J.; et al. Altered fecal microbiota composition in patients with major depressive disorder. *Brain Behav. Immun.* **2015**, *48*, 186–194. [CrossRef]
62. Szczesniak, O.; Hestad, K.A.; Hanssen, J.F.; Rudi, K. Isovaleric acid in stool correlates with human depression. *Nutr. Neurosci.* **2016**, *19*, 279–283. [CrossRef]

63. Ogyu, K.; Kubo, K.; Noda, Y.; Iwata, Y.; Tsugawa, S.; Omura, Y.; Wada, M.; Tarumi, R.; Plitman, E.; Moriguchi, S.; et al. Kynurenine pathway in depression: A systematic review and meta-analysis. *Neurosci. Biobehav. Rev.* **2018**, *90*, 16–25. [CrossRef]
64. Schwarz, E.; Maukonen, J.; Hyytiäinen, T.; Kieseppä, T.; Orešič, M.; Sabunciyan, S.; Mantere, O.; Saarela, M.; Yolken, R.; Suvisaari, J. Analysis of microbiota in first episode psychosis identifies preliminary associations with symptom severity and treatment response. *Schizophr. Res.* **2018**, *192*, 398–403. [CrossRef]
65. Shen, Y.; Xu, J.; Li, Z.; Huang, Y.; Yuan, Y.; Wang, J.; Zhang, M.; Hu, S.; Liang, Y. Analysis of gut microbiota diversity and auxiliary diagnosis as a biomarker in patients with schizophrenia: A cross-sectional study. *Schizophr. Res.* **2018**. [CrossRef]
66. Evans, S.J.; Bassis, C.M.; Hein, R.; Assari, S.; Flowers, S.A.; Kelly, M.B.; Young, V.B.; Ellingrod, V.E.; McInnis, M.G. The gut microbiome composition associates with bipolar disorder and illness severity. *J. Psychiatr. Res.* **2017**, *87*, 23–29. [CrossRef]
67. Painold, A.; Mörkl, S.; Kashofer, K.; Halwachs, B.; Dalkner, N.; Bengesser, S.; Birner, A.; Fellendorf, F.; Platzer, M.; Queissner, R.; et al. A step ahead: Exploring the gut microbiota in inpatients with bipolar disorder during a depressive episode. *Bipolar Disord.* **2018**. [CrossRef]
68. Keshavarzian, A.; Green, S.J.; Engen, P.A.; Voigt, R.M.; Naqib, A.; Forsyth, C.B.; Mutlu, E.; Shannon, K.M. Colonic bacterial composition in Parkinson's disease. *Mov. Disord.* **2015**, *30*, 1351–1360. [CrossRef]
69. De Angelis, M.; Francavilla, R.; Piccolo, M.; De Giacomo, A.; Gobbetti, M. Autism spectrum disorders and intestinal microbiota. *Gut Microbes* **2015**, *6*, 207–213. [CrossRef]
70. Kushak, R.I.; Winter, H.S.; Buie, T.M.; Cox, S.B.; Phillips, C.D.; Ward, N.L. Analysis of the Duodenal Microbiome in Autistic Individuals: Association With Carbohydrate Digestion. *J. Pediatr. Gastroenterol. Nutr.* **2017**, *64*, 110–116. [CrossRef]
71. Lee, Y.; Park, J.-Y.; Lee, E.-H.; Yang, J.; Jeong, B.-R.; Kim, Y.-K.; Seoh, J.-Y.; Lee, S.; Han, P.-L.; Kim, E.-J. Rapid assessment of microbiota changes in individuals with autism spectrum disorder using bacteria-derived membrane vesicles in urine. *Exp. Neurobiol.* **2017**, *26*, 307–317. [CrossRef]
72. Strati, F.; Cavalieri, D.; Albanese, D.; De Felice, C.; Donati, C.; Hayek, J.; Jousson, O.; Leoncini, S.; Renzi, D.; Calabrò, A.; et al. New evidences on the altered gut microbiota in autism spectrum disorders. *Microbiome* **2017**, *5*, 24. [CrossRef]
73. Bryn, V.; Verkerk, R.; Skjeldal, O.H.; Saugstad, O.D.; Ormstad, H. Kynurenine pathway in autism spectrum disorders in children. *Neuropsychobiology* **2017**, *76*, 82–88. [CrossRef]
74. Aarts, E.; Ederveen, T.H.A.; Naaijen, J.; Zwiers, M.P.; Boekhorst, J.; Timmerman, H.M.; Smeekens, S.P.; Netea, M.G.; Buitelaar, J.K.; Franke, B.; et al. Gut microbiome in ADHD and its relation to neural reward anticipation. *PLoS ONE* **2017**, *12*, e0183509. [CrossRef]
75. Cattaneo, A.; Cattane, N.; Galluzzi, S.; Provasi, S.; Lopizzo, N.; Festari, C.; Ferrari, C.; Guerra, U.P.; Paghera, B.; Muscio, C.; et al. Association of brain amyloidosis with pro-inflammatory gut bacterial taxa and peripheral inflammation markers in cognitively impaired elderly. *Neurobiol. Aging* **2017**, *49*, 60–68. [CrossRef]
76. Vogt, N.M.; Kerby, R.L.; Dill-McFarland, K.A.; Harding, S.J.; Merluzzi, A.P.; Johnson, S.C.; Carlsson, C.M.; Asthana, S.; Zetterberg, H.; Blennow, K.; et al. Gut microbiome alterations in Alzheimer's disease. *Sci Rep.* **2017**, *7*, 13537. [CrossRef]
77. Cekanaviciute, E.; Yoo, B.B.; Runia, T.F.; Debelius, J.W.; Singh, S.; Nelson, C.A.; Kanner, R.; Bencosme, Y.; Lee, Y.K.; Hauser, S.L.; et al. Gut bacteria from multiple sclerosis patients modulate human T cells and exacerbate symptoms in mouse models. *Proc. Natl. Acad. Sci. USA* **2017**, *114*, 10713–10718. [CrossRef]
78. Schwensen, H.F.; Kan, C.; Treasure, J.; Høiby, N.; Sjögren, M. A systematic review of studies on the faecal microbiota in anorexia nervosa: Future research may need to include microbiota from the small intestine. *Eat. Weight Disord.* **2018**, *23*, 399–418. [CrossRef]
79. Bailey, M.T.; Dowd, S.E.; Galley, J.D.; Hufnagle, A.R.; Allen, R.G.; Lyte, M. Exposure to a social stressor alters the structure of the intestinal microbiota: Implications for stressor-induced immunomodulation. *Brain Behav. Immun.* **2011**, *25*, 397–407. [CrossRef]
80. Zijlmans, M.A.C.; Korpela, K.; Riksen-Walraven, J.M.; de Vos, W.M.; de Weerth, C. Maternal prenatal stress is associated with the infant intestinal microbiota. *Psychoneuroendocrinology* **2015**, *53*, 233–245. [CrossRef]
81. Yarandi, S.S.; Peterson, D.A.; Treisman, G.J.; Moran, T.H.; Pasricha, P.J. modulatory effects of gut microbiota on the central nervous system: how gut could play a role in neuropsychiatric health and diseases. *J. Neurogastroenterol. Motil.* **2016**, *22*, 201–212. [CrossRef]

82. Kelly, J.R.; Kennedy, P.J.; Cryan, J.F.; Dinan, T.G.; Clarke, G.; Hyland, N.P. Breaking down the barriers: The gut microbiome, intestinal permeability and stress-related psychiatric disorders. *Front. Cell. Neurosci.* **2015**, *9*, 392. [CrossRef]
83. Ait-Belgnaoui, A.; Bradesi, S.; Fioramonti, J.; Theodorou, V.; Bueno, L. Acute stress-induced hypersensitivity to colonic distension depends upon increase in paracellular permeability: Role of myosin light chain kinase. *Pain* **2005**, *113*, 141–147. [CrossRef]
84. Winter, G.; Hart, R.A.; Charlesworth, R.P.G.; Sharpley, C.F. Gut microbiome and depression: What we know and what we need to know. *Rev. Neurosci.* **2018**, *29*, 629–643. [CrossRef]
85. Bauer, M.E.; Teixeira, A.L. Inflammation in psychiatric disorders: What comes first? *Ann. N. Y. Acad. Sci.* **2018**. [CrossRef]
86. Spiller, R.; Lam, C. An Update on Post-infectious Irritable Bowel Syndrome: Role of Genetics, Immune Activation, Serotonin and Altered Microbiome. *J. Neurogastroenterol. Motil.* **2012**, *18*, 258–268. [CrossRef]
87. Futagami, S.; Itoh, T.; Sakamoto, C. Systematic review with meta-analysis: Post-infectious functional dyspepsia. *Aliment. Pharmacol. Ther.* **2015**, *41*, 177–188. [CrossRef]
88. Neuendorf, R.; Harding, A.; Stello, N.; Hanes, D.; Wahbeh, H. Depression and anxiety in patients with Inflammatory Bowel Disease: A systematic review. *J. Psychosom. Res.* **2016**, *87*, 70–80. [CrossRef]
89. Ratajczak, M.Z.; Pedziwiatr, D.; Cymer, M.; Kucia, M.; Kucharska-Mazur, J.; Samochowiec, J. Sterile inflammation of brain, due to activation of innate immunity, as a culprit in psychiatric disorders. *Front. Psychiatry* **2018**, *9*. [CrossRef]
90. Kahn, M. Wnt signaling in stem cells and cancer stem cells: A tale of two coactivators. *Prog. Mol. Biol. Transl. Sci.* **2018**, *153*, 209–244. [CrossRef]
91. Kabiri, Z.; Greicius, G.; Zaribafzadeh, H.; Hemmerich, A.; Counter, C.M.; Virshup, D.M. Wnt signaling suppresses MAPK-driven proliferation of intestinal stem cells. *J. Clin. Invest.* **2018**, *128*, 3806–3812. [CrossRef]
92. Xing, L.; Anbarchian, T.; Tsai, J.M.; Plant, G.W.; Nusse, R. Wnt/β-catenin signaling regulates ependymal cell development and adult homeostasis. *Proc. Natl. Acad. Sci. USA* **2018**, *115*, 5954–5962. [CrossRef]
93. Ratajczak, M.Z.; Liu, R.; Marlicz, W.; Blogowski, W.; Starzynska, T.; Wojakowski, W.; Zuba-Surma, E. Identification of very small embryonic/epiblast-like stem cells (VSELs) circulating in peripheral blood during organ/tissue injuries. *Methods Cell. Biol.* **2011**, *103*, 31–54. [CrossRef]
94. Wojakowski, W.; Tendera, M.; Kucia, M.; Zuba-Surma, E.; Paczkowska, E.; Ciosek, J.; Hałasa, M.; Król, M.; Kazmierski, M.; Buszman, P.; et al. Mobilization of bone marrow-derived Oct-4+ SSEA-4+ very small embryonic-like stem cells in patients with acute myocardial infarction. *J. Am. Coll. Cardiol.* **2009**, *53*, 1–9. [CrossRef]
95. Paczkowska, E.; Kucia, M.; Koziarska, D.; Halasa, M.; Safranow, K.; Masiuk, M.; Karbicka, A.; Nowik, M.; Nowacki, P.; Ratajczak, M.Z.; et al. Clinical evidence that very small embryonic-like stem cells are mobilized into peripheral blood in patients after stroke. *Stroke* **2009**, *40*, 1237–1244. [CrossRef]
96. Drukała, J.; Paczkowska, E.; Kucia, M.; Młyńska, E.; Krajewski, A.; Machaliński, B.; Madeja, Z.; Ratajczak, M.Z. Stem cells, including a population of very small embryonic-like stem cells, are mobilized into peripheral blood in patients after skin burn injury. *Stem Cell. Rev.* **2012**, *8*, 184–194. [CrossRef]
97. Marlicz, W.; Zuba-Surma, E.; Kucia, M.; Blogowski, W.; Starzynska, T.; Ratajczak, M.Z. Various types of stem cells, including a population of very small embryonic-like stem cells, are mobilized into peripheral blood in patients with Crohn's disease. *Inflamm. Bowel Dis.* **2012**, *18*, 1711–1722. [CrossRef]
98. Stonesifer, C.; Corey, S.; Ghanekar, S.; Diamandis, Z.; Acosta, S.A.; Borlongan, C.V. Stem cell therapy for abrogating stroke-induced neuroinflammation and relevant secondary cell death mechanisms. *Prog. Neurobiol.* **2017**, *158*, 94–131. [CrossRef]
99. Ratajczak, J.; Zuba-Surma, E.; Paczkowska, E.; Kucia, M.; Nowacki, P.; Ratajczak, M.Z. Stem cells for neural regeneration—A potential application of very small embryonic-like stem cells. *J. Physiol. Pharmacol.* **2011**, *62*, 3–12.
100. Kim, C.; Schneider, G.; Abdel-Latif, A.; Mierzejewska, K.; Sunkara, M.; Borkowska, S.; Ratajczak, J.; Morris, A.J.; Kucia, M.; Ratajczak, M.Z. Ceramide-1-phosphate regulates migration of multipotent stromal cells and endothelial progenitor cells–implications for tissue regeneration. *Stem Cells* **2013**, *31*, 500–510. [CrossRef]
101. Jabłoński, M.; Mazur, J.K.; Tarnowski, M.; Dołęgowska, B.; Pędziwiatr, D.; Kubiś, E.; Budkowska, M.; Sałata, D.; Wysiecka, J.P.; Kazimierczak, A.; et al. Mobilization of peripheral blood stem cells and changes in the concentration of plasma factors influencing their movement in patients with panic disorder. *Stem Cell. Rev.* **2017**, *13*, 217–225. [CrossRef]

102. Adamiak, M.; Bujko, K.; Cymer, M.; Plonka, M.; Glaser, T.; Kucia, M.; Ratajczak, J.; Ulrich, H.; Abdel-Latif, A.; Ratajczak, M.Z. Novel evidence that extracellular nucleotides and purinergic signaling induce innate immunity-mediated mobilization of hematopoietic stem/progenitor cells. *Leukemia* **2018**, *32*, 1920–1931. [CrossRef]
103. Ratajczak, M.Z.; Kim, C.; Ratajczak, J.; Janowska-Wieczorek, A. Innate immunity as orchestrator of bone marrow homing for hematopoietic stem/progenitor cells. *Adv. Exp. Med. Biol.* **2013**, *735*, 219–232.
104. Ratajczak, M.Z.; Ratajczak, J. extracellular microvesicles as game changers in better understanding the complexity of cellular interactions-from bench to clinical applications. *Am. J. Med. Sci.* **2017**, *354*, 449–452. [CrossRef]
105. Kucharska-Mazur, J.; Tarnowski, M.; Dołęgowska, B.; Budkowska, M.; Pędziwiatr, D.; Jabłoński, M.; Pełka-Wysiecka, J.; Kazimierczak, A.; Ratajczak, M.Z.; Samochowiec, J. Novel evidence for enhanced stem cell trafficking in antipsychotic-naïve subjects during their first psychotic episode. *J. Psychiatr. Res.* **2014**, *49*, 18–24. [CrossRef]
106. Hunter, S.F.; Bowen, J.D.; Reder, A.T. The direct effects of fingolimod in the central nervous system: Implications for relapsing multiple sclerosis. *CNS Drugs* **2016**, *30*, 135–147. [CrossRef]
107. Mutneja, H.R.; Arora, S.; Vij, A. Ozanimod treatment for ulcerative colitis. *N. Engl. J. Med.* **2016**, *375*, e17. [CrossRef]
108. Szulińska, M.; Łoniewski, I.; van Hemert, S.; Sobieska, M.; Bogdański, P. Dose-dependent effects of multispecies probiotic supplementation on the lipopolysaccharide (LPS) level and cardiometabolic profile in obese postmenopausal women: A 12-week randomized clinical trial. *Nutrients* **2018**, *10*, 773. [CrossRef]
109. Marlicz, W.; Loniewski, I.; Grimes, D.S.; Quigley, E.M. Nonsteroidal anti-inflammatory drugs, proton pump inhibitors, and gastrointestinal injury: Contrasting interactions in the stomach and small intestine. *Mayo Clin. Proc.* **2014**, *89*, 1699–1709. [CrossRef]
110. Le Bastard, Q.; Al-Ghalith, G.A.; Grégoire, M.; Chapelet, G.; Javaudin, F.; Dailly, E.; Batard, E.; Knights, D.; Montassier, E. Systematic review: Human gut dysbiosis induced by non-antibiotic prescription medications. *Aliment. Pharmacol. Ther.* **2018**, *47*, 332–345. [CrossRef]
111. Utzeri, E.; Usai, P. Role of non-steroidal anti-inflammatory drugs on intestinal permeability and nonalcoholic fatty liver disease. *World J. Gastroenterol.* **2017**, *23*, 3954–3963. [CrossRef]
112. Wallace, J.L.; Syer, S.; Denou, E.; de Palma, G.; Vong, L.; McKnight, W.; Jury, J.; Bolla, M.; Bercik, P.; Collins, S.M.; et al. Proton pump inhibitors exacerbate NSAID-induced small intestinal injury by inducing dysbiosis. *Gastroenterology* **2011**, *141*. [CrossRef]
113. Maier, L.; Pruteanu, M.; Kuhn, M.; Zeller, G.; Telzerow, A.; Anderson, E.E.; Brochado, A.R.; Fernandez, K.C.; Dose, H.; Mori, H.; et al. Extensive impact of non-antibiotic drugs on human gut bacteria. *Nature* **2018**, *555*, 623–628. [CrossRef]
114. Koliada, A.; Syzenko, G.; Moseiko, V.; Budovska, L.; Puchkov, K.; Perederiy, V.; Gavalko, Y.; Dorofeyev, A.; Romanenko, M.; Tkach, S.; et al. Association between body mass index and Firmicutes/Bacteroidetes ratio in an adult Ukrainian population. *BMC Microbiol.* **2017**, *17*. [CrossRef]
115. Davey, K.J.; O'Mahony, S.M.; Schellekens, H.; O'Sullivan, O.; Bienenstock, J.; Cotter, P.D.; Dinan, T.G.; Cryan, J.F. Gender-dependent consequences of chronic olanzapine in the rat: Effects on body weight, inflammatory, metabolic and microbiota parameters. *Psychopharmacology (Berl.)* **2012**, *221*, 155–169. [CrossRef]
116. Davey, K.J.; Cotter, P.D.; O'Sullivan, O.; Crispie, F.; Dinan, T.G.; Cryan, J.F.; O'Mahony, S.M. Antipsychotics and the gut microbiome: Olanzapine-induced metabolic dysfunction is attenuated by antibiotic administration in the rat. *Transl. Psychiatry* **2013**, *3*, 309. [CrossRef]
117. Bahr, S.M.; Weidemann, B.J.; Castro, A.N.; Walsh, J.W.; deLeon, O.; Burnett, C.M.L.; Pearson, N.A.; Murry, D.J.; Grobe, J.L.; Kirby, J.R. Risperidone-induced weight gain is mediated through shifts in the gut microbiome and suppression of energy expenditure. *EBioMedicine* **2015**, *2*, 1725–1734. [CrossRef]
118. Morgan, A.P.; Crowley, J.J.; Nonneman, R.J.; Quackenbush, C.R.; Miller, C.N.; Ryan, A.K.; Bogue, M.A.; Paredes, S.H.; Yourstone, S.; Carroll, I.M.; et al. The antipsychotic olanzapine interacts with the gut microbiome to cause weight gain in mouse. *PLoS ONE* **2014**, *9*, e115225. [CrossRef]
119. Castaner, O.; Goday, A.; Park, Y.-M.; Lee, S.-H.; Magkos, F.; Shiow, S.-A.T.E.; Schröder, H. The Gut Microbiome Profile in Obesity: A Systematic Review. Available online: https://www.hindawi.com/journals/ije/2018/4095789/ (accessed on 8 October 2018).

120. Bahr, S.M.; Tyler, B.C.; Wooldridge, N.; Butcher, B.D.; Burns, T.L.; Teesch, L.M.; Oltman, C.L.; Azcarate-Peril, M.A.; Kirby, J.R.; Calarge, C.A. Use of the second-generation antipsychotic, risperidone, and secondary weight gain are associated with an altered gut microbiota in children. *Transl. Psychiatry* **2015**, *5*, 652. [CrossRef]
121. Flowers, S.A.; Evans, S.J.; Ward, K.M.; McInnis, M.G.; Ellingrod, V.L. Interaction between atypical antipsychotics and the gut microbiome in a bipolar disease cohort. *Pharmacotherapy* **2017**, *37*, 261–267. [CrossRef]
122. Yuan, X.; Zhang, P.; Wang, Y.; Liu, Y.; Li, X.; Kumar, B.U.; Hei, G.; Lv, L.; Huang, X.-F.; Fan, X.; et al. Changes in metabolism and microbiota after 24-week risperidone treatment in drug naïve, normal weight patients with first episode schizophrenia. *Schizophr. Res.* **2018**. [CrossRef]
123. Skonieczna-Żydecka, K.; Łoniewski, I.; Misera, A.; Stachowska, E.; Maciejewska, D.; Marlicz, W.; Galling, B. Second-generation antipsychotics and metabolism alterations: A systematic review of the role of the gut microbiome. *Psychopharmacology* **2018**. [CrossRef]
124. Lei, B.; Wei, C.J.; Tu, S.C. Action mechanism of antitubercular isoniazid activation by *Mycobacterium* tuberculosis KatG, isolation, and characterization of inha inhibitor. *J. Biol. Chem.* **2000**, *275*, 2520–2526. [CrossRef]
125. Jena, L.; Waghmare, P.; Kashikar, S.; Kumar, S.; Harinath, B.C. Computational approach to understanding the mechanism of action of isoniazid, an anti-TB drug. *Int. J. Mycobacteriol.* **2014**, *3*, 276–282. [CrossRef]
126. Csiszar, K.; Molnar, J. Mechanism of action of tricyclic drugs on *Escherichia coli* and *Yersinia enterocolitica* plasmid maintenance and replication. *Anticancer Res.* **1992**, *12*, 2267–2272.
127. Binding of Tricyclic Antidepressant Drugs to Trophozoites of Giardia Lamblia. Available online: http://jglobal.jst.go.jp/en/public/20090422/200902093831082291 (accessed on 29 September 2018).
128. Antiplasmid Activity of Tricyclic Compounds. Available online: https://www.ncbi.nlm.nih.gov/pubmed/3047509 (accessed on 29 September 2018).
129. Bitonti, A.J.; Sjoerdsma, A.; McCann, P.P.; Kyle, D.E.; Oduola, A.M.; Rossan, R.N.; Milhous, W.K.; Davidson, D.E. Reversal of chloroquine resistance in malaria parasite Plasmodium falciparum by desipramine. *Science* **1988**, *242*, 1301–1303. [CrossRef]
130. Antidepressants Cause Lethal Disruption of Membrane Function in the Human Protozoan Parasite Leishmania. Available online: http://science.sciencemag.org/content/226/4677/977 (accessed on 29 September 2018).
131. Munoz-Bellido, J.L.; Munoz-Criado, S.; Garcìa-Rodrìguez, J.A. Antimicrobial activity of psychotropic drugs: Selective serotonin reuptake inhibitors. *Int. J. Antimicrob. Agents* **2000**, *14*, 177–180. [CrossRef]
132. Ayaz, M.; Subhan, F.; Ahmed, J.; Khan, A.-U.; Ullah, F.; Ullah, I.; Ali, G.; Syed, N.-I.-H.; Hussain, S. Sertraline enhances the activity of antimicrobial agents against pathogens of clinical relevance. *J. Biol. Res. (Thessalon)* **2015**, *22*, 4. [CrossRef]
133. Coban, A.Y.; Tanriverdi Cayci, Y.; Keleş Uludağ, S.; Durupinar, B. Investigation of antibacterial activity of sertralin. *Mikrobiyol. Bul.* **2009**, *43*, 651–656.
134. Kruszewska, H.; Zareba, T.; Tyski, S. Examination of antimicrobial activity of selected non-antibiotic medicinal preparations. *Acta Pol. Pharm.* **2012**, *69*, 1368–1371.
135. Bohnert, J.A.; Szymaniak-Vits, M.; Schuster, S.; Kern, W.V. Efflux inhibition by selective serotonin reuptake inhibitors in Escherichia coli. *J. Antimicrob. Chemother.* **2011**, *66*, 2057–2060. [CrossRef]
136. Begec, Z.; Yucel, A.; Yakupogullari, Y.; Erdogan, M.A.; Duman, Y.; Durmus, M.; Ersoy, M.O. The antimicrobial effects of ketamine combined with propofol: An in vitro study. *Braz J. Anesthesiol.* **2013**, *63*, 461–465. [CrossRef]
137. Felice, V.D.; O'Mahony, S.M. The microbiome and disorders of the central nervous system. *Pharmacol. Biochem. Behav.* **2017**, *160*, 1–13. [CrossRef]
138. Mörkl, S.; Wagner-Skacel, J.; Lahousen, T.; Lackner, S.; Holasek, S.J.; Bengesser, S.A.; Painold, A.; Holl, A.K.; Reininghaus, E. The role of nutrition and the gut-brain axis in psychiatry: A review of the literature. *Neuropsychobiology* **2018**, 1–9. [CrossRef]
139. Liang, S.; Wu, X.; Jin, F. Gut-Brain Psychology: Rethinking psychology from the microbiota–gut–brain axis. *Front. Integr. Neurosci.* **2018**, *12*. [CrossRef]
140. Tilg, H.; Schmiderer, A.; Djanani, A. Gut microbiome-immune crosstalk affects progression of cancer. *Transl. Gastroenterol. Hepatol.* **2018**, *3*. [CrossRef]

141. Tilg, H.; Grander, C. Microbiota and diabetes: An increasingly relevant association. *Pol. Arch. Int. Med.* **2018**, *128*, 333–335. [CrossRef]
142. Adolph, T.E.; Grander, C.; Moschen, A.R.; Tilg, H. Liver–microbiome axis in health and disease. *Trends Immunol.* **2018**, *39*, 712–723. [CrossRef]
143. Quigley, E.M.M. Prebiotics and probiotics in digestive health. *Clin. Gastroenterol. Hepatol.* **2018**. [CrossRef]
144. WGO Practice Guideline —Probiotics and Prebiotics. Available online: http://www.worldgastroenterology.org/guidelines/global-guidelines/probiotics-and-prebiotics (accessed on 5 October 2018).
145. Dinan, T.G.; Stanton, C.; Cryan, J.F. Psychobiotics: A novel class of psychotropic. *Biol. Psychiatry* **2013**, *74*, 720–726. [CrossRef]
146. Sarkar, A.; Lehto, S.M.; Harty, S.; Dinan, T.G.; Cryan, J.F.; Burnet, P.W.J. Psychobiotics and the manipulation of bacteria-gut-brain signals. *Trends Neurosci.* **2016**, *39*, 763–781. [CrossRef]
147. Hill, C.; Guarner, F.; Reid, G.; Gibson, G.R.; Merenstein, D.J.; Pot, B.; Morelli, L.; Canani, R.B.; Flint, H.J.; Salminen, S.; et al. Expert consensus document: The International Scientific Association for Probiotics and Prebiotics consensus statement on the scope and appropriate use of the term probiotic. *Nat. Rev. Gastroenterol. Hepatol.* **2014**, *11*, 506–514. [CrossRef]
148. Misra, S.; Mohanty, D. Psychobiotics: A new approach for treating mental illness? *Crit. Rev. Food Sci. Nutr.* **2017**, 1–7. [CrossRef]
149. Ait-Belgnaoui, A.; Colom, A.; Braniste, V.; Ramalho, L.; Marrot, A.; Cartier, C.; Houdeau, E.; Theodorou, V.; Tompkins, T. Probiotic gut effect prevents the chronic psychological stress-induced brain activity abnormality in mice. *Neurogastroenterol. Motil.* **2014**, *26*, 510–520. [CrossRef]
150. Ait-Belgnaoui, A.; Payard, I.; Rolland, C.; Harkat, C.; Braniste, V.; Théodorou, V.; Tompkins, T.A. *Bifidobacterium longum* and *Lactobacillus helveticus* synergistically suppress stress-related visceral hypersensitivity through hypothalamic-pituitary-adrenal axis modulation. *J. Neurogastroenterol. Motil.* **2018**, *24*, 138–146. [CrossRef]
151. Gareau, M.G.; Jury, J.; MacQueen, G.; Sherman, P.M.; Perdue, M.H. Probiotic treatment of rat pups normalises corticosterone release and ameliorates colonic dysfunction induced by maternal separation. *Gut* **2007**, *56*, 1522–1528. [CrossRef]
152. Gareau, M.G.; Wine, E.; Reardon, C.; Sherman, P.M. Probiotics prevent death caused by citrobacter rodentium infection in neonatal mice. *J. Infect. Dis.* **2010**, *201*, 81–91. [CrossRef]
153. Diop, L.; Guillou, S.; Durand, H. Probiotic food supplement reduces stress-induced gastrointestinal symptoms in volunteers: A double-blind, placebo-controlled, randomized trial. *Nutr. Res.* **2008**, *28*, 1–5. [CrossRef]
154. Messaoudi, M.; Lalonde, R.; Violle, N.; Javelot, H.; Desor, D.; Nejdi, A.; Bisson, J.-F.; Rougeot, C.; Pichelin, M.; Cazaubiel, M.; et al. Assessment of psychotropic-like properties of a probiotic formulation (*Lactobacillus helveticus* R0052 and *Bifidobacterium longum* R0175) in rats and human subjects. *Br. J. Nutr.* **2011**, *105*, 755–764. [CrossRef]
155. Steenbergen, L.; Sellaro, R.; van Hemert, S.; Bosch, J.A.; Colzato, L.S. A randomized controlled trial to test the effect of multispecies probiotics on cognitive reactivity to sad mood. *Brain Behav. Immun.* **2015**, *48*, 258–264. [CrossRef]
156. Allen, A.P.; Hutch, W.; Borre, Y.E.; Kennedy, P.J.; Temko, A.; Boylan, G.; Murphy, E.; Cryan, J.F.; Dinan, T.G.; Clarke, G. Bifidobacterium longum 1714 as a translational psychobiotic: Modulation of stress, electrophysiology and neurocognition in healthy volunteers. *Transl. Psychiatry* **2016**, *6*, 939. [CrossRef]
157. Kato-Kataoka, A.; Nishida, K.; Takada, M.; Kawai, M.; Kikuchi-Hayakawa, H.; Suda, K.; Ishikawa, H.; Gondo, Y.; Shimizu, K.; Matsuki, T.; et al. Fermented milk containing *Lactobacillus casei* strain shirota preserves the diversity of the gut microbiota and relieves abdominal dysfunction in healthy medical students exposed to academic stress. *Appl. Environ. Microbiol.* **2016**, *82*, 3649–3658. [CrossRef]
158. Lv, F.; Chen, S.; Wang, L.; Jiang, R.; Tian, H.; Li, J.; Yao, Y.; Zhuo, C. The role of microbiota in the pathogenesis of schizophrenia and major depressive disorder and the possibility of targeting microbiota as a treatment option. *Oncotarget* **2017**, *8*, 100899–100907. [CrossRef]
159. Huang, R.; Wang, K.; Hu, J. Effect of probiotics on depression: A systematic review and meta-analysis of randomized controlled trials. *Nutrients* **2016**, *8*, 483. [CrossRef]

160. McKean, J.; Naug, H.; Nikbakht, E.; Amiet, B.; Colson, N. Probiotics and subclinical psychological symptoms in healthy participants: a systematic review and meta-analysis. *J. Altern Complement. Med.* **2017**, *23*, 249–258. [CrossRef]
161. Ng, Q.X.; Peters, C.; Ho, C.Y.X.; Lim, D.Y.; Yeo, W.-S. A meta-analysis of the use of probiotics to alleviate depressive symptoms. *J. Affect. Disord.* **2018**, *228*, 13–19. [CrossRef]
162. Kazemi, A.; Noorbala, A.A.; Azam, K.; Eskandari, M.H.; Djafarian, K. Effect of probiotic and prebiotic vs placebo on psychological outcomes in patients with major depressive disorder: A randomized clinical trial. *Clin. Nutr.* **2018**. [CrossRef]
163. Reininghaus, E.Z.; Wetzlmair, L.-C.; Fellendorf, F.T.; Platzer, M.; Queissner, R.; Birner, A.; Pilz, R.; Hamm, C.; Maget, A.; Koidl, C.; et al. The impact of probiotic supplements on cognitive parameters in euthymic individuals with bipolar disorder: A pilot study. *Neuropsychobiology* **2018**, 1–8. [CrossRef]
164. Citi, S. Intestinal barriers protect against disease. *Science* **2018**, *359*, 1097–1098. [CrossRef]
165. Zhou, L.; Foster, J.A. Psychobiotics and the gut-brain axis: In the pursuit of happiness. *Neuropsychiatr Dis. Treat.* **2015**, *11*, 715–723. [CrossRef]
166. Nishida, K.; Sawada, D.; Kawai, T.; Kuwano, Y.; Fujiwara, S.; Rokutan, K. Para-psychobiotic Lactobacillus gasseri CP2305 ameliorates stress-related symptoms and sleep quality. *J. Appl. Microbiol.* **2017**, *123*, 1561–1570. [CrossRef]
167. Barichella, M.; Pacchetti, C.; Bolliri, C.; Cassani, E.; Iorio, L.; Pusani, C.; Pinelli, G.; Privitera, G.; Cesari, I.; Faierman, S.A.; et al. Probiotics and prebiotic fiber for constipation associated with Parkinson disease: An RCT. *Neurology* **2016**, *87*, 1274–1280. [CrossRef]
168. Tamtaji, O.R.; Taghizadeh, M.; Daneshvar Kakhaki, R.; Kouchaki, E.; Bahmani, F.; Borzabadi, S.; Oryan, S.; Mafi, A.; Asemi, Z. Clinical and metabolic response to probiotic administration in people with Parkinson's disease: A randomized, double-blind, placebo-controlled trial. *Clin. Nutr.* **2018**. [CrossRef]
169. Ticinesi, A.; Tana, C.; Nouvenne, A.; Prati, B.; Lauretani, F.; Meschi, T. Gut microbiota, cognitive frailty and dementia in older individuals: A systematic review. *Clin. Interv. Aging* **2018**, *13*, 1497–1511. [CrossRef]
170. Agahi, A.; Hamidi, G.A.; Daneshvar, R.; Hamdieh, M.; Soheili, M.; Alinaghipour, A.; Esmaeili Taba, S.M.; Salami, M. Does severity of Alzheimer's disease contribute to its responsiveness to modifying gut microbiota? A double blind clinical trial. *Front. Neurol.* **2018**, *9*, 662. [CrossRef]
171. Patusco, R.; Ziegler, J. Role of probiotics in managing gastrointestinal dysfunction in children with autism spectrum disorder: An update for practitioners. *Adv. Nutr.* **2018**, *9*, 637–650. [CrossRef]
172. Rudzki, L.; Ostrowska, L.; Pawlak, D.; Małus, A.; Pawlak, K.; Waszkiewicz, N.; Szulc, A. Probiotic *Lactobacillus plantarum* 299v decreases kynurenine concentration and improves cognitive functions in patients with major depression: A double-blind, randomized, placebo controlled study. *Psychoneuroendocrinology* **2018**, *100*, 213–222. [CrossRef]

15

Examining the Association and Directionality between Mental Health Disorders and Substance Use among Adolescents and Young Adults in the U.S. and Canada

Sarvenaz Esmaeelzadeh [1], John Moraros [1], Lilian Thorpe [2] and Yelena Bird [1,*]

1 School of Public Health, University of Saskatchewan, Saskatoon, SK S7N 2Z4, Canada; sarv.esmaeelzadeh@usask.ca (S.E.); john.moraros@usask.ca (J.M.)
2 FRCP, Faculty, Community Health and Epidemiology, University of Saskatchewan, Saskatoon, SK S7N 2Z4, Canada; lilian.thorpe@usask.ca
* Correspondence: yelena.bird@usask.ca;

Abstract: Background: The purpose of this systematic review was to examine the association and directionality between mental health disorders and substance use among adolescents and young adults in the U.S. and Canada. Methods: The following databases were used: Medline, PubMed, Embase, PsycINFO, and Cochrane Library. Meta-analysis used odds ratios as the pooled measure of effect. Results: A total of 3656 studies were screened and 36 were selected. Pooled results showed a positive association between depression and use of alcohol (odds ratio (OR) = 1.50, 95% confidence interval (CI): 1.24–1.83), cannabis (OR = 1.29, 95% CI: 1.10–1.51), and tobacco (OR = 1.65, 95% CI: 1.43–1.92). Significant associations were also found between anxiety and use of alcohol (OR = 1.54, 95% CI: 1.19–2.00), cannabis (OR = 1.36, 95% CI: 1.02–1.81), and tobacco (OR = 2.21, 95% CI: 1.54–3.17). A bidirectional relationship was observed with tobacco use at baseline leading to depression at follow-up (OR = 1.87, CI = 1.23–2.85) and depression at baseline leading to tobacco use at follow-up (OR = 1.22, CI = 1.09–1.37). A unidirectional relationship was also observed with cannabis use leading to depression (OR = 1.33, CI = 1.19–1.49). Conclusion: This study offers insights into the association and directionality between mental health disorders and substance use among adolescents and young adults. Our findings can help guide key stakeholders in making recommendations for interventions, policy and programming.

Keywords: depression; anxiety; alcohol; cannabis; tobacco; adolescents; young adults; U.S.; Canada

1. Background

Mental health disorders and substance use are important problems and relatively common among adolescents and young adults [1]. These two conditions are the leading cause of years lived with disability worldwide [2]. People are more likely to initiate substance use during adolescence, a critical period in one's life as they transition from childhood to adulthood [3]. It is estimated that 50% of all mental health disorders start by the age of 14 years old and 75% by the age of 25 years old [4]. Mental health disorders and substance use problems are closely linked, and both conditions can share similar biological and environmental components [5,6].

Mental health disorders contribute significantly to the burden of disease [2]. Globally, approximately one in five adolescents experience a mental health disorder each year [7]. Depressive and anxiety disorders are quite prevalent among adolescents and young adults. In the U.S., 8.4% of adolescents were diagnosed with either anxiety or depression in their lifetime [8]. In Canada, 5% of adolescents were diagnosed with an anxiety disorder and 6.3% with a mood disorder, mainly depression [9]. Despite the magnitude of the problem posed by mental health disorders among adolescents and young adults in the U.S. and Canada, frequently they are undiagnosed and when diagnosed not treated properly [10].

Adolescents and young adults with mental health disorders are at an increased risk of many negative health and social outcomes including self-harm and suicide [11], poor academic performance [12], and involvement in risky behaviors and poor sexual health [13]. It is reported that there is a link between adverse life events such as maltreatment and violence, loss, intra-familial problems, and school and interpersonal problems and suicidal behavior among young people. Also, the number of negative life events experienced by a young individual is reported to have a positive dose–response relation to suicidal behavior [14]. Risk factors for mental health disorders include biological factors (such as genetic tendency, head trauma, and substance abuse), psychological factors (such as maladaptive personality traits, difficult temperament, and physical/sexual abuse), and social factors (such as family conflict, loss of a loved one, bullying, and academic failure) [15].

Substance use among adolescents and young adults is a growing public health concern in developed countries such as the U.S. and Canada. Alcohol, cannabis, and tobacco are the substances most commonly used by adolescents and young adults. In Canada, the highest prevalence of alcohol (83%), cannabis (30%), and tobacco (18%) use was seen among young adults aged 20 to 24 years old followed by adolescents aged 15 to 19 years old (alcohol: 59%, cannabis: 21%, and tobacco: 10%) [16]. Similar trends in the prevalence of substance use were seen in the U.S. [17]. The magnitude of substance use among adolescents and young adults represents a major public health concern.

Substance use among adolescents and young adults is associated with many negative health, social, and economic consequences. These vary from suicidal behaviors [18] to low academic performance and school dropout [19], employment problems later in life [20], and risky behaviors [21]. Moreover, initiation of substance use in adolescence may be associated with the development of substance abuse and substance dependence later in life [22]. Risk factors associated with substance use are found at the individual (such as age, sex, personality and family history of substance use), interpersonal (such as relationship with parents, siblings, and peer pressure), and environmental (such as social norms, availability and accessibility of substance) levels [23].

Evidence suggests a complex interplay between substance use and vulnerability to mental health disorders [23,24]. Mental health disorders and substance use can co-occur due to a variety of reasons, including but not limited to: (1) common risk factors (such as environmental, genetic, personality, biological factors or traumatic events); (2) self-medication hypothesis (coping with psychological pressures and stressors as they relate to maturation, untreated traumas, and underlying conditions may lead to substance use and related risky behaviours); (3) substance use-induced mental health problems (individuals may develop a mental health problem as a direct (i.e., pharmacogenic) consequence of their substance use); and (4) substance use-related mental health problems (individuals may develop a mental health problem as an indirect (i.e., socio-economic stressors, unemployment, dysfunctional relationships) consequence of their substance use) [23,24].

Previous studies have been conducted examining the relationship between mental health disorders and substance use. Some studies have suggested that an association exists between depression and/or anxiety and alcohol, cannabis or tobacco use [25–30]. However, findings in the literature have been inconsistent [31–36]. Due to the high prevalence of mental health disorders and substance use among adolescents and young adults and the high potential of co-occurrence, further research in this important area is warranted. The purpose of this study was to examine the association and directionality between the three most common substances used (alcohol, cannabis, and tobacco) and two mental health disorders (depression and anxiety) among adolescents and young adults in the U.S. and Canada. Specifically, its objectives aimed to determine and quantify the association and directionality between: (1) depression and alcohol use, (2) depression and cannabis use, (3) depression and tobacco use,

(4) anxiety and alcohol use, (5) anxiety and cannabis use, and (6) anxiety and tobacco use among adolescents and/or young adults.

2. Methods

2.1. Data Sources

We conducted an extensive systematic literature review on the following electronic databases: Medline, PubMed, Cochrane Library, Embase, and PsycINFO. Our searches consisted of two major categories (substance use behaviors and mental health disorders) and their corresponding Medical Subject Headings (MeSH) terms and keywords: Subject OR Title (alcohol drinking or alcohol use or cannabis or marijuana smoking or marijuana use or smoking or tobacco smoking or tobacco use) AND Subject OR Title (depression or depressive disorders or major depressive disorder or anxiety or anxiety disorders or mood disorders). Snowball method (reference tracking) was also used to scan the reference lists of retrieved full-text articles and then to search manually for additional relevant literature.

2.2. Eligibility Criteria, Data Extraction and Analysis

The inclusion criteria for this review centered on the following: (1) English language peer-reviewed articles, available in full text, with human studies, published from 2000 to 2017. All study designs were eligible except for case series and case report. Newspaper, conference posters, dissertations were excluded; (2) depression/anxiety symptoms or disorders (major depressive disorder, panic disorder, social anxiety disorder, specific phobias, generalized anxiety disorder) data measured by using standardized scales, diagnostic criteria, self-reported surveys or diagnosed by healthcare professionals; (3) substance use (alcohol, cannabis, or tobacco) or disorder data presented, analyzed, and discussed; (4) target population that included adolescents and/or young adults; (5) only studies conducted in the US or Canada; and (6) data was either presented as an odds ratio (OR) or permitted the OR to be calculated.

Two screeners, independently, reviewed the list of identified articles to assess eligibility for inclusion in our study. Any disagreements were resolved by a tiebreaker vote. Extraction criteria included: year of publication, study design, sample size, target population, country where the study was conducted, measurement instrument used for substance use and mental health disorders, effect measure, covariates, and results. The effect measures examined the association between any of the following categories: (1) depression and alcohol use; (2) depression and cannabis use; (3) depression and tobacco use; (4) anxiety and alcohol use; (5) anxiety and cannabis use, and (6) anxiety and tobacco use. If a study discussed more than one of these categories, we extracted and analyzed all relevant effect measures separately.

2.3. Definitions of Mental Health Disorders and Substance Use

Overall, the definitions and measurements of mental health disorders and substance use in the various studies included in our review were heterogeneous. When multiple measures were used, we selected the most standardized and commonly used measure in order to maximize comparability between studies (Appendix A) [25–60].

Standardized scales for depression or anxiety symptoms, instruments measuring depression or anxiety disorders using diagnostic criteria, and diagnosis of depression or anxiety by healthcare professionals were used by the various studies to define and select for mental health disorders. Certain studies examined subgroups of anxiety disorders such as social phobia or panic attack. We counted these subgroups as anxiety disorders and included them in our analysis. Similarly, a variety of well-established definitions and measurements were employed by a number of studies for substance use. For example, some studies defined participants as current users, whereas others as regular, daily, or ever users in their measurement categories (tobacco, alcohol and/or cannabis use). Appendix A provides the details for the definitions of mental health disorders and substance use employed by the various studies that were included in our analysis.

2.4. Quality Assessment

The modified Newcastle-Ottawa Scale (NOS) was used to assess the quality of both cross-sectional and longitudinal study designs. This scale includes three components and 8 items: (1) selection of study groups (4 items); (2) comparability of the groups (1 item); and the (3) ascertainment of the outcomes of interest (3 items) [61]. To assess the quality of the studies a star system was used. The quality of each study was determined by assigning it to one of three subgroups: (1) good (≥2 stars for selection of study groups, 1 star for comparability of the groups, and 3 stars for ascertainment of the outcomes of interest components); (2) fair (1 star for selection of study groups and 2 stars for ascertainment of the outcomes of interest components); or (3) poor (0 stars for selection of study groups, 0 stars for comparability of the groups, and ≤1 star for ascertainment of the outcomes of interest components). Risk of bias was designated as: low, if there was good quality in all components; unclear/moderate, if there was fair quality in one or more components without poor quality in any components; or high, if there was poor quality in any one of the components.

2.5. Meta-Analysis

Statistical analysis was completed using the Comprehensive Meta-Analysis software version 3 (Biostat Inc., Englewood, NJ, USA). For pooled mean effect size, random-effects models were used because differences were expected in the methodology and the samples of selected studies [62]. The primary outcome measure was odds ratio (OR). ORs and 95% confidence intervals (CI) were either extracted from the articles or calculated by the authors using the quantitative data provided in the studies. Six separate meta-analyses were conducted. Q-statistics and I^2 were used to examine the heterogeneity among studies. Publication bias was assessed by graphing funnel plots to visualize any possible asymmetries and Duval and Tweedie's trim and fill test was conducted to adjust the results in case of publication bias [63]. Sensitivity analysis was done using one-study removed analysis. Moreover, subgroup analysis was performed using moderator variables including point estimate (crude or adjusted), target population (adolescents and young adults), severity of mental health disorders (symptoms and disorders), and intensity of substance use behavior (definitions).

3. Results

3.1. Study Selection and Characteristics

In total, 3656 articles (Medline (n = 945), PubMed (n = 883), Cochrane Library (n = 41), Embase (n = 1618), and PsycINFO (n = 169)) were identified by our initial search. After removing studies prior to the year 2000 and duplicates, 2341 articles remained. Title and abstract screening excluded 2177 articles, leaving 164 for full-text screening. After the full-text screening, 30 articles remained. Six additional articles were manually added by use of the snowball method.

In completing the title, abstract, and full-text screening, studies were excluded, if they were related to: (1) exposures other than those of interest in this study, such as cessation/withdrawal from substances, use of e-cigarettes, opiates, cocaine, methamphetamine, sedative, and hallucinogens; (2) outcomes other than those of interest in this study, such as suicide ideations, bipolar disorder, mania, postpartum depression, and hypomania; (3) the recruited population was other than that of interest in this study, such as adults, participants who were pregnant, specific ethnic groups or gender, military veterans, participants with comorbid chronic medical illnesses such as diabetes, cardiovascular or lung diseases.

All 36 selected articles used either a cross-sectional (n = 19) or longitudinal (n = 17) study design. The summary of our study selection is shown in a PRISMA diagram (Figure 1). Study characteristics are presented in Table 1. The quality of studies was assessed using a modified Newcastle-Ottawa scale (NOS), which found 5 studies with a low, 27 with a moderate, and 4 with a high risk of bias.

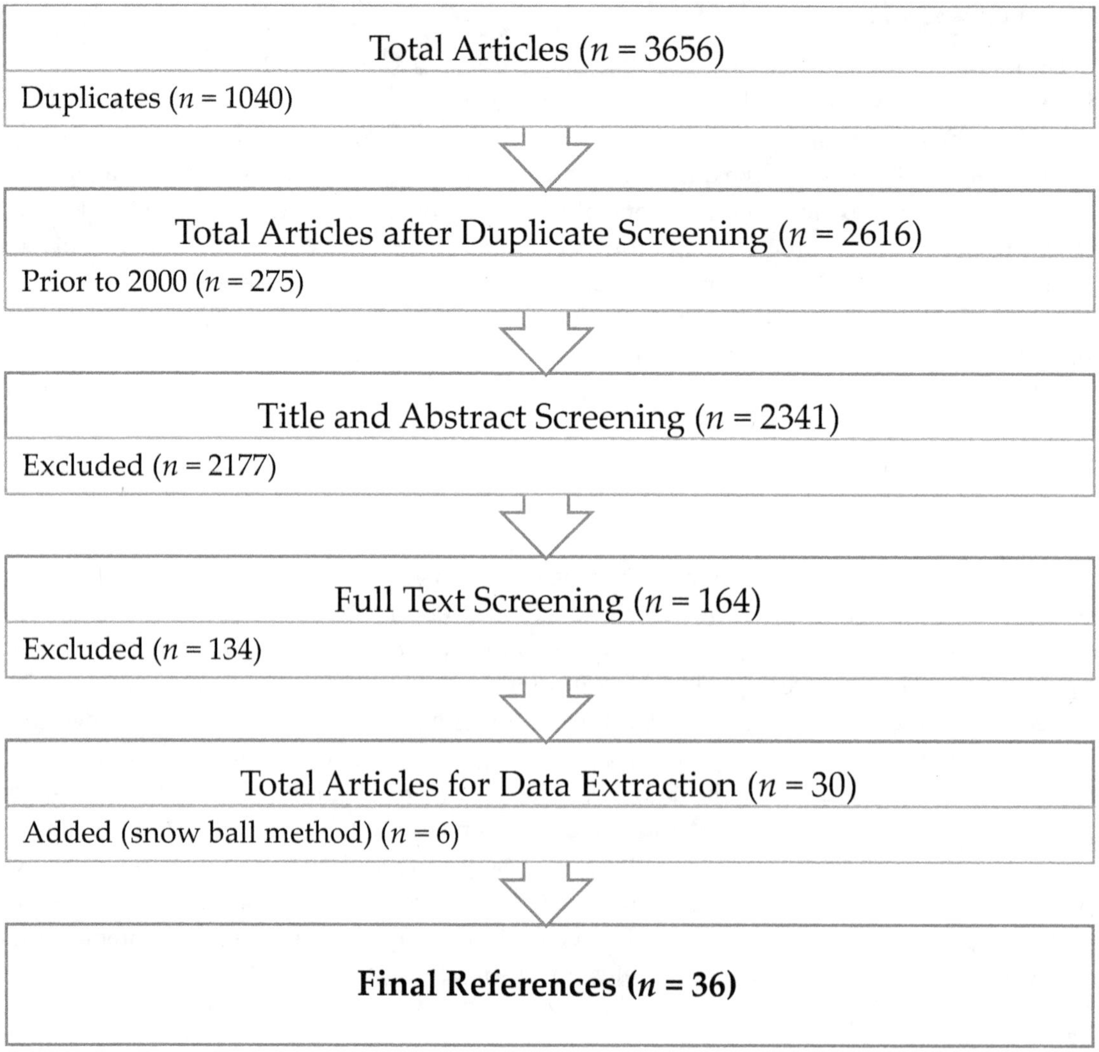

Figure 1. PRISMA diagram.

Table 1. Characteristics and associations of selected studies.

First Author's Name, Year, Country	Sample Size	Target Population	Substance Use Measure	Mental Health Disorders Assessment	% of Depressive Participants	Controlled Variables	OR (95% CI)
Association between Depression and Alcohol Use							
Cross-Sectional Studies							
Elissa Weitzman, 2004, U.S. [55]	27,687	College students aged 18–24	Binge/non-drinkers	Depressive symptoms: The 5-item subscale of SF36	4.9%	Age, sex, ethnicity	Adjusted: 1.05 (0.96–1.14)
Martha Kubik, 2005, U.S. [33]	3466	Grade 7 students	Heavy/non-drinkers	Depressive symptoms: CES-D, cut-off point of 16.	35%	Age, ethnicity, socioeconomic status (SES), smoking, cannabis, and inhalants use	Adjusted: 2.03 (1.30–3.17)
Susan Roberts, 2009, U.S. [32]	418	College students	Binge/non-drinkers	Depressive symptoms: BDI-II, cut-off point of 20	22%	-	Crude: 0.99 (0.61–1.58)
Elisabeth Simantov, 2000, U.S. [48]	5513	Grade 7–12 students	Regular/non-drinkers	Depressive symptoms: Modified version of CDI, cut-off point of 9	18.2%	-	Crude: 2.08 (1.79–2.42)
Linda Richter, 2015, U.S. [26]	24,445	Adolescents aged 12–20	Binge/non-drinkers	Major depressive disorder: Diagnosed depression (self-reported)	-	Sex, ethnicity, and age	Adjusted: 1.45 (1.11–1.91)
Eleanor Hanna, 2001, U.S. [31]	2001	Adolescents aged 12–16	Moderate/non-drinkers	Major depressive disorder: Diagnostic interview schedule, DSM-III	9%	Age, sex, ethnicity, family poverty level, school problem, smoking status	Adjusted: 3.31 (1.39–7.90)
Longitudinal Studies: Alcohol Use (Exposure) → Depression (Outcome)							
Mallie Paschall, 2005, U.S. [44]	13,892	Grade 6–12 students	Moderate/non-drinkers	Depressive symptoms: CES-D, cut-off point of 16.	5.3%	-	Crude: 1.17 (1.11–1.23)
David Brook, 2002, U.S. [52]	736	Adolescents aged 14, 13-year follow-up	Ever/never alcohol users	Major depressive disorder: Modified version of CIDI	8.3%	Age, sex, parental educational level, family income, prior psychiatric disorders	Adjusted: 1.72 (1.35–2.20)
Longitudinal Study: Depression (Exposure) → Alcohol Use (Outcome)							
Kiyuri Naicker, 2012, Canada [51]	1027	Adolescents aged 16–17, 10-year follow-up	Heavy/non-drinkers	Major Depressive Disorder: CIDI-SF, cut-off point of 5	6.9%	Sex and SES	Adjusted: 1.78 (1.10–2.88)

Table 1. *Cont.*

First Author's Name, Year, Country	Sample Size	Target Population	Substance Use Measure	Mental Health Disorders Assessment	% of Depressive Participants	Controlled Variables	OR (95% CI)
Association between Depression and Cannabis Use							
Cross-Sectional Studies							
Lee Ridner, 2005, U.S. [40]	895	College students aged 18–24	Current/non- cannabis users	Depressive symptoms: CES-D, cut-off point of 16	-	-	Crude: 1.27 (1.00–1.61)
Susan Roberts, 2009, U.S. [32]	418	College students	Current/non- cannabis users	Depressive symptoms: BDI-II, cut-off point of 20	22%	-	Crude: 1.99 (1.23–3.22)
Martha Kubik, 2005, U.S. [33]	3466	Grade 7 students	Current/non- cannabis users	Depressive symptoms: CES-D, cut-off point of 16	35%	Age, ethnicity, SES, smoking, alcohol, and inhalants use.	Adjusted: 1.02 (0.66–1.57)
Longitudinal Studies: Cannabis Use (Exposure) → Depression (Outcome)							
Daniel Rasic, 2012, Canada [27]	976	Grade 10 students, 2-year follow-up	Current/non- cannabis users	Depressive symptoms: CES-D, cut-off point of 22 (M) and 24 (F)	20%	Sex	Adjusted: 1.24 (1.05–1.46)
Katholiki Georgiades, 2007, Canada [50]	1282	Adolescents aged 12–16, 14-year follow-up	Past 6-month/non- cannabis users	Major depressive disorder: CIDI-SF	11.8%	Physical health, life satisfaction, personal income, years of education	Adjusted: 1.97 (0.81–4.81)
David Brook, 2002, U.S. [52]	736	Adolescents aged 14, 10-year follow-up	Ever/never cannabis users	Major depressive disorder: Modified version of CIDI	8.3%	Age, sex, parental educational level, family income, prior psychiatric disorders	Adjusted: 1.36 (1.14–1.62)
Naomi Marmorstein, 2011, U.S. [56]	1252	Adolescents aged 17, A 6-year follow-up	CUD/non- cannabis users	Major depressive disorder: The structured clinical interview for DSM-III-R.	13.9%	MDD by age 17 and gender	Adjusted: 1.86 (1.11–3.11),
Valerie Harder, 2008, U.S. [53]	1494	Adolescents aged 12–16, 7-year follow-up	CUD/non- cannabis users	Major depressive disorder: CIDI, DSM IV diagnostic criteria	6%	Ethnicity, family income, free lunch, tobacco, alcohol, and other illegal drug use, parental monitoring, concentration, behavior problems, shyness, anxiety symptoms, intervention status	Adjusted: 1.33 (0.70–2.53)

Table 1. *Cont.*

First Author's Name, Year, Country	Sample Size	Target Population	Substance Use Measure	Mental Health Disorders Assessment	% of Depressive Participants	Controlled Variables	OR (95% CI)
Longitudinal Study: Depression (Exposure) → Cannabis Use (Outcome)							
Cynthia Suerken, 2014, U.S. [45]	3146	College students, A 6-month follow-up	Ever/never cannabis users	Depressive symptoms: CES-D, Iowa short form	-	Sex, ethnicity, parental education and spending money available, varsity athlete, club, intramural sports, member of a sorority/fraternity, attend religious services, live on campus, relationship status, current use of tobacco, alcohol, and lifetime use of other illicit drugs	Crude: 1.03 (1.01–1.05)
Association between Depression and Tobacco Use							
Cross-Sectional Studies							
Lee Ridner, 2005, U.S. [40]	895	College students aged 18–24	Current/non-tobacco users	Depressive symptoms: CES-D, cut-off point of 16	-	-	Crude: 1.49 (1.18–1.90)
Susan Roberts, 2009, U.S. [32]	418	College students, aged 18–21	Current/non- tobacco users	Depressive symptoms: BDI-II, cut-off point of 20	22%	-	Crude: 2.08 (1.29–3.36)
Elisabeth Simantov, 2000, U.S. [48]	5513	Grade 7–12 students	Regular/non- tobacco users	Depressive symptoms: Modified version of CDI, cut-off point of 9	18.2%	-	Crude: 2.47 (2.06–2.97)
Sung Chung, 2014, U.S. [25]	11,848	Grade 9–11 students	Current/non- tobacco users	Depressive symptoms: 1 item question	28.4%	-	Crude: 1.33 (1.16–1.53)
Shahm Martini, 2002, U.S. [46]	11,201	Adolescents aged 12–17	Current/non- tobacco users	Depressive symptoms: YSR, cut-off point of 3	-	Age, ethnicity, school attendance, site, substance use behaviors	Crude: 1.83 (1.67–2.01)
Carla Berg, 2008, U.S. [47]	299	Adolescents aged 10–19	Current/non- tobacco users	Depressive symptoms: A 5-item question, cut-off point of 21	12%	Age, sex, ethnicity, church attendance, perceived parental attitude	Crude: 3.83 (1.65–8.88)
Martha Kubik, 2005, U.S. [33]	3466	Grade 7 students	Current/non- tobacco users	Depressive symptoms: CES-D, cut-off point of 16	35%	Age, ethnicity, SES, all other substance use behaviors	Adjusted: 1.56 (1.14–2.14)
Gilat Grunau, 2009, Canada [28]	6943	Students aged 13–18	Current/non- tobacco users	Major depressive disorder: Prescribed depression medications	2.2%	Age, sex, ethnicity, parent(s), sibling(s), peer(s) smokes, anxiety	Adjusted: 2.59 (1.79–3.73)

Table 1. *Cont.*

First Author's Name, Year, Country	Sample Size	Target Population	Substance Use Measure	Mental Health Disorders Assessment	% of Depressive Participants	Controlled Variables	OR (95% CI)
Amanda Richardson, 2012, U.S. [49]	1884	Adolescents aged 12–15	Ever/never tobacco users	Major depressive disorder: NIMH-DISC-IV	-	Age, ethnicity, attending school, poverty index ratio, live with smokers, anxiety disorders	Adjusted: 2.80 (1.13–6.91)
Eleanor Hanna, 2001, U.S. [31]	719	Adolescents aged 12–16	Current/non- tobacco users	Major depressive disorder: Diagnostic interview schedule, DSM-III	9%	Age, sex, ethnicity, family poverty status, school problem, drinking status	Adjusted: 0.98 (0.33–2.90)
Longitudinal Studies: Tobacco Use (Exposure) → Depression (Outcome)							
Brian Duncan, 2005, U.S. [41]	13,068	Students grade 7–12, 1-year follow-up	Current/non- tobacco users	Depressive symptoms: CES-D, cut-off point of 22 (M) and 24 (F)	-	Disability, age, ethnicity, household, parental education, county-level variables	Crude: 2.37 (2.02–2.77)
Elizabeth Goodman, 2000, U.S. [42]	8704	Adolescents aged 11–22, 1-year follow-up	Current/non- tobacco users	Depressive symptoms: CES-D, cut-off point of 22 (M) and 24 (F)	6.4%	Age, sex, ethnicity, parental education	Crude: 2.31 (1.83–2.92)
Katholiki Georgiades, 2007, Canada [50]	1282	Adolescents aged 12–16, 14-year follow-up	Daily/non- tobacco users	Major depressive disorder: CIDI-SF	11.8%	Physical health, life satisfaction, personal income, years of education	Adjusted: 1.93 (1.01–3.70)
David Brook, 2002, U.S. [52]	736	Adolescents aged 14, A 13-year follow-up	Ever/never tobacco users	Major depressive disorder: Modified version of CIDI	8.3%	Age, sex, parental educational level, family income, prior psychiatric disorders	Adjusted: 1.18 (1.01–1.39)
Longitudinal Studies: Depression (Exposure) → Tobacco Use (Outcome)							
Elizabeth Goodman, 2000, U.S. [42]	6947	Adolescents aged 11–22, 1-year follow-up	Current/non- tobacco users	Depressive symptoms: CES-D, cut-off point of 22 (M) and 24 (F)	6.4%	Age, sex, ethnicity, education	Crude: 2.81 (1.67–4.74)
Kiyuri Naicker, 2012, Canada [51]	681	Adolescents aged 16–17, 10-year follow-up	Daily/non- tobacco users	Major depressive disorder: CIDI-SF, cut-off point of 5	6.9%	Sex and SES	Adjusted: 2.89 (1.53–5.45)
Jie Wu Weiss, 2004, U.S. [37]	1699	Grade 6 students, A 1-year follow-up	Ever/never tobacco users	Depressive symptoms: CES-D, cut-off point of 16	-	change in depression and hostility, sex, ethnicity, SES	Adjusted: 1.76 (1.30–2.38)

Table 1. *Cont.*

First Author's Name, Year, Country	Sample Size	Target Population	Substance Use Measure	Mental Health Disorders Assessment	% of Depressive Participants	Controlled Variables	OR (95% CI)
Jennifer Mendel, 2012, U.S. [38]	1205	Grade 10–11 students, A 5-year follow-up	Ever/never tobacco users	Depressive symptoms: CES-D, cut-off point of 16	-	Sex, parental marital status, family income, education level, marital status, children, GPA, delinquency, stressful life events, family support, quality of friendship, parental smoking, adolescent alcohol, cannabis use, extent of alcohol problems, peers who drink or use drugs, change in CESD and alcohol use	Adjusted: 0.97 (0.92–1.03)
Jennifer O'Loughlin, 2016, Canada [54]	690	Grade 5 students, 7-year follow-up	Ever/never tobacco users	Depressive symptoms: 6-item question	-	Age, sex, mother's education	Adjusted: 1.34 (1.16–1.56)
Marcus Munafo, 2007, U.S. [39]	12,149	Grade 7–12 students, 1-year follow-up	Ever/never tobacco users	Depressive symptoms: CES-D, cut-off point of 22 (M) and 24 (F)	-	Age, sex, ethnicity, depressed mood, parental/peer tobacco, alcohol use, delinquency score	Adjusted: 1.13 (1.03–1.25)
William Lechner, 2016, U.S. [43]	2460	Grade 9 students, A 1-year follow-up	Ever/never tobacco users	Depressive symptoms: CES-D, cut-off point of 22 (M) and 24 (F)	-	Age, sex, ethnicity, school, living situation, parental education, use of alcohol and other tobacco products	Adjusted: 1.02 (1.01–1.04)
First author's name, year, country	**Sample size**	Target population	**Substance use measure**	**Mental health disorders assessment**	**% of participants with anxiety**	**Controlled variables**	**OR (95% CI)**
Association between Anxiety and Alcohol Use							
Cross-Sectional Studies							
Margo Villarosa, 2014, U.S. [29]	532	College students aged 18–22	Alcohol Use Disorder: AUDIT	Social anxiety symptoms: SIAS	-	-	Crude: 1.61 (1.29–2.00)
Meade Eggleston, 2003, U.S. [57]	284	College students aged 17–23	Binge/non-drinkers	Social anxiety symptoms: SIAS	-	-	Crude: 1.55 (1.15–2.10)
Esther Strahan, 2010, U.S. [58]	697	College students aged 17–27	Alcohol Use Disorder: AUDIT	Social anxiety symptoms: SIAS	-	-	Crude: 1.04 (1.01–1.08)

Table 1. *Cont.*

First Author's Name, Year, Country	Sample Size	Target Population	Substance Use Measure	Mental Health Disorders Assessment	% of Depressive Participants	Controlled Variables	OR (95% CI)
Ping Wu, 2009, U.S. [59]	781	Adolescents aged 13–17	Frequent, heavy/non-drinkers	Any anxiety disorders: DISC	18.4%	Age, ethnicity, public assistance, not living with parents, parental drug/alcohol problems, site	Adjusted: 1.74 (1.07–2.81)
Linda Richter, 2015, U.S. [26]	24,445	Adolescents aged 12–20	Binge/non-drinkers	Any anxiety disorders: Diagnosed anxiety (self-reported)	-	Age, sex, ethnicity	Adjusted: 1.54 (1.12–2.12)
Robert Roberts, 2007, U.S. [35]	4175	Adolescents aged 11–17	Alcohol Use Disorder: AUD	Any anxiety disorders: DISC-IV	6.9%	Mood, conduct oppositional, and ADHD disorders.	Crude: 1.57 (0.72–3.40)
Nancy Low, 2008, U.S. [36]	632	Adolescents aged 13–19	Alcohol Use Disorder: AUD	Any Anxiety Disorders: PRIME-MD	7%	Age, sex, ethnicity, sample site, mood disorders	Adjusted: 3.80 (1.21–11.91)
Longitudinal Study: Anxiety (Exposure) → Alcohol Use (Outcome)							
Julia Buckner, 2008, U.S. [60]	816	Students aged 15–17, 14-year follow-up	Alcohol Use Disorder: AUD	Any anxiety disorders: K-SADS	-	Sex, conduct, mood, CUDs, T1 AUD excluded	Adjusted: 2.16 (0.82–5.69)
Association between Anxiety and Cannabis Use							
Cross-Sectional Studies							
Julia Buckner, 2008, U.S. [30]	337	College students aged 18–26	Frequent/non-cannabis users	Social anxiety symptoms: SIAS	18.8%	-	Crude: 1.23 (0.88–1.73)
Robert Roberts, 2007, U.S. [35]	4175	Adolescents aged 11–17	Cannabis Use Disorder: CUD	Any anxiety disorder: DISC-IV	6.9%	Mood, conduct oppositional, and ADHD disorders	Crude: 1.38 (0.70–2.75)
Nancy Low, 2008, U.S. [36]	632	Adolescents aged 13–19	Cannabis Use Disorder: CUD	Any anxiety disorder: PRIME-MD	7%	Age, sex, ethnicity, sample site, mood disorders	Crude: 1.40 (0.40–4.70)
Longitudinal Study: Anxiety (Exposure) → Cannabis Use (Outcome)							
Julia Buckner, 2008, U.S. [60]	816	Students aged 15–17, 14-year follow-up	Cannabis Use Disorder: CUD	Social anxiety disorder: K-SADS	-	Sex, conduct, mood, AUDs, T1 CUD excluded	Adjusted: 3.28 (1.14–9.40)

Table 1. *Cont.*

First Author's Name, Year, Country	Sample Size	Target Population	Substance Use Measure	Mental Health Disorders Assessment	% of Depressive Participants	Controlled Variables	OR (95% CI)
Association between Anxiety and Cannabis Use							
Cross-Sectional Studies							
Gilat Grunau, 2009, Canada [28]	6943	Students aged 13–18	Current/non-cannabis users	Any anxiety disorder: Prescribed anxiety medications	0.6%	Sex, ethnicity, age, parent(s), sibling(s), peer(s) smokes, depression	Adjusted: 1.83 (1.05–3.22)
Ping Wu, 2009, U.S. [59]	781	Adolescents aged 13–17	Daily/non- cannabis users	Any anxiety disorders: DISC	18.4%	Age, ethnicity, public assistance, not living with parents, parental drug/alcohol problems, site.	Adjusted: 3.14 (1.69–5.81)
Amanda Richardson, 2012, U.S. [49]	1884	Adolescents aged 12–15	Ever/never cannabis users	Any anxiety disorder: NIMH-DISC-IV	-	Age, ethnicity, attending school, poverty index ratio, live with smokers, depressive disorder	Adjusted: 4.70 (1.61–13.75)
Longitudinal Study: Tobacco Use (Exposure) → Anxiety (Outcome)							
Renee Goodwin, 2005, U.S. [34]	940	Students aged 14–18, anxiety: young adults mean age 24.2	Ever/never cannabis users	Any anxiety disorders: K-SADS	-	-	Crude: 1.88 (1.47–2.41)
Longitudinal Study: Anxiety (Exposure) → Tobacco Use (Outcome)							
Renee Goodwin, 2005, U.S. [34]	940	Students aged 14–18, tobacco use: young adults mean age 24.2	Ever/Never cannabis users	Any anxiety disorders: K-SADS	-	-	Crude: 1.38 (0.83–2.29)

All terms/acronyms used in Table 1 are fully defined in Appendix A.

3.2. Synthesis of Results

The results of the meta-analysis found significant positive associations between depression and alcohol use (OR = 1.50, 95% CI: 1.24–1.83), cannabis use (OR = 1.29, 95% CI: 1.10–1.51) and tobacco use (OR = 1.65, 95% CI: 1.43–1.92). Similarly, significant positive associations were found between anxiety and alcohol use (OR = 1.54, 95% CI: 1.19–2.00), cannabis use (OR = 1.36, 95% CI: 1.02–1.81) and tobacco use (OR = 2.21, 95% CI: 1.54–3.17) (Table 2).

Table 2. Overall pooled estimates for mental health disorders and substance use.

Topics	Study Designs	n	OR (95% CI)	I^2% and p-Value
Depression and Alcohol use	Overall	9	1.50 (1.24–1.83)	90.54, <0.001
	Cross-Sectional	6	1.57 (1.09–2.26)	92.89, <0.001
	Longitudinal: Alcohol use at baseline	2	1.39 (0.95–2.03)	89.24, <0.001
	Longitudinal: Depression at baseline	1	1.78 (1.10–2.88)	n/a
Depression and Cannabis use	Overall	9	1.29 (1.10–1.51)	74.79, <0.01
	Cross-Sectional	3	1.34 (0.97–1.84)	53.26, 0.12
	Longitudinal: Cannabis use at baseline	5	1.33 (1.19–1.49)	0.00, 0.53
	Longitudinal: Depression at baseline	1	1.03 (1.01–1.05)	n/a
Depression and Tobacco use	Overall	20	1.65 (1.43–1.92)	96.23, <0.01
	Cross-Sectional	10	1.87 (1.55–2.25)	78.60, <0.01
	Longitudinal: Tobacco use at baseline	4	1.87 (1.23–2.85)	92.95, <0.01
	Longitudinal: Depression at baseline	7	1.22 (1.09–1.37)	89.56, <0.001
Anxiety and Alcohol use	Overall	8	1.54 (1.19–2.00)	81.52, <0.001
	Cross-Sectional	7	1.51 (1.16–1.97)	83.28, <0.001
	Longitudinal: Alcohol use at baseline	-	-	-
	Longitudinal: Anxiety at baseline	1	2.16 (0.82–5.69)	n/a
Anxiety and Cannabis use	Overall	4	1.36 (1.02–1.81)	0.39, 0.39
	Cross-Sectional	3	1.27 (0.94–1.70)	0.00, 0.94
	Longitudinal: Cannabis use at baseline	-	-	-
	Longitudinal: Anxiety at baseline	1	3.28 (1.14–9.40)	n/a
Anxiety and Tobacco use	Overall	4	2.21 (1.54–3.17)	46.17, 0.13
	Cross-Sectional	3	2.67 (1.62–4.37)	33.12, 0.22
	Longitudinal: Tobacco use at baseline	1	1.88 (1.47–2.41)	n/a
	Longitudinal: Anxiety at baseline	1	1.38 (0.83–2.29)	n/a

3.3. Analysis of the Directionality

The directionality of the association between each relevant category was assessed by pooled analysis of the longitudinal studies. Results showed that there was a significant positive bi-directional association between tobacco use at baseline leading to depression at follow-up (OR = 1.87, CI = 1.23–2.85) and depression at baseline leading to tobacco use at follow-up (OR = 1.22, CI = 1.09–1.37). Cannabis use at baseline was significantly associated with depression at follow-up (OR = 1.33, CI = 1.19–1.49) (Figure 2).

Subgraph A: The association between tobacco use at baseline and depression at follow-up

Study name	Statistics for each study		
	Odds ratio	Lower limit	Upper limit
R. Duncan et al. 2005	2.37	2.02	2.77
D. Brook et al. 2002	1.18	1.01	1.39
E. Goodman et al. 2000	2.31	1.83	2.92
K. Georgiades et al. 2007	1.93	1.01	3.70
	1.87	1.23	2.85

Odds ratio and 95% CI

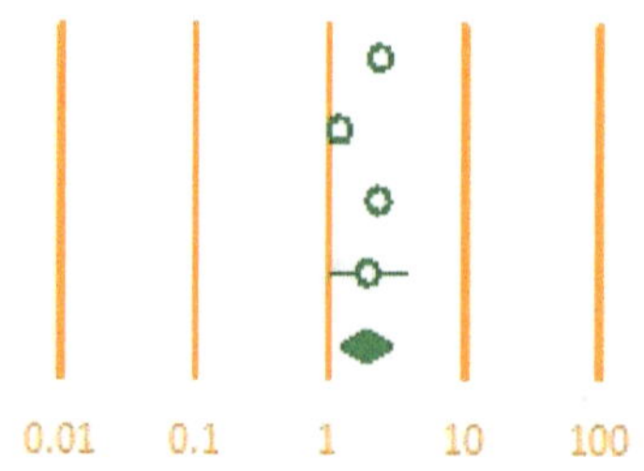

Figure 2. *Cont.*

Subgraph B: The association between depression at baseline and tobacco use at follow up

Study name	Odds ratio	Lower limit	Upper limit
E. Goodman et al. 2000	2.81	1.67	4.74
J. O'Loughlin et al. 2016	1.34	1.16	1.56
J. Mendel et al. 2012	0.97	0.92	1.03
J. Weiss et al. 2004	1.76	1.30	2.38
K. Naicker et al. 2012	2.89	1.53	5.45
M. Munafo et al. 2007	1.13	1.03	1.25
W. Lechner et al. 2016	1.02	1.01	1.04
	1.22	1.09	1.37

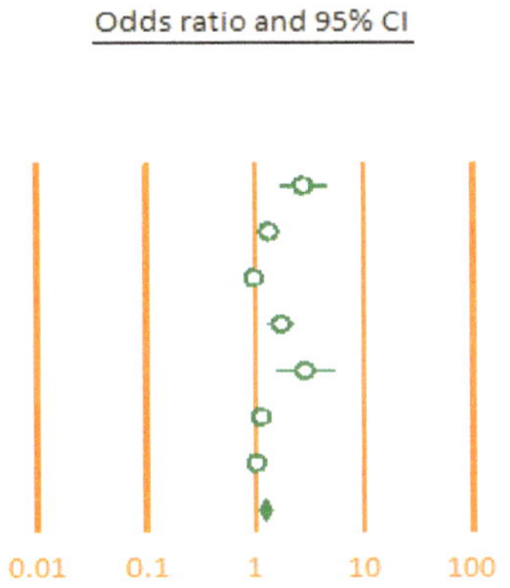

Subgraph C: The association between cannabis use at baseline and depression at follow up

Study name	Odds ratio	Lower limit	Upper limit
D. Rasic et al. 2012	1.24	1.05	1.46
D. Brook et al. 2002	1.36	1.14	1.62
K. Georgiades et al. 2007	1.97	0.81	4.81
N. Marmorstein et al. 2011	1.86	1.11	3.11
V. Harder et al. 2008	1.33	0.70	2.53
	1.33	1.19	1.49

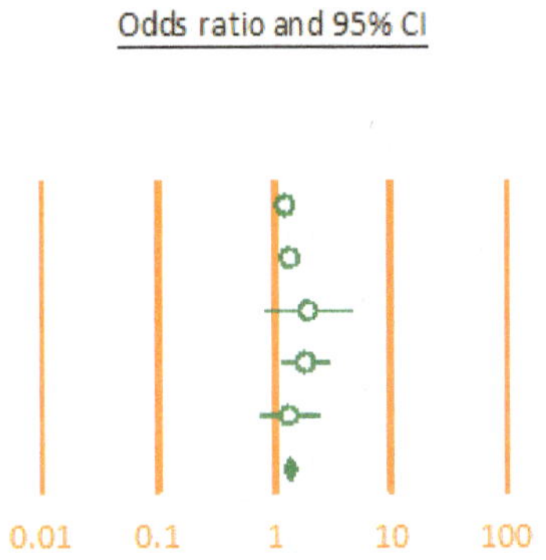

Figure 2. Examining the directionality in longitudinal studies (forest plots A–C).

3.4. Subgroup Analysis

Due to the heterogeneity detected upon pooled analysis, subgroup analysis was conducted to examine whether the differences within categories could be attributed to specific moderators (age group, measures of mental health disorder, and severity of substance use). Results of our subgroup analysis are summarized in Table 3. Results from the subgroup analysis by age group including adolescents (aged 10 to 18 years old) and young adults (aged 18 to 24 years old) found that the association between mental health disorders and substance use remained significant among adolescents but not among young adults. Subgroup analysis based on severity of mental health disorders showed a consistently higher point estimate for clinically diagnosed mental health disorder patients. Finally, subgroup analysis based on the intensity of substance use showed a recurring theme, whereby, as severity increased, mental health disorders also increased (Table 3).

Table 3. Subgroup analysis for mental health disorders and substance use.

	Subgroup Analysis		n	OR (95% CI)	I^2% and p-Value	p-Value
Depression and Alcohol use	Point Estimate	Crude	3	1.37 (0.87–2.18)	96.08, <0.001	0.56
		Adjusted	6	1.62 (1.19–2.19)	84.60, <0.001	
	Target Population	Adolescents	7	1.69 (1.28–2.25)	90.63, <0.001	0.28
		Young adults	3	1.28 (0.83–1.97)	82.52, <0.001	
	Severity of MHDs [1]	Symptoms	5	1.37 (1.08–1.75)	94.04, <0.001	0.21
		Disorders	4	1.67 (1.38–2.02)	14.68, 0.32	
	Intensity of substance use	Not binge drinkers	6	1.61 (1.29–2.01)	79.79, <0.001	0.06
		Binge drinkers	6	1.21 (0.99–1.47)	87.67, <0.001	
Depression and Cannabis use	Point Estimate	Crude	3	1.27 (0.95–1.69)	80.29, <0.001	0.85
		Adjusted	6	1.31 (1.17–1.46)	0.00, 0.48	
	Target Population	Adolescents	6	1.34 (1.17–1.54)	9.96, 0.35	0.46
		Young adults	4	1.22 (0.99–1.51)	72,62, 0.01	
	Severity of MHDs	Symptoms	5	1.20 (1.01–1.42)	73.16, <0.001	0.16
		Disorders	4	1.41 (1.21–1.65)	0.00, 0.60	
	Intensity of substance use	Cannabis use	7	1.25 (1.06–1.47)	77.10, <0.001	0.23
		CUD [2]	2	1.63 (1.09–2.44)	0.00, 0.42	
Depression and Tobacco use	Point Estimate	Crude	8	1.99 (1.65–2.40)	86.62, <0.001	<0.001
		Adjusted	12	1.30 (1.16–1.45)	87.12, <0.001	
	Target Population	Adolescents	18	1.67 (1.43–1.96)	96.56, <0.001	0.40
		Young adults	3	1.37 (0.89–2.12)	84.18, <0.001	
	Severity of MHDs	Symptoms	14	1.61 (1.36–1.89)	97.18, <0.001	0.48
		Disorders	6	1.91 (1.22–2.97)	78.86, <0.001	
	Intensity of substance use	Ever smokers	7	1.14 (1.04–1.25)	84.89, <0.001	<0.001
		Current smokers	14	1.90 (1.62–2.23)	82.65, <0.001	
Anxiety and Alcohol use	Point Estimate	Crude	4	1.37 (1.00–1.88)	86.27, <0.001	0.3
		Adjusted	4	1.70 (1.32–2.18)	0.00, 0.47	
	Target Population	Adolescents	5	1.69 (1.33–2.14)	0.00, 0.64	0.29
		Young adults	3	1.35 (0.96–1.90)	90.40, <0.001	
	Severity of MHDs	Symptoms	3	1.35 (0.96–1.90)	90.40, <0.001	0.29
		Disorders	5	1.69 (1.33–2.14)	0.00, 0.64	
	Intensity of substance use	Alcohol use	6	1.49 (1.26–1.76)	0.00, 0.88	0.59
		AUD [3]	5	1.71 (1.05–2.79)	83.88, <0.001	
Anxiety and Cannabis use	Point Estimate	Crude	2	1.26 (0.93–1.71)	0.00, 0.76	0.19
		Adjusted	2	2.28 (1.00–5.20)	5.37, 0.30	
	Target Population	Adolescents	3	1.71 (1.02–2.89)	0.00, 0.38	0.29
		Young adults	1	1.23 (0.88–1.73)	n/a	
	Severity of MHDs			n/a		
	Intensity of substance use	Cannabis use	1	1.23 (0.88–1.73)	n/a	0.29
		CUD	3	1.71 (1.02–2.89)	0.00, 0.38	
Anxiety and Tobacco use	Point Estimate	Crude	1	1.78 (1.42–2.22)	n/a	0.14
		Adjusted	3	2.67 (1.62–4.37)	33.125, 0.22	
	Target Population			n/a		
	Severity of MHDs			n/a		
	Intensity of substance use	Ever	3	1.62 (0.67–3.92)	69.87, 0.04	0.58
		Current	4	2.10 (1.69–2.62)	0.00, 0.52	

[1] Mental Health Disorders, [2] Cannabis Use Disorder, [3] Alcohol Use Disorder.

3.5. Publication Bias

Funnel plots showed no evidence of publication bias in the included studies that examined the association between depression and alcohol use; depression and cannabis use; depression and tobacco use; anxiety and alcohol use; and anxiety and tobacco use. However, there was evidence of publication bias in the included studies which examined the association between anxiety and cannabis use. Therefore, in these instances, a Duval and Tweedie's trim and fill method was used to test and adjust for the publication bias in our meta-analysis.

4. Discussion

Our findings suggest that a significant association exists between depression and the use of alcohol, cannabis, and tobacco. Similarly, significant associations were found to exist between anxiety and the use of alcohol, cannabis, and tobacco. A bidirectional relationship was observed between depression and the use of tobacco. Additionally, we found evidence that cannabis use at baseline led to depression at follow-up. The results of our study were consistent with those reported in previous systematic reviews [64–66] and provide additional evidence in support of the inter-association between mental health disorders and substance use.

Harmful alcohol use, which has been defined as heavy episodic or binge drinking, is an important health issue among adolescents and young adults in the U.S. [67]. The adolescent/young adult brain is still developing, and there is evidence to suggest that frequent use of alcohol at this age may lead to mental health disorders including depression [68,69]. Our results support these findings. We found that alcohol use was a significant predictor of higher levels of depression among adolescents and young adults. However, further research is needed in this area with more longitudinal studies, using longer follow-up periods.

A systematic review conducted by Lev-Ran et al. found a positive association between cannabis use at baseline and the development of depression [70]. Our results corroborate these findings and demonstrate that the overall pooled estimate for depression among heavy cannabis users was higher, compared to light users. Another systematic review by Number-Kedzior et al. found a significant positive association between cannabis use at baseline and anxiety at follow-up [66]. In our study, it was not possible to infer whether such a causal relationship exists due to the lack of sufficient studies on this topic, which fit our inclusion criteria. Proposed mechanisms for the association between cannabis and depression could be due to biological effects from the alteration in neurotransmitters such as serotonin in the brain [71] and its impact on developing depression and mediating psychosocial factors such as unemployment and educational failure [50]. We observed that when adjusting for personal income and years of education, the association between cannabis use and depression was reduced [50].

In our study, we found a stronger pooled estimate for tobacco use predicting depression, compared to depression predicting tobacco use. Moreover, a stronger pooled estimate was observed in those studies that used a clinical measure of depression rather than depressive symptoms. Although, our study was limited in investigating the associations rather than the causality between mental health disorders and substance use, our results are biologically plausible. For instance, the association between tobacco use and anxiety or depression may be due to the effect of nicotine on the central neurotransmitter systems and peripheral circulating stress hormones [72]. In the brain, the primary target of nicotine (the addictive substance found in tobacco) is the neuronal nicotinic acetylcholine receptors (nACHRs). The nACHRs have a large number of subtypes responsible for the regulation of different neurotransmitter systems. Nicotine can make alterations in the balance of these neurotransmitter systems by activating or inactivating the receptors responsible for release of stimulatory (glutamate), inhibitory (GABA), and modulatory (dopamine, norepinephrine, and serotonin) neurotransmitters in different brain regions. Thus, different behavioral outputs such as depression or anxiety may occur [72]. The ability of nicotine to act as an anxiolytic or anxiogenic and depressant or anti-depressant agent is complex and may dependent on the severity and duration of its use, the route of administration, and the genetic and behavioral state of the individual user [72].

The effects of nicotine on the hypothalamic pituitary adrenal (HPA) axis are centrally mediated by the stimulation of neurotransmitter systems [73]. Acute nicotine exposure can result in increase in basal level of stress hormones by stimulating the HPA axis [73]. The anxiogenic effect of nicotine may be explained by the acute peripheral effect of tobacco smoking such as the increases observed in blood pressure, heart rate, and cortisol output. Also, nicotine increases corticosteroids in the amygdala, a brain area critical for emotionality. With chronic use of tobacco, nicotine alters activity of the HPA axis. The HPA axis in combination with genetic factors may be involved in producing tolerance to the effects of nicotine. Thus, this might predispose smokers to depressive episodes during withdrawal [72,74].

The association between anxiety and tobacco use might be explained by the negative effect of tobacco use on different brain pathways such as neurotransmitter systems, inflammation and the immune system, oxidative and nitrosative stress pathways, neurotrophins and neurogenesis regulations, mitochondrial function, and epigenetic influences. Alteration in abovementioned pathways can also play a role in development of anxiety disorders [75].

4.1. Strengths and Limitations

Our study has several strengths. There is a high level of congruence between our findings and those reported in the existing literature. However, this systematic review is unique because: (1) it incorporates only studies originating in the U.S. and Canada, (2) it focuses on the adolescent and young adult population, and (3) it examines the associations and directionality between depression or anxiety and alcohol, cannabis, or tobacco use, separately.

Our study also has some limitations. We found that certain factors such as the study design (longitudinal vs. cross-sectional), the intensity of substance use (light vs. heavy), and the variation in clinical diagnosis (depressive and anxiety disorders vs. symptoms) affect the outcomes of our study. Participant's age (adolescents vs. young adults) also influenced the inter-association between substance use behaviors and mental health disorders. In our review, several of our included studies used different instruments to measure depression and anxiety and a broad spectrum of measurements for substance use, making the results difficult to compare due to their heterogeneity. When extracting data, we were unable to calculate the unadjusted odds ratio from all included studies. Different studies varied in the degree to which they controlled for potential confounders. Variation in the population sampled, length of follow-up in longitudinal studies, and different sample sizes also added to the variability.

4.2. Implications for Practice, Research and Policy

The co-occurrence of mental health disorders and/or substance use presents complex challenges in their prevention, diagnosis, and treatment. If left untreated, these conditions may result in loss of productivity, poor educational outcomes, increased psychiatric hospitalizations/emergency department visits, inefficient use of limited healthcare resources, and a higher prevalence of chronic diseases. By affecting change at the personal (increase awareness), interpersonal (decrease stigma), and societal (policies and interventions) levels, we can assist adolescents and young adults to make better choices, seek support as needed, and live healthier and well-adjusted lives.

Overall, our systematic review and meta-analysis found a clear association between depression/anxiety and substance use, regardless of the severity of the mental health disorder or the intensity of substance use. These findings have significant implications and may impact:

(1) Practice: our study helps highlight the importance of addressing adolescents and young adults' mental health (depression/anxiety) and substance use behaviors (drinking, smoking, cannabis use) early, concurrently and with an integrated clinical approach through the use of timely screening, team-based diagnosis, patient-oriented treatment and effective interventions. These observations underscore the need for a shift in our collective perspective, when implementing integrated services for patients with co-occurring disorders.

(2) Research: our findings corroborate and expand those reported in previous studies and provide invaluable insight and guidance to future rigorous, longitudinal research that aims to widen our knowledge of psychopathology by elucidating the associated links and delineating best practices in the prevention, diagnosis, and treatment of co-occurring mental health disorders and substance use. Additionally, it will be of keen scientific interest to investigate and determine whether substance use cessation treatments lead to reduction and/or remission of depression/anxiety or whether the treatment of depression/anxiety leads to reduction and/or cessation of substance use among adolescents and young adults.

(3) Policy: our results demonstrate that integrated treatment approaches and health education campaigns are needed to improve quality of care and increase awareness among the public and healthcare practitioners of the associations between depression/anxiety and substance use among adolescents and young adults. School-based intervention programs, in particular, hold much promise as they could encourage adolescents and young adults to seek professional help safely and in a supportive environment.

4.3. Recommendations

Given the findings of our study, it is important that patients diagnosed with mental health disorder and/or a substance use problems be evaluated, screened, and if need be, treated for both conditions. To assist in this regard, the following recommendations are proposed:

(1) Bilateral cooperation between the U.S. and Canada: along with sharing the longest international boarder, the two countries share many common socio-cultural factors, demonstrate similar patterns in the prevalence of mental health disorders and substance use, and report common health priorities (i.e., advancement of mental health and substance use services) [76,77]. Therefore, it would be beneficial for key stakeholders at educational settings in both the U.S. and Canada to collaborate and exchange information and ideas on how to further improve their health education and promotion programs.

(2) Implementation of the quadrants of care model (the New York Model): in our systematic review, it became apparent that as the severity of mental health disorders and intensity of substance use varied, different approaches to their healthcare management were needed. Thus, the potential usefulness of the quadrants of care model to most appropriately direct the efforts of healthcare professionals [78]. Individuals treated simultaneously by two or more healthcare providers at one point of entry may receive an integrated treatment plan for both conditions. By following this model, individuals will receive an appropriate level of care based on their needs, and this will ensure the efficient use of available resources.

(3) Reforming the healthcare system: healthcare reforms are needed to make the necessary changes from the current parallel and independent practice sectors towards coordinated systems of care. Coordinated practice sectors will require sharing funds, developing mandates in concert, and treating affected individuals collaboratively. Reforms should be broad and encompass all levels of service delivery including health promotion and prevention, diagnosis, treatment, and research.

(4) Efficient use of limited resources: preventive interventions, early detection, diagnosis, and treatment of the co-occurrence of mental health disorders and substance use, can improve the quality of life of adolescents and young adults. Addressing this issue upstream will reduce the associated healthcare costs and permit the efficient use of limited resources, including the need for frequent psychiatric hospitalizations, over-use of emergency departments, and ambulatory care.

(5) Training of healthcare providers: it is essential to cross-train healthcare providers from different sectors to increase their awareness of the existing association between mental health disorders and substance use. There is a need for the characterization of patient risk profiles, the use of valid assessment tools, and updated diagnostic and treatment guidelines to help improve outcomes for these two conditions among adolescents and young adults.

5. Conclusions

This study offers significant insight into the association and directionality between substance use (alcohol, cannabis, and tobacco) and mental health disorders (depression and anxiety) among adolescents and young adults in the U.S. and Canada. Our findings can help guide key stakeholders (school administrators, nurses, physicians, public health professionals, and policymakers) in making evidence-based recommendations for school-based interventions, policy, and programming. It is increasingly evident that adolescents and young adults with substance use issues may also suffer from co-occurring mental health disorders. However, they are frequently undiagnosed and, consequently, they do not receive the specialized cross-treatment needed to address both conditions. To be most effective, school-based substance use and mental health programmes should consider integrating and expanding their services for patients with dual disorders. Further research is needed to help guide evidence-based treatment and initiatives for this vulnerable population.

Author Contributions: J.M., S.E., Y.B., and L.T. were involved in the study conception and design. J.M. and S.E. were responsible for the data analysis. All authors contributed to the discussion, interpreted the findings, helped write and reviewed/edited the manuscript for intellectual content, and read and approved the final manuscript.

Acknowledgments: We gratefully acknowledge the support of Rita Hanoski, Health Education and Promotion Coordinator and Jocelyn Orb, Manager, Student Health Services, University of Saskatchewan.

Appendix A. Definitions of Mental Health Disorders and Substance Use

Depression
The center for epidemiologic studies depression scale (CES-D) [27,33,37–45]
Beck depression inventory-II (BDI-II) [32]
One item question: Whether respondents felt so sad or hopeless almost daily for two consecutive weeks that usual activities were interrupted [25]
Youth self-report checklist (8 self-reported symptoms of depression within the past 6 months): I feel guilty, I cry a lot, I deliberately try to hurt myself, I think of killing myself, I feel lonely, I am unhappy, I feel that no one loves me, and I feel worthless (YSR) [46]
A five-item question: within the past 12 months how often have you felt too tired to do things? Felt unhappy, sad, or depressed? Felt hopeless about the future? Felt nervous or tense? And worried too much about things? [47]
Modified version of the children depression inventory (CDI) [48]
Depression medication prescribed by a doctor or a nurse in the last 12 months [28]
National institute of mental health diagnostic interview schedule for children version IV (NIMH-DISC, version IV): A structured diagnostic interview administered by lay interviewers to assess diagnostic criteria for mental disorders in children and adolescents, in accordance with the diagnostic and statistical manual of mental disorders, fourth edition (DSM-IV) [49]
CIDI-SF: 12-month prevalence of major depressive disorder (MDD), based on the Composite International Diagnostic Interview–Short Form [50,51]
The university of Michigan composite international diagnostic interview (CIDI): A highly structured research diagnostic instrument developed for use by trained lay interviewers to assess the most common diagnoses among children, adolescents, and young adults as described in the DSM-III-R [52,53]
A 6-item question: During the past 3-month how often you have felt too tired to do things; had trouble going to sleep or staying asleep; felt unhappy, sad or depressed; felt hopeless about the future; felt nervous or tense; worried too much about things [54]
Major depressive episode diagnosis: self-reported depression diagnosed by a medical professional with the past year [26]
The short-form (36) health survey (SF-36) [55]
Mental health component of national health and nutrition examination survey (NHANES), assess diagnostic criteria for mental disorders in children and adolescents, in accordance with the diagnostic and statistical manual of mental disorders, third edition (DSM-III) [31,56]
Anxiety
Social interaction anxiety scale (SIAS) [29,30,57,58]
Diagnostic interview schedule for children, version IV (DISC-IV) [26,35,59]
Primary care evaluation of mental disorders (PRIME-MD) [36]

Schedule for affective disorders and schizophrenia for school-age children (K-SADS) [34,60]
Anxiety medication prescribed by a doctor or a nurse in the last 12 months [28]
National Institute of Mental Health Diagnostic Interview for children (NIMHD) [49]
Alcohol
Ever drinkers: Drinking at least once within a lifetime [52]
Light drinkers: Consuming less than three drinks per week [31]
Moderate drinkers: Drinking without engaging in heavy episodic or binge drinking in the past two weeks [55]
Moderate drinkers: Drinking no more than 1 to 2 drinks per occasion in the past year, and no intoxication or heavy drinking in the past year [26,44]
Moderate to heavy drinkers: Consuming more than 3 drinks per week [31]
Regular drinkers: Drink at least once a month or more frequently and consume at least three to four drinks when drinking [48]
Current drinkers: Drinking at least one time during the past 30 days [33]
Daily drinking questionnaire (DDQ): The total number of standard alcoholic drinks consumed during the past week by summing the number of drinks reported for each day [29]
Frequent/heavy drinkers: Those who over the past 6 months had a drink at least once a week or had been drunk at least once [59]
Binge drinkers: Men/women as drinking five/four or more drinks per drinking occasion at least once in the past two weeks [26,32,33,44,51,55,57]
Alcohol use disorders identification test (AUDIT) [29,58]
Diagnostic interview schedule for children, version IV, alcohol use disorder (DISC-IV, AUD) [35]
Primary care evaluation for mental disorders, alcohol use disorder (PRIME-MD, AUD) [36]
Longitudinal interval follow-up evaluation and structured clinical interview for DSM-IV, non-patient version, alcohol use disorder (LIFE and SCID-I/NP, AUD) [60]
Cannabis
Ever cannabis users: Using cannabis at least once within a lifetime [45,52]
Any use of cannabis or hashish in the past six months [50]
Infrequent cannabis users: Using cannabis at least once per year but not more than once per month [56]
Infrequent cannabis users: Less than weekly cannabis use [30]
Frequent cannabis users: Weekly or more cannabis use [30]
Current cannabis users: Cannabis use at least one time during the past 30 days [27,32,33,40]
The substance abuse module of the composite international diagnostic interview, cannabis use disorder (CIDI-SAM, CUD) [35,36,53,56,60]
Tobacco
Ever smokers: Smoking at least once within a lifetime [34,37–39,52]
Current smokers: Smoking at least one time during the past 30 days [25,31–33,40–43,46,47]
Regular smokers: Smoking several cigarettes or more per week [48]
Regular smokers: Self-report measure: I'm a regular smoker/I'm a heavy smoker [28]
Daily smokers: Daily consumption of cigarettes or cigars for a continuous 30-day period or longer [28,34,50,51,59]

References

1. Pearson, C.; Janz, T.; Ali, J. *Health at a Glance: Mental and Substance Use Disorders in Canada*; Statistics Canada: Ottawa, Canada, 2013.
2. Whiteford, H.A.; Ferrari, A.J.; Degenhardt, L.; Feigin, V.; Vos, T. The global burden of mental, neurological and substance use disorders: An analysis from the Global Burden of Disease Study 2010. *PLoS ONE* **2015**, *10*, e0116820. [CrossRef] [PubMed]
3. Canadian Centre on Substance Abuse. Substance Abuse in Canada: Youth in Focus. Available online: http://www.ccsa.ca/Resource%20Library/ccsa-011521-2007-e.pdf (accessed on 9 September 2018).
4. Kessler, R.C.; Amminger, G.P.; Aguilar-Gaxiola, S.; Alonso, J.; Lee, S.; Ustün, T.B. Age of onset of mental disorders: A review of recent literature. *Curr. Opin. Psychiatry* **2007**, *20*, 359–364. [CrossRef] [PubMed]
5. Mueser, K.T.; Drake, R.E.; Wallach, M.A. Dual diagnosis: A review of etiological theories. *Addict. Behav.* **1998**, *23*, 717–734. [CrossRef]
6. Canadian Centre on Substance Abuse. Substance Abuse in Canada: Concurrent Disorders. Available online: http://www.ccsa.ca/Resource%20Library/ccsa-011811-2010.pdf (accessed on 9 September 2018).
7. World Health Organization. Caring for Children and Adolescents with Mental Disorders: Setting WHO Directions. Available online: http://www.who.int/mental_health/media/en/785.pdf (accessed on 9 September 2018).
8. Bitsko, R.H.; Holbrook, J.R.; Ghandour, R.M.; Blumberg, S.J.; Visser, S.N.; Perou, R.; Walkup, J.T. Epidemiology and impact of health care provider-diagnosed anxiety and depression among US children. *J. Dev. Behav. Pediatr.* **2018**, *39*, 395–403. [CrossRef] [PubMed]
9. Public Health Agency of Canada. Chapter 3: The Chief Public Health Officer's Report on the State of Public Health in Canada 2011—The Health and Well-Being of Canadian Youth and Young Adults. Available online: https://www.canada.ca/en/public-health/corporate/publications/chief-public-health-officer-reports-state-public-health-canada/chief-public-health-officer-report-on-state-public-health-canada-2011/chapter-3.html (accessed on 10 September 2018).
10. Demyttenaere, K.; Bruffaerts, R.; Posada-Villa, J.; Gasquet, I.; Kovess, V.; Lepine, J.; Angermeyer, M.C.; Bernert, S.; Morosini, P.; Polidori, G.; et al. Prevalence, severity, and unmet need for treatment of mental disorders in the World Health Organization World Mental Health Surveys. *JAMA* **2004**, *291*, 2581–2590. [PubMed]
11. Holmes, A.; Silvestri, R. Rates of mental illness and associated academic impacts in Ontario's College students. *Can. J. Sch. Psychol.* **2016**, *31*, 27–46. [CrossRef]
12. Gallagher, M.; Prinstein, M.J.; Simon, V.; Spirito, A. Social anxiety symptoms and suicidal ideation in a clinical sample of early adolescents: Examining loneliness and social support as longitudinal mediators. *J. Abnorm. Child Psychol.* **2014**, *42*, 871–883. [CrossRef] [PubMed]
13. Shrier, L.A.; Harris, S.; Sternberg, M.; Beardslee, W.R. Associations of depression, self-esteem, and substance use with sexual risk among adolescents. *Prev. Med.* **2001**, *33*, 179–189. [CrossRef] [PubMed]
14. Serafini, G.; Muzio, C.; Piccinini, G.; Flouri, E.; Ferrigno, G.; Pompili, M.; Girardi, P.; Amore, M. Life adversities and suicidal behavior in young individuals: A systematic review. *Eur. Child Adolesc. Psychiatry* **2015**, *24*, 1423–1446. [CrossRef] [PubMed]
15. Patel, V.; Flisher, A.J.; Hetrick, S.; McGorry, P. Mental health of young people: A global public-health challenge. *Lancet* **2007**, *369*, 1302–1313. [CrossRef]
16. Health Canada. Canadian Tobacco Alcohol and Drugs (CTADS): 2015 Summary. Available online: https://www.canada.ca/en/health-canada/services/canadian-tobacco-alcohol-drugs-survey/2015-summary.html (accessed on 9 September 2018).
17. Banken, J.A. Drug abuse trends among youth in the United States. *Ann. N.Y. Acad. Sci.* **2004**, 465–471. [CrossRef] [PubMed]
18. Nock, M.K.; Green, J.G.; Hwang, I.; McLaughlin, K.A.; Sampson, N.A.; Zaslavsky, A.M.; Kessler, R.C. Prevalence, correlates, and treatment of lifetime suicidal behavior among adolescents: Results from the National Comorbidity Survey Replication Adolescent Supplement. *JAMA Psychiatry* **2013**, *70*, 300–310. [CrossRef] [PubMed]
19. Townsend, L.; Flisher, A.J.; King, G. A systematic review of the relationship between high school dropout and substance use. *Clin. Child Fam. Psychol. Rev.* **2007**, *10*, 295–317. [CrossRef] [PubMed]

20. Henkel, D. Unemployment and substance use: A review of the literature (1990–2010). *Curr. Drug Abuse Rev.* **2011**, *4*, 4–27. [CrossRef] [PubMed]
21. Ritchwood, T.D.; Ford, H.; DeCoster, J.; Sutton, M.; Lochman, J.E. Risky sexual behavior and substance use among adolescents: A meta-analysis. *Child Youth Serv. Rev.* **2015**, *52*, 74–88. [CrossRef] [PubMed]
22. Jordan, C.J.; Andersen, S.L. Sensitive periods of substance abuse: Early risk for the transition to dependence. *Dev. Cogn. Neurosci.* **2017**, *25*, 29–44. [CrossRef] [PubMed]
23. Sadock, B.J.; Sadock, V.A.; Ruiz, P. *Kaplan and Sadock's Concise Textbook of Clinical Psychiatry*, 4th ed.; Wolters Kluwer: Philadelphia, PA, USA, 2016.
24. Khantzian, E.J. The self-medication hypothesis of substance use disorders: A reconsideration and recent applications. *Harv. Rev. Psychiatry* **1997**, *4*, 231–244. [CrossRef]
25. Chung, S.S.; Joung, K.H. Risk factors for current smoking among American and South Korean adolescents. 2005–2011. *J. Nurs. Scholarsh.* **2014**, *46*, 408–415. [CrossRef]
26. Richter, L.; Pugh, B.S.; Peters, E.A.; Vaughan, R.D.; Foster, S.E. Underage drinking: Prevalence and correlates of risky drinking measures among youth aged 12–20. *Am. J. Drug Alcohol Abuse* **2016**, *42*, 385–394. [CrossRef]
27. Rasic, D.; Weerasinghe, S.; Asbridge, M.; Langille, D.B. Longitudinal associations of cannabis and illicit drug use with depression, suicidal ideation, and suicidal attempts among Nova Scotia high school students. *Drug Alcohol Depend.* **2013**, *129*, 49–53. [CrossRef]
28. Grunau, G.L.; Ratner, P.A.; Hossain, S.; Johnson, J.L. Depression and anxiety as possible mediators of the association between smoking and attention deficit hyperactivity disorder. *Int. J. Ment. Health Addict.* **2010**, *8*, 595–607. [CrossRef]
29. Villarosa, M.C.; Madson, M.B.; Zeigler-Hill, V.; Noble, J.J.; Mohn, R.S. Social anxiety symptoms and drinking behaviors among college students: The mediating effects of drinking motives. *Psychol. Addict. Behav.* **2014**, *28*, 710–718. [CrossRef] [PubMed]
30. Buckner, J.D.; Schmidt, N.B. Marijuana effect expectancies: Relations to social anxiety and marijuana use problems. *Addict. Behav.* **2008**, *33*, 1477–1483. [CrossRef] [PubMed]
31. Hanna, E.Z.; Yi, H.Y.; Dufour, M.C.; Whitmore, C.C. The relationship of early-onset regular smoking to alcohol use, depression, illicit drug use, and other risky behaviors during early adolescence: Results from the youth supplement to the third national health and nutrition examination survey. *J. Subst. Abuse* **2001**, *13*, 265–282. [CrossRef]
32. Roberts, S.J.; Glod, C.A.; Kim, R.; Hounchell, J. Relationships between aggression, depression, and alcohol, tobacco: Implications for healthcare providers in student health. *J. Am. Acad. Nurse Pract.* **2010**, *22*, 369–375. [CrossRef] [PubMed]
33. Kubik, M.Y.; Lytle, L.A.; Birnbaum, A.S.; Murray, D.M.; Perry, C.L. Prevalence and correlates of depressive symptoms in young adolescents. *Am. J. Health Behav.* **2003**, *27*, 546–553. [CrossRef]
34. Goodwin, R.D.; Lewinsohn, P.M.; Seeley, J.R. Cigarette smoking and panic attacks among young adults in the community: The role of parental smoking and anxiety disorders. *Biol. Psychiatry* **2005**, *58*, 686–693. [CrossRef]
35. Roberts, R.E.; Roberts, C.R.; Xing, Y. Comorbidity of substance use disorders and other psychiatric disorders among adolescents: Evidence from an epidemiologic survey. *Drug Alcohol Depend.* **2007**, *88*, S4–S13. [CrossRef]
36. Low, N.C.; Lee, S.S.; Johnson, J.G.; Williams, J.B.; Harris, E.S. The association between anxiety and alcohol versus cannabis abuse disorders among adolescents in primary care settings. *Fam. Pract.* **2008**, *25*, 321–327. [CrossRef]
37. Weiss, J.W.; Mouttapa, M.; Chou, C.P.; Nezami, E.; Johnson, C.A.; Palmer, P.H.; Cen, S.; Gallaher, P.; Ritt-Olson, A.; Azen, S.; et al. Hostility, depressive symptoms, and smoking in early adolescence. *J. Adolesc.* **2005**, *28*, 49–62. [CrossRef]
38. Mendel, J.R.; Berg, C.J.; Windle, R.C.; Windle, M. Predicting young adulthood smoking among adolescent smokers and non-smokers. *Am. J. Health Behav.* **2012**, *36*, 542–554. [CrossRef] [PubMed]
39. Munafò, M.R.; Hitsman, B.; Rende, R.; Metcalfe, C.; Niaura, R. Effects of progression to cigarette smoking on depressed mood in adolescents: Evidence from the National Longitudinal Study of Adolescent Health. *Addiction* **2008**, *103*, 162–171. [CrossRef]
40. Ridner, S.L.; Staten, R.R.; Danner, F.W. Smoking and depressive symptoms in a college population. *J. Sch. Nurs.* **2005**, *21*, 229–235. [CrossRef] [PubMed]

41. Duncan, B.; Rees, D.I. Effect of smoking on depressive symptomatology: A re-examination of data from the National Longitudinal Study of Adolescent Health. *Am. J. Epidemiol.* **2005**, *162*, 461–470. [CrossRef] [PubMed]
42. Goodman, E.; Capitman, J. Depressive symptoms and cigarette smoking among teens. *Pediatrics* **2000**, *106*, 748–755. [CrossRef] [PubMed]
43. Lechner, W.V.; Janssen, T.; Kahler, C.W.; Audrain-McGovern, J.; Leventhal, A.M. Bi-directional associations of electronic and combustible cigarette use onset patterns with depressive symptoms in adolescents. *Prev. Med.* **2017**, *96*, 73–78. [CrossRef] [PubMed]
44. Paschall, M.J.; Freisthler, B.; Lipton, R.I. Moderate alcohol use and depression in young adults: Findings from a national longitudinal study. *Am. J. Public Health* **2005**, *95*, 453–457. [CrossRef] [PubMed]
45. Suerken, C.K.; Reboussin, B.A.; Sutfin, E.L.; Wagoner, K.G.; Spangler, J.; Wolfson, M. Prevalence of marijuana use at college entry and risk factors for initiation during freshman year. *Addict. Behav.* **2014**, *39*, 302–307. [CrossRef] [PubMed]
46. Martini, S.; Wagner, F.A.; Anthony, J.C. The association of tobacco smoking and depression in adolescence: Evidence from the United States. *Subst. Use Misuse* **2002**, *37*, 1853–1867. [CrossRef] [PubMed]
47. Berg, C.; Choi, W.S.; Kaur, H.; Nollen, N.; Ahluwalia, J.S. The roles of parenting, church attendance, and depression in adolescent smoking. *J. Community Health* **2009**, *34*, 56–63. [CrossRef] [PubMed]
48. Simantov, E.; Schoen, C.; Klein, J.D. Health-compromising behaviors: Why do adolescents smoke or drink? Identifying underlying risk and protective factors. *Arch. Pediatr. Adolesc. Med.* **2000**, *154*, 1025–1033. [CrossRef] [PubMed]
49. Richardson, A.; He, J.P.; Curry, L.; Merikangas, K. Cigarette smoking and mood disorders in U.S. adolescents: Sex-specific associations with symptoms, diagnoses, impairment and health services use. *J. Psychosom. Res.* **2012**, *72*, 269–275. [CrossRef]
50. Georgiades, K.; Boyle, M.H. Adolescent tobacco and cannabis use: Young adult outcomes from the Ontario Child Health Study. *J. Child Psychol. Psychiatry* **2007**, *48*, 724–731. [CrossRef] [PubMed]
51. Naicker, K.; Galambos, N.L.; Zeng, Y.; Senthilselvan, A.; Colman, I. Social, demographic, and health outcomes in the 10 years following adolescent depression. *J Adolesc. Heal.* **2013**, *52*, 533–538. [CrossRef] [PubMed]
52. Brook, D.W.; Brook, J.S.; Zhang, C.; Cohen, P.; Whiteman, M. Drug use and the risk of major depressive disorder, alcohol dependence, and substance use disorders. *Arch. Gen. Psychiatry* **2002**, *59*, 1039–1044. [CrossRef] [PubMed]
53. Harder, V.S.; Stuart, E.A.; Anthony, J.C. Adolescent cannabis problems and young adult depression: Male-female stratified propensity score analyses. *Am. J. Epidemiol.* **2008**, *168*, 592–601. [CrossRef] [PubMed]
54. O'Loughlin, J.; O'Loughlin, E.K.; Wellman, R.J.; Sylvestre, M.P.; Dugas, E.N.; Chagnon, M.; Dutczak, H.; Laguë, J.; McGrath, J.J. Predictors of cigarette smoking initiation in early, middle, and late adolescence. *J. Adolesc. Health* **2017**, *61*, 363–370. [CrossRef] [PubMed]
55. Weitzman, E.R. Poor mental health, depression, and associations with alcohol consumption, harm, and abuse in a national sample of young adults in college. *J. Nerv. Ment. Dis.* **2004**, *192*, 269–277. [CrossRef] [PubMed]
56. Marmorstein, N.R. Anxiety disorders and substance use disorders: Different associations by anxiety disorder. *J. Anxiety Disord.* **2012**, *26*, 88–94. [CrossRef]
57. Meade, E.A.; Woolaway-Bickel, K.; Schmidt, N.B. Social anxiety and alcohol use: Evaluation of the moderating and mediating effects of alcohol expectancies. *J. Anxiety Disord.* **2004**, *18*, 33–49. [CrossRef]
58. Strahan, E.Y.; Panayiotou, G.; Clements, R.; Scott, J. Beer, wine, and social anxiety: Testing the "self-medication hypothesis" in the US and Cyprus. *Addict. Res. Theory* **2011**, *19*, 302–311. [CrossRef]
59. Wu, P.; Goodwin, R.D.; Fuller, C.; Liu, X.; Comer, J.S.; Cohen, P.; Hoven, C.W. The relationship between anxiety disorders and substance use among adolescents in the community: Specificity and gender differences. *J. Youth Adolesc.* **2010**, *39*, 177–188. [CrossRef] [PubMed]
60. Buckner, J.D.; Schmidt, N.B.; Lang, A.R.; Small, J.W.; Schlauch, R.C.; Lewinsohn, P.M. Specificity of social anxiety disorder as a risk factor for alcohol and cannabis dependence. *J. Psychiatr. Res.* **2008**, *42*, 230–239. [CrossRef] [PubMed]
61. Wells, G.; Shea, B.; O'Connell, D.; Peterson, J.; Welch, V.; Losos, M.; Tugwell, P. *The Newcastle-Ottawa Scale (NOS) for Assessing the Quality of Nonrandomised Studies in Meta-Analyses*; Ottawa Health Research Institute: Ottawa, ON, Canada, 1999.

62. Hedges, L.V.; Vevea, J.L. Fixed and random effects models in meta-analysis. *Psychol. Methods* **1998**, *3*, 486–504. [CrossRef]
63. Duval, S.; Tweedie, R. Trim and fill: A simple funnel-plot-based method of testing and adjusting for publication bias in meta-analysis. *Biometrics* **2000**, *56*, 455–463. [CrossRef] [PubMed]
64. Chaiton, M.O.; Cohen, J.E.; O'Loughlin, J.; Rehm, J. A systematic review of longitudinal studies on the association between depression and smoking in adolescents. *BMC Public Health* **2009**, *9*, 356. [CrossRef] [PubMed]
65. Moore, T.H.; Zammit, S.; Lingford-Hughes, A.; Barnes, T.R.; Jones, P.B.; Burke, M.; Lewis, G. Cannabis use and risk of psychotic or affective mental health outcomes: A systematic review. *Lancet* **2007**, *370*, 319–328. [CrossRef]
66. Kedzior, K.K.; Laeber, L.T. A positive association between anxiety disorders and cannabis use or cannabis use disorders in the general population- a meta-analysis of 31 studies. *BMC Psychiatry* **2014**, *14*, 136. [CrossRef] [PubMed]
67. Windle, M. Alcohol use among adolescents and young adults. *Alcohol Res. Health* **2003**, *27*, 79–85. [PubMed]
68. Brière, F.N.; Rohde, P.; Seeley, J.R.; Klein, D.; Lewinsohn, P.M. Comorbidity between major depression and alcohol use disorder from adolescence to adulthood. *Compr. Psychiatry* **2014**, *55*, 526–533. [CrossRef] [PubMed]
69. Rohde, P.; Lewinsohn, P.M.; Kahler, C.W.; Seeley, J.R.; Brown, R.A. Natural course of alcohol use disorders from adolescence to young adulthood. *J. Am. Acad. Child Adolesc. Psychiatry* **2001**, *40*, 83–90. [CrossRef] [PubMed]
70. Lev-Ran, S.; Roerecke, M.; Le Foll, B.; George, T.P.; McKenzie, K.; Rehm, J. The association between cannabis use and depression: A systematic review and meta-analysis of longitudinal studies. *Psychol. Med.* **2014**, *44*, 797–810. [CrossRef] [PubMed]
71. Degenhardt, L.; Hall, W.; Lynskey, M. Exploring the association between cannabis use and depression. *Addiction* **2003**, *98*, 1493–1504. [CrossRef]
72. Picciotto, M.R.; Brunzell, D.H.; Caldarone, B.J. Effect of nicotine and nicotinic receptors on anxiety and depression. *Neuroreport* **2002**, *13*, 1097–1106. [CrossRef] [PubMed]
73. Tweed, J.O.; Hsia, S.H.; Lutfy, K.; Friedman, T.C. The endocrine effects of nicotine and cigarette smoke. *Trends Endocrinol. Metab.* **2012**, *23*, 334–342. [CrossRef] [PubMed]
74. Kassel, J.D.; Stroud, L.R.; Paronis, C.A. Smoking, stress, and negative affect: Correlation, causation, and context across stages of smoking. *Psychol. Bull.* **2003**, *129*, 270–304. [CrossRef] [PubMed]
75. Moylan, S.; Jacka, F.N.; Pasco, J.A.; Berk, M. How cigarette smoking may increase the risk of anxiety symptoms and anxiety disorders: A critical review of biological pathways. *Brain Behav.* **2013**, *3*, 302–326. [CrossRef]
76. American College Health Association. *American College Health Association-National College Health Assessment II: Canadian Reference Group Executive Summary Spring 2016*; American College Health Association: Hanover, MD, USA, 2016.
77. American College Health Association. *American College Health Association-National College Health Assessment II: U.S. Reference Group Executive Summary Spring 2016*; American College Health Association: Hanover, MD, USA, 2016.
78. National Association of State Mental Health Program Directors and National Association of State Alcohol and Drug Abuse Directors. *National Dialogue on Co-Occurring Mental Health and Substance Abuse Disorders*; National Association of State Alcohol and Drug Abuse Directors: Washington, DC, USA, 1999.

16

Evaluating the Effectiveness of Clinical Pharmacy Consultations on Nutrition, Physical Activity, and Sleep in Improving Patient-Reported Psychiatric Outcomes for Individuals with Mental Illnesses

Jennifer Bingham [1,*], David R. Axon [2], Nicole Scovis [1] and Ann M. Taylor [2]

[1] SinfoníaRx, Tucson, AZ 85701, USA; NScovis@sinfoniarx.com
[2] College of Pharmacy, University of Arizona, Tucson, AZ 85721, USA; Axon@pharmacy.arizona.edu (D.R.A.); Taylor@pharmacy.arizona.edu (A.M.T.)
* Correspondence: JMBingham@sinfoniarx.com;

Abstract: One fifth of U.S. adults have a current mental illness. Nutrition, physical activity, and sleep are critical to physical health; any related deficiencies may worsen existing mental health conditions. Little is known about the impact of clinical pharmacist assessment and consultation in improving physical and mental health outcomes. The study objective was to determine whether patients' mental health status improved following clinical pharmacist consultation. This pilot study involved clinical pharmacist-delivered services at an integrated medical behavioral health clinic in June 2018. Inclusion criteria required adults aged 18 years older, an established mental health diagnosis, and taking $\geq$2 prescribed psychotropic medications. One pharmacist conducted telephonic, medical, and psychiatric health risk assessment and counseling to improve nutrition, physical activity, and sleep status, both initially and at two-week follow-up. The Duke Health Profile (Duke) physical, anxiety, depression, and anxiety-depression scores measured patients' pre/post changes. Participants ($n = 20$) experienced higher Duke physical scores ($p = 0.007$) and significantly lower anxiety ($p = 0.025$), depression ($p = 0.001$) and anxiety-depression scores ($p = 0.005$) at follow-up. This pilot study provides preliminary evidence for pharmacist-led, targeted, telephonic counseling in improving short-term physical and mental Duke health scores. Further research evaluating the impact of clinical pharmacists' role in improving physical and behavioral health outcomes is warranted.

Keywords: pharmacist; education; Duke; nutrition; exercise; sleep

1. Introduction

Mental health conditions are prevalent in the United States (U.S.), with 55% of the population expected to experience a mental health illness during their lifetime [1]. The 2015 National Survey on Drug Use and Health estimated that roughly one in five U.S. adults had a current mental illness [2]. Of these, approximately 22% (9.7 million) of adults did not receive mental health care [3]. Individuals with mental illness have decreased access to healthcare and monitoring services for physical health conditions [4]. Additionally, the deficit in mental health professionals has forced patients to seek psychiatric care from their primary care providers [3]. Thus, a gap exists in service provisions to address patients' physical and mental well-being, which is critical to one's overall health.

The effects of mental illness are far-reaching, affecting many facets of patients' lives. Specifically, these patients are at increased risk of physical health problems [5], and of experiencing increased morbidity and mortality secondary to preventable conditions with modifiable factors, including alcohol consumption, smoking, poor nutrition, and lack of exercise [4]. Furthermore, an interrelationship exists between psychiatric outcomes and lifestyle habits, such as diet, exercise, and sleep [6–8]. Several neurotransmitters (e.g., serotonin and norepinephrine) require intake of essential dietary amino acids, vitamins and adequate sleep for synthesis to occur, as well as physical activity for their release. Inadequate consumption of appropriate foods may worsen anxiety, depression, and insomnia [7,8], while physical activity can reduce their severity [9].

Lifelong preventive care is critical to guide appropriate nutrition, physical activity, and sleep to prevent negative health outcomes, whereas improved health outcomes typically are influenced by positive lifestyle habits. To date, a few studies have investigated the impact of pharmacists' role in mental health care. Integration of a clinical pharmacist into a collaborative care model in combination with direct, patient-centered counseling and education can improve health outcomes [10,11]. Yet, little is known about pharmacists' involvement in preventive strategies to improve diet; assess deficiency of essential amino acids, vitamins, and minerals; encourage more physical activity; and recommend adequate daily sleep.

To address this gap in service provision, a clinical pharmacist developed a pilot program to offer preventive mental health care services to patients. The pharmacist assessed patients' current nutrition, physical activity, and sleep status; subsequent counseling and education were provided as deemed appropriate.

The study objective was to determine whether clinical pharmacist consultation improved patients' mental health status, measured via the Duke Health Profile (Duke) mental health scales (anxiety, depression, anxiety-depression) two weeks after the clinical pharmacist consultation.

2. Materials and Methods

2.1. Study Design

This pilot program involved a retrospective record review of patients who participated in a pharmacist-delivered program designed for individuals with mental health conditions; the program was conducted at an integrated medical behavioral health clinic. The program was designed specifically to optimize management of mental health conditions by focusing on patients' nutritional intake, physical activity level, and sleep quality and quantity. The Institutional Review Board approved this study (protocol number 1804441035, approved 20 April 2018).

2.2. Study Sample

Eligible individuals met these study criteria: 18 years of age or older; an established (receiving care for at least a year) patient at the clinic; designation of general mental health condition by the Arizona Health Care Cost Containment System (Arizona's Medicaid program); and were taking at least two chronic, psychotropic medications (e.g., alpha-2 antagonist, antipsychotics, second-generation atypical antipsychotics, monoamine oxidase inhibitors, non-dopamine reuptake inhibitors, nefazodone, serotonin reuptake inhibitors, selective serotonin reuptake inhibitors, and U.S. Food and Drug Administration (FDA)-labeled mood stabilizers). The sampling method was based on the primary investigator requesting clinic records for patients meeting the study inclusion criteria. Individuals were excluded if they were less than 18 years of age, had developmental disabilities, had a documented inpatient hospitalization within the last 90 days, or were enrolled in an existing wellness program at the clinic. Participants voluntarily enrolled in an existing wellness program at the participating site were excluded to avoid confounding by providing duplicative clinical services.

2.3. Initial Consultation (Intervention)

The initial assessment and consultation, utilizing a standardized call script (see Appendix A), was conducted via telephone, and consisted of multiple components. First, the pharmacist reconciled the patient's medication list, reviewed allergies, assessed adherence to medications, and assessed nutritional intake, physical activity, and sleep quality. Next, the pharmacist provided standardized educational counseling on strategies to improve dietary precursors for targeted neurotransmitters, specific to the patient's medications' mechanism(s) of action. The pharmacist then addressed barriers (e.g., access to appropriate food) to physical, nutritional, and sleep adherence recommendations; pharmacist-delivered patient education was based on relevant guidelines [e.g., Recommended Dietary Allowances (RDA), American Academy of Sleep Medicine and Sleep Research Society, Centers for Disease Control and Prevention (for sleep hygiene), Office of Disease Promotion and Health Promotion (for physical activity)] [12–15]. Finally, the pharmacist identified psychotropic medications' targeted neurotransmitter(s) (e.g., serotonin, norepinephrine, and dopamine), based on the mechanism of action. This information, in combination with the patient's status (e.g., chronic conditions, self-reported dietary and supplement intake), assisted the pharmacist in determining the proteins essential for achieving nutritional intake of neurotransmitter precursors (e.g., L-tryptophan for serotonin, phenylalanine for norepinephrine, and dopamine).

2.4. *Physical and Mental Health Assessment*

The Duke instrument assessed patient health status. The 17-item instrument measures general, mental, physical, social, and perceived health, plus anxiety, depression, pain, disability and self-esteem [11]. This study only assessed patient's physical and mental health. Both high Duke physical scores (0 = poorest health, and 100 = best health) and low anxiety, depression, and anxiety-depression scores (0 = best health, and 100 = poorest health) represented better controlled conditions [16].

Variables included the physical Duke score, anxiety Duke score, depression Duke score, anxiety-depression combined Duke score. The pharmacist reviewed baseline Duke scores prior to the initial consultation; the scores were provided to the pharmacist by the clinic staff who obtained the data from the electronic health record. At the two-week follow up, the pharmacist conducted the assessment with the patient. Follow-up scores were collected from the electronic health record software program that housed a built-in Duke health survey; however, the research team did not have access to these scores in the electronic system. Baseline and follow-up scores were compared to assess changes in physical and mental health status scores, after the pharmacist intervention.

The pharmacist conducted comprehensive reviews, during the intial and follow-up consultations, to address each of the following:

2.4.1. General Nutrition Counseling

- Assess patient dietary and supplement intake of essential nutrients required for optimal absorption, based on patient recall of a typical daily meal plan. Address apparent deficit(s) and make recommendations to supplement patient's intake of these nutrients.
- Identify strategies (e.g., educate patient on integrating good food sources of essential nutrients or encourage tracking intake of essential nutrients) for achieving the Acceptable Macronutrient Distribution Range of 10–35% of healthy complete protein daily and creating individualized meal plans through open discussion, based on patient dietary restrictions, comorbidities, and financial barriers [12].
- Recommend smaller, more frequent meals throughout the day, when appropriate.
- Ensure alignment with prescribed medications for achieving optimal mental health status.

2.4.2. Serotonin-Targeting Psychotropic Medications

- Assess sources of complete protein, including all nine essential amino acids and L-tryptophan (e.g., meat, poultry, fish, dairy, eggs); sources containing all essential amino acids were deemed necessary for patients taking a serotonin-targeting psychotropic medication [17].

- Evaluate dietary intake of vitamins B6, B9, B12, and D3, as well as omega fatty acids for enzyme activation of tryptophan hydroxylase [17]. In cases where the patient reported dietary intolerance or avoidance of complete proteins, the pharmacist emphasized these precursors.

2.4.3. Norepinephrine and Dopamine-Targeting Psychotropic Medications

- Assess nutritional intake of essential amino acids phenylalanine and tyrosine, as well as vitamins B6, B9, B12, D3, and iron (for dopamine) for tyrosine hydroxylase activation.
- Encourage consumption of incomplete proteins containing phenylalanine and tyrosine (e.g., nuts, grains, beans, legumes, soy, or animal-based complete proteins).

2.4.4. Sleep Counseling

- Assess sleep quality and quantity based on the amount of patient-reported uninterrupted sleep received each night. Patients were advised to sleep at least seven hours per night, according to consensus guidelines [13].
- Educate on sleep hygiene, including the importance of maintaining a consistent routine (e.g., rising and going to bed at same time daily); removing distractions (i.e., computers, electronic devices, televisions, cellular phones); and avoiding large meals, physical activity, and stimulants (e.g., smoking, caffeine) before bedtime, per the Centers for Disease Control and Prevention recommendations [14].

2.4.5. Physical Activity Counseling

- Assess physical activity level. Patients were advised to engage in 150 minutes of physical activity each week per the Office of Disease Prevention and Health Promotion guidelines [15]. A personalized plan was created after the pharmacist and patient mutually agreed on a physical activity schedule that aligned with the patient's normal routine (e.g., shorter sessions throughout the day if needed).
- Recommend consulting with their healthcare provider before starting a new program, and selecting physical activities of interest to help increase motivation and maintenance.

2.5. Follow-up Consultation (Intervention)

During this telephonic consultation, the pharmacist revisited follow-up points from the initial call, assessing changes in nutrition, physical activity, and sleep habits using a standardized call script. The pharmacist also conducted a Duke assessment with the patient.

2.6. Data Collection and Statistical Analysis

Data from the clinic's electronic health record and the Duke instrument were used to assess the impact of the pharmacist interventions on respective physical and mental health. At the beginning of the initial telephone call, the primary investigator (PI) briefly described the study; if the patient chose to participate, he or she provided verbal consent to the PI at that time. Participants also were mailed a waiver of consent document outlining pertinent information related to the research project. Patient confidentiality and anonymity was maintained throughout the study.

The baseline scores were collected in the electronic health record (EHR) by clinic staff and provided to the pharmacist just prior to the initial consultation; the PI/pharmacist did not have access to the patient's EHR during the study. To minimize bias, the baseline outcome data (i.e., DUKE scores) were entered and stored in Research Data Electronic Capture (REDCap) secure web application (Vanderbilt University Medical Center, Version 8.10.0, Nashville, TN, United States) [18]. The follow-up data was collected initially by the pharmacist in an Excel tracking spreadsheet (Microsoft Office 360 Plus) containing labels (no identifiers). The pharmacist became aware of the relationship between the baseline data (e.g., Duke scores) upon entering the follow-up data in REDCap, after completing the telephonic follow-up consultation. To ensure data security and integrity, the PI was HIPAA-certified and the only person who had access to the final coded dataset. Physical and mental health (anxiety, depression, and anxiety-depression) scores were reported at the initial and follow-up consultations and compared using paired t-tests. An alpha of 0.05 was set a priori. Analyses were conducted using SPSS (IBM Corp., Version 21, Armonk, NY, United States).

3. Results

A total of 267 eligible patients met the inclusion criteria for this pilot study. Of these, 34 participated in the program, and 20 (59%) received both the initial and follow-up consultations (see Figure 1). Participants were typically female (60%), white (60%), non-Hispanic or Latino (60%), and younger (less than 40 years old, 60%), although all age groups were well represented in this study. Interestingly, 40% of participants were 31 to 40 years of age, while one fifth were less than 30 years of age. Additionally, seven participants did not report their race nor ethnicity. All participants had Medicaid as both their primary and secondary healthcare insurance. For further details, see Table 1.

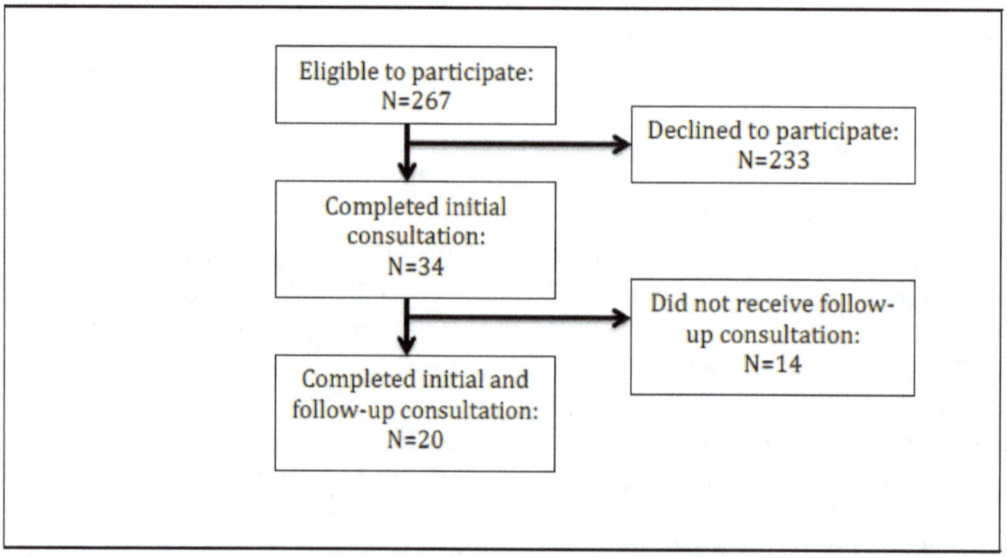

Figure 1. Flowchart showing the number of individuals in the study.

Table 1. Demographic characteristics of participants (N = 20) participating in a pharmacist-delivered program for Medicaid patients with mental illness.

Characteristic	*N* (%)
Age (in years)	
20–30	4 (20)
31–40	8 (40)
41–50	6 (30)
≥51	2 (10)
Gender	
Female	12 (60)
Male	8 (40)
Ethnicity	
Not Hispanic or Latino	12 (60)
Race	
American Indian or Alaska Native	0 (0)
White	12 (60)
Asian	0 (0)
Black or African American	1 (5)
Unknown	7 (35)

There were significant improvements in both the physical and mental health Duke measures. The physical scores increased from baseline to follow-up, indicating improvements in lifestyle habits. Furthermore, significant reductions were observed in the anxiety ($p < 0.025$), depression ($p < 0.001$), and anxiety-depression ($p < 0.005$) scores between initial and follow-up consultations. For further details, see Table 2.

From the initial to follow-up measurement, there was a larger change among females compared to males for depression score (mean change -32.5 ± 26.3 versus -7.5 ± 19.8, respectively; $p = 0.035$) and depression-anxiety score (mean change -31.0 ± 28.0 versus -3.6 ± 21.6 respectively; $p = 0.031$). Likewise, there was a larger change among those reporting their race as white compared to their non-white counterparts for the anxiety score (mean change -25.0 ± 22.5 versus 3.1 ± 19.9 respectively; $p = 0.010$), depression score (mean change -33.3 ± 22.7 versus -6.25 ± 24.5, respectively; $p = 0.021$) and depression-anxiety score (mean change -33.3 ± 24.4 versus 0.1 ± 22.6, respectively; $p = 0.006$).

Table 2. Differences between Duke Health Profile Scores of participants at baseline and follow-up ($n = 20$).

Profile Scale Scores	Baseline Mean (SD)	Follow up Mean (SD)	*p*-value
Physical	54.5 (21.9)	74.5 (17.9)	0.007
Mental			
Anxiety	49.6 (26.1)	35.8 (17.7)	0.025
Depression	53.5 (31.2)	31.0 (18.3)	0.001
Anxiety-depression scale	49.3 (31.8)	29.3 (18.4)	0.005
Overall	50.8 (29.7)	32.0 (18.1)	0.010

Key: SD: standard deviation. The level of significance was set at <0.05.

4. Discussion

These pilot study findings provide preliminary evidence to support the value of pharmacist-led consultations for underserved patients with mental health conditions. Specifically, patients with mental health conditions often require additional health care services [4,5], and the pharmacist is uniquely positioned to help address, and ultimately improve those patients' health outcomes [10].

The pilot program demonstrated a larger change among females versus males for depression scores. This parallels other models that found telephonic consultations improved the management of depression [19].

The majority of participants in this mental health pilot study were female, suggesting that they may be more likely than males to seek [20] and utilize mental health services [21,22]. White, non-Latino individuals represented the majority of patients in this study, which aligns with research reported by others regarding help-seeking behavior for mental health conditions [23]. This may speak to the reluctance of some groups of individuals (e.g., African Americans, non-white Hispanics) to seek mental healthcare services. To that end, African-Americans and Hispanics (e.g., non-white Latinos) may be less likely to perceive the need for help [24]. Additionally, African-Americans are more likely to believe that mental conditions will improve on their own [25], relying more on informal support systems compared to non-Latino whites. Furthermore, minority groups typically underutilize mental health services [26–29].

With regard to race/ethnicity, the current study demonstrated a larger change in Duke scores among those reporting their race as white compared to non-whites for anxiety, depression, and depression-anxiety. Other factors (e.g., mental health literacy, economic resouces) may partially explain some of these differences in Duke scores. For example, some non-white groups may experience disparities (e.g., limited access and ability to incorporate better food sources of essential amino acids), potentially affecting their response and ability to engage in more positive health behaviors [23].

The telepharmacist was board-certified in ambulatory care pharmacy, experienced in the provision of medication therapy management consultations, and had completed a psychiatric pharmacy certificate program. While this pharmacist had considerable advanced education and training, it is important that appropriate academic and lifelong programs are developed, evaluated, and available to support pharmacists in providing these specialized services. Further research is needed to determine pharmacists' perceptions regarding their ability to provide counseling services to patients with mental health conditions, and more specifically, after participating in programs designed to address the health care needs of these underserved patients.

Furthermore, the pharmacist's role was critical in the provision of medication management, and in particular, for psychotropic medications. With added emphasis on lifestyle habits, the pharmacist was key in addressing patients' needs and providing expertise and medication support in light of the apparent provider shortage. Providing personalized care during the consultations was critical to improved outcomes, yet was quite time-consuming. However, the average time spent on each consultation was not documented for this study. Tracking of the pharmacist-related resources necessary for implementing this integrated model in other clinical settings is warranted in future studies.

Further expansion of the current pilot study is of interest, specifically to include investigation of this populations' vulnerability to substance abuse. This could provide valuable insight for researchers with regard to these vulnerable individuals. Additionally, this sample population included younger patients with mental health challenges, all of whom were receiving healthcare benefits through Arizona's managed care Medicaid benefit. However, future work could include implementing this integrated model in a subset of patients with anxiety disorders (e.g., agoraphobia and those susceptible to isolation), to better understand the pharmacist's role in helping these patients adhere to their medical appointments, and thus improve their health outcomes.

It is critical to build in longer-term patient follow-up to study the effects of the pharmacist's interventions on self-reported health outcomes. Moreover, integrating an interprofessional coordinator in to programs such as this is vital to implement strategies for increasing patient engagement and reducing attrition (e.g., contacting patients for telephonic pharmacist consultation appointments); to serve as a liaison to enhance patient–provider–pharmacist communication; and to improve overall program efficiency.

While the pharmacist assessed dietary and supplement intake, more accurate measures of consumption are warranted. For instance, a tracking log or diet records could provide insight regarding the exact sources of protein. Utilizing a food frequency questionnaire, designed specifically to measure protein intake, could assist the pharmacist in assessing average consumption over time (e.g., months rather than days) [30], as well as providing valuable information to integrate into the pharmacist's patient-related recommendations during the consultations. Additionally, the pharmacist's medication reconciliation was based on patient-reported information, given that EHR was not granted to study personnel. Future work must include capturing this valuable medication data to enrich the reportable results.

Preventive care is an established benefit of physical health care, especially given that diet and exercise are routinely discussed during half of primary care visits [31]. However, less is known about the benefits of preventive care in the behavioral health setting. The results of this study lend evidence to the value of routinely incorporating prevention when caring for individuals with behavioral health needs.

Limitations

This pilot study had its limitations. First, a substantial number of patients ($n = 14$; 41%) were lost at the follow-up, considerably affecting the sample size. Second, patients were only followed for two weeks before the second measures were taken, preventing the ability to draw long-term conclusions. Third, all data collected was self-reported by the participant, and was therefore susceptible to bias. Fourth, the consultation was conducted via telephone, and presented challenges with monitoring consumption and adherence to interventions. Fifth, the fact that the pilot program did not capture patients' medications in the dataset is a study limitation; in hindsight, having this information could provide valuable insight. This study was only conducted in one outpatient clinic setting with Medicaid patients, thus limiting its generalizability to other settings and populations.

5. Conclusions

This pilot study provides preliminary evidence regarding the benefits of pharmacist-provided lifestyle counseling in improving participants' Duke physical and mental (anxiety, depression, anxiety-depression) health scores at the two-week follow up. These results highlight the value of the pharmacist's involvement, suggesting the potential for improved nutrition, physical activity, and sleep for patients with mental health conditions, at least in the short term. However, more research is warranted to determine the impact of similar pharmacist interventions on medical and behavioral outcomes and long-term health benefits, as well as integrating such a concept into accredited pharmacy education programs.

Author Contributions: Methodology: J.B. and N.S.; validation: D.A; formal analysis: D.R.A.; investigation: J.B.; resources: A.M.T.; writing—original draft preparation: A.M.T., J.B.; writing—review and editing: J.B., N.S., D.R.A., and A.M.T.; supervision: N.S.; project administration: J.B.

Acknowledgments: The authors would like to thank Dr. George Parkerson for his permission to use and cite the Duke Health Profile (Duke). The authors would also like to thank Martha Fankhauser for her assistance with the manuscript preparation.

Appendix A : Call Scripts

Nutrition

The pharmacist researcher will reconcile the medication list with the patient. After reviewing their entire medication list, they will identify the specific neurotransmitter that applies to their regimen and follow the appropriate script below:

- Serotonin helps with your mood. It is also what makes you feel happy. Your [medication name] needs serotonin to work.
- Norepinephrine helps with your response to stressful situations. It can also help with depression. Your [medication name] needs norepinephrine to work.
- Dopamine helps with your emotional response and mental focus. Your [medication name] needs dopamine to work.

"I am going to ask you some questions about your diet to see if you are getting enough of the right foods for your body to build [serotonin/norepinephrine/dopamine]."
"What does your daily meal plan look like?" Review with patient. Identify strengths within diet to build positive foundation. Identify/address cost-related barriers.
"How often do you eat? It is recommended to eat every couple of hours during the day. Do not skip meals, particularly breakfast. When you eat, try to eat slowly over 30 minutes. It will allow your body time to absorb the nutrients better."
"Do you know which foods are classified as complete proteins? The greatest building blocks for [serotonin/norepinephrine] are things that you might already have in your kitchen. You can find them in beef, venison, buffalo, pork, fish, shellfish, cheese, cottage cheese, milk, yogurt, and eggs."
"Do you know which foods are classified as incomplete proteins? The building blocks for [norepinephrine/dopamine] are also found in your kitchen. In addition to eating complete proteins,

it's also important to eat incomplete proteins as well. You can find these in nuts, grains, beans, legumes, and soy."

"How many servings of protein do you eat in a day? Now that we know what types of protein you eat, it is important to talk about how much you consume to make sure you are getting enough to allow your medications to work their best." Review with patient. Identify methods to achieve 3–4 servings of healthy protein daily intake.

"What else is included on your meal plan?" Based on patient's medication regimen, the pharmacist will follow the appropriate script below:

"When we think about serotonin building blocks, key vitamins play an important role as well. Vitamin B6 is a great nutritional source of this vitamin, and is found in whole grains, vegetables, and nuts. Vitamin B12 is found in meats, fish, liver, and milk. Folic acid and Vitamin D3 are often found in fortified foods like dairy products, orange juice, and yogurt. Omega-3 Fatty Acids are found in fish, dairy products, and grains."

"When we think about norepinephrine building blocks, key vitamins play an important role as well. Folic acid is often found in fortified foods like dairy products, orange juice, and yogurt. Vitamin B12 is found in meats, fish, liver, and milk."

"When we think about dopamine building blocks, key vitamins play an important role as well. Vitamin B6 is a great nutritional source of this vitamin, and is found in whole grains, vegetables, and nuts. Folic acid is often found in fortified foods like dairy products, orange juice, and yogurt. Vitamin B12 is found in meats, fish, liver, and milk. Iron is also a key player. It is found in beans, leafy greens, and fortified cereals."

Sleep

"How many hours of sleep do you get on average per night?" Adults 18 to 60 years should sleep at least seven hours per night.

"Do you have trouble with sleeping?" If patient answers yes, ask for more details. Review relevant sleep hygiene tips (online: https://www.cdc.gov/sleep/about_sleep/sleep_hygiene.html).

Physical Activity

"How would you describe your physical activity? Being physically active is important not only for heart health, but also for mental health. It is recommended to be physically active for 30 minutes a day, five times a week. Another option is to break it up. If you have a busy schedule, try dividing your time into two or three segments of 10 to 15 minutes per day. Do not start a new exercise program without talking with their doctor first." Ask the patient what types of physical activity they like to do. Motivational counseling.

References

1. Kessler, R.C.; Angermeyer, M.; Anthony, J.C.; DEGraaf, R.; Demyttenaere, K.; Gasquet, I.; DEGirolamo, G.; Gluzman, S.; Gureje, O.; Haro, J.M.; et al. Lifetime prevalence and age-of-onset distributions of mental disorders in the World Health Organization's World Mental Health Survey Initiative. *World Psychiatry* **2007**, *6*, 168–176. [PubMed]
2. National Institute of Mental Health. Available online: https://www.nimh.nih.gov/health/statistics/mental-illness.shtml (accessed on 8 August 2018).
3. Results from the 2016 National Survey on Drug Use and Health. Available online: https://www.samhsa.gov/data/sites/default/files/NSDUH-FFR1-2016/NSDUH-FFR1-2016.htm (accessed on 8 August 2018).
4. National Association of State Mental Health Program Directors. Available online: https://www.nasmhpd.org/sites/default/files/Mortality%20and%20Morbidity%20Final%20Report%208.18.08.pdf (accessed on 8 August 2018).
5. Reeves, W.; Strine, T.; Pratt, L.; Thompson, W.; Ahluwalia, I.; Dhingra, S.; McKnight-Eily, L.; Harrison, L.; D'Angelo, D.V.; Williams, L.; et al. CDC Report: Mental Illness Surveillance Among Adults in the United States. *MMWR Morb. Mortal. Wkly. Rep.* **2011**, *60*, 1–32.

6. Kline, C. The bidirectional relationship between exercise and sleep: Implications for exercise adherence and sleep improvement. *Am. J. Lifestyle Med.* **2014**, *8*, 375–379. [CrossRef] [PubMed]
7. Lopresti, A.L.; Hood, S.D.; Drummond, P.D. A review of lifestyle factors that contribute to important pathways associated with major depression: Diet, sleep and exercise. *J. Affect. Disord.* **2013**, *148*, 12–27. [CrossRef] [PubMed]
8. Rössler, W. Nutrition, sleep, physical exercise: Impact on mental health. *J. Eur. Psychol.* **2016**, *33*, S12. [CrossRef]
9. Mayo Clinic. Available online: https://www.mayoclinic.org/diseases-conditions/depression/in-depth/depression-and-exercise/art-20046495 (accessed on 8 August 2018).
10. Finley, P.; Crismon, M.; Rush, A. Evaluating the impact of pharmacists in mental health: A systematic review. *Pharmacotherapy* **2003**, *23*, 1634–1644. [CrossRef] [PubMed]
11. Parkerson, G.R., Jr.; Broadhead, W.E.; Tse, C.K. The Duke Health Profile. A 17-item measure of health and dysfunction. *Med. Care* **1990**, *28*, 1056–1072. [CrossRef] [PubMed]
12. Wolfe, R.R.; Cifelli, A.M.; Kostas, G.; Kim, I.-Y. Optimizing Protein Intake in Adults: Interpretation and Application of the Recommended Dietary Allowance Compared with the Acceptable Macronutrient Distribution Range. *Adv. Nutr.* **2017**, *8*, 266–275. [CrossRef]
13. Watson, N.F.; Badr, M.S.; Belenky, G.; Bliwise, D.L.; Buxton, O.M.; Buysse, D.; Dinges, D.F.; Gangwisch, J.; Grandner, M.A.; Kushida, C.; et al. Recommended amount of sleep for a healthy adult: A joint consensus statement of the American Academy of Sleep Medicine and Sleep Research Society. *Sleep* **2015**, *38*, 843–844. [CrossRef]
14. Centers for Disease Control and Prevention. Available online: https://www.cdc.gov/sleep/about_sleep/sleep_hygiene.html (accessed on 8 August 2018).
15. Office of Disease Promotion and Health Promotion. Available online: https://health.gov/paguidelines/guidelines/adults.aspx (accessed on 8 August 2018).
16. Duke Community & Family Medicine. Available online: https://cfm.duke.edu/research/duke-health-measures (accessed on 26 September 2018).
17. Bingham, J. What You Need to Know about Behavioral Health Medications. WellRx. Available online: https://news.wellrx.com/2017/07/24/what-you-need-to-know-about-behavioral-health-medications/ (accessed on 2 December 2018).
18. REDCap. Available online: https://projectredcap.org/ (accessed on 13 December 2018).
19. Simon, G.E.; VonKorff, M.; Rutter, C.; Wagner, E. Randomised trial of monitoring, feedback, and management of care by telephone to improve treatment of depression in primary care. *BMJ* **2000**, *320*, 550–554. [CrossRef]
20. Gonzalez, J.M.; Alegría, M.; Prihoda, T.J.; Copeland, L.A.; Zeber, J.E. How the Relationship of Attitudes toward Mental Health Treatment and Service Use Differs by Age, Gender, Ethnicity/Race and Education. *Soc. Psychiatry Psychiatr. Epidemiol.* **2011**, *46*, 45–57. [CrossRef] [PubMed]
21. Ojeda, V.D.; McGuire, T.G. Gender and Racial/Ethnic Differences in Use of Outpatient Mental Health and Substance Use Services by Depressed Adults. *Psychiatr. Q.* **2006**, *77*, 211–222. [CrossRef] [PubMed]
22. Wang, P.S.; Lane, M.; Olfson, M.; Pincus, H.A.; Wells, K.B.; Kessler, R.C. Twelve-month Use of Mental Health Services in the United States: Results from the National Comorbidity Survey Replication. *Arch. Gen. Psychiatry* **2005**, *62*, 629–640. [CrossRef] [PubMed]
23. Villatoro, A.P.; Mays, V.M.; Ponce, N.A.; Aneshensel, C.S. Perceived Need for Mental Health Care: The Intersection of Race, Ethnicity, Gender, and Socioeconomic Status. *Soc. Ment. Health* **2018**, *8*, 1–24. [CrossRef]
24. Jang, Y.; Park, N.S.; Young Kang, S.; Chiriboga, D.A. Racial/Ethnic Differences in the Association between Symptoms of Depression and Self-rated Mental Health among Older Adults. *Community Ment. Health J.* **2014**, *50*, 325–330. [CrossRef]
25. Anglin, D.M.; Albertic, P.M.; Link, B.G.; Phelan, J.C. Racial Differences in Beliefs about the Effectiveness and Necessity of Mental Health Treatment. *Am. J. Community Psychol.* **2008**, *42*, 17–24. [CrossRef]
26. Jimenez, D.E.; Bartels, S.J.; Cardenas, V.; Dhaliwal, S.S.; Alegría, M. Cultural Beliefs and Mental Health Treatment Preferences of Ethnically Diverse Older Adult Consumers in Primary Care. *Am. J. Geriatr. Psychiatry* **2012**, *20*, 533–542. [CrossRef]
27. Taylor, R.J.; Woodward, A.T.; Chatters, L.M.; Mattis, J.S.; Jackson, J.B. Seeking Help from Clergy among Black Caribbeans in the United States. *Race Soc. Probl.* **2011**, *3*, 241–251. [CrossRef]

28. Woodward, A.T.; Chatters, L.M.; Taylor, R.J.; Neighbors, H.W.; Jackson, J.S. Differences in Professional and Informal Help Seeking among Older African Americans. Black Caribbeans, and Non-Hispanic Whites. *J. Soc. Soc. Work Res.* **2010**, *1*, 124–139. [CrossRef]
29. Cook, B.L.; Zuvekas, S.H.; Carson, N.; Wayne, G.F.; Vesper, A.; McGuire, T.G. Assessing Racial/Ethnic. Disparities in Treatment across Episodes of Mental Health Care. *Health Serv. Res.* **2014**, *49*, 206–221. [CrossRef]
30. Morin, P.; Herrmman, F.; Ammann, P.; Uebelhart, B.; Rizzoli, R. A rapid self-administered food frequency questionnaire for the evaluation of dietary protein intake. *Clin. Nutr.* **2005**, *24*, 768–774. [CrossRef] [PubMed]
31. Smith, A.W.; Borowski, L.A.; Liu, B.; Galuska, D.A.; Signore, C.; Klabunde, C.; Huang, T.T.-K.; Krebs-Smith, S.M.; Frank, E.; Pronk, N.; et al. U.S. Primary Care Physicians' Diet, Physical Activity, and Weight-Related Care of Adult Patients. *Am. J. Prev. Med.* **2011**, *41*, 33–42. [CrossRef] [PubMed]

Permissions

All chapters in this book were first published by MDPI; hereby published with permission under the Creative Commons Attribution License or equivalent. Every chapter published in this book has been scrutinized by our experts. Their significance has been extensively debated. The topics covered herein carry significant findings which will fuel the growth of the discipline. They may even be implemented as practical applications or may be referred to as a beginning point for another development.

The contributors of this book come from diverse backgrounds, making this book a truly international effort. This book will bring forth new frontiers with its revolutionizing research information and detailed analysis of the nascent developments around the world.

We would like to thank all the contributing authors for lending their expertise to make the book truly unique. They have played a crucial role in the development of this book. Without their invaluable contributions this book wouldn't have been possible. They have made vital efforts to compile up to date information on the varied aspects of this subject to make this book a valuable addition to the collection of many professionals and students.

This book was conceptualized with the vision of imparting up-to-date information and advanced data in this field. To ensure the same, a matchless editorial board was set up. Every individual on the board went through rigorous rounds of assessment to prove their worth. After which they invested a large part of their time researching and compiling the most relevant data for our readers.

The editorial board has been involved in producing this book since its inception. They have spent rigorous hours researching and exploring the diverse topics which have resulted in the successful publishing of this book. They have passed on their knowledge of decades through this book. To expedite this challenging task, the publisher supported the team at every step. A small team of assistant editors was also appointed to further simplify the editing procedure and attain best results for the readers.

Apart from the editorial board, the designing team has also invested a significant amount of their time in understanding the subject and creating the most relevant covers. They scrutinized every image to scout for the most suitable representation of the subject and create an appropriate cover for the book.

The publishing team has been an ardent support to the editorial, designing and production team. Their endless efforts to recruit the best for this project, has resulted in the accomplishment of this book. They are a veteran in the field of academics and their pool of knowledge is as vast as their experience in printing. Their expertise and guidance has proved useful at every step. Their uncompromising quality standards have made this book an exceptional effort. Their encouragement from time to time has been an inspiration for everyone.

The publisher and the editorial board hope that this book will prove to be a valuable piece of knowledge for researchers, students, practitioners and scholars across the globe.

List of Contributors

Emma Rose
Lancaster Institute for the Contemporary Arts, Lancaster University, Lancaster LA1 4YW, UK

Amanda Bingley
Division of Health Research, Lancaster University, Lancaster LA1 4YG, UK

Macarena Rioseco
Lancaster Institute for the Contemporary Arts, Lancaster LA1 4YW, UK

Kirsten Lamb
Freedom from Torture, Manchester M1 1JU, UK

Vijay Kumar Chattu and Soosanna Kumary
Faculty of Medical Sciences, The University of the West Indies, St. Augustine, Trinidad and Tobago

Md. Dilshad Manzar
Department of Nursing, College of Applied Medical Sciences, Majmaah University, Majmaah 11952

Deepa Burman
School of Medicine, University of Pittsburgh, 4200 Fifth Ave, Pittsburgh, PA 15260, USA

David Warren Spence
Independent Researcher, 652 Dufferin Street, Toronto, ON M6K 2B4, Canada

Seithikurippu R. Pandi-Perumal
Somnogen Canada Inc., College Street, Toronto, ON M1H 1C5, Canada

Sara Thomée
Department of Psychology, University of Gothenburg, 405 30 Gothenburg, Sweden

Hongyu Guan, Kang Du, Jin Zhao and Yaojiang Shi
Center for Experimental Economics in Education, Shaanxi Normal University, Xi'an 710127, China

Huan Wang and Matthew Boswell
Freeman Spogli Institute for International Studies, Stanford University, Stanford, CA 94305, USA

Yiwei Qian
Department of Economics, University of Southern California, Los Angeles, CA 90089, USA

Chulhwan Choi
Department of Golf Industry, College of Physical Education, Kyung Hee University, Seocheon-dong 1, Giheung-gu, Yongin-si, Gyeonggi-do 17104, Korea

Mary A. Hums
Department of Health and Sport Science, University of Louisville, SAC East 104Q, University of Louisville, Louisville, KY 40292, USA

Chul-Ho Bum
Department of Sports Taekwondo, Graduate School of Physical Education, Kyung Hee University, Seocheon-dong 1, Giheung-gu, Yongin-si, Gyeonggi-do 17104, Korea

Regina Winzer
Department of Public Health Sciences, Karolinska Institutet, 17165 Stockholm, Sweden
Department of Living Conditions and Lifestyles, Public Health Agency of Sweden, 17182 Solna, Sweden

Kimmo Sorjonen
Department of Clinical Neuroscience, Karolinska Institutet, 17165 Stockholm, Sweden

Keyu Zhai and Geng Wang
School of Education, University of Glasgow, Glasgow G12 8QQ, UK

Lene Lindberg
Department of Public Health Sciences, Karolinska Institutet, 17165 Stockholm, Sweden
Center for Epidemiology and Community Medicine, Stockholm County Council, 10431 Stockholm, Sweden

Xing Gao
The Bartlett School of Planning, University College London, London WC1E 6BT, UK

Sunil Kumar and Ilyoung Chong
Department of Information and Communications Engineering, Hankuk University of Foreign Studies, Seoul 02450, Korea

Jerrod Brown
Pathways Counseling Center, Inc., St. Paul, MN 55104, USA
Department of Human Services, College of Humanities and Social Sciences, Concordia University, St. Paul, MN 55104, USA
American Institute for the Advancement of Forensic Studies, St. Paul, MN 55104, USA

Diane Harr
Department of Graduate Teacher Education, College of Education, Concordia University, St. Paul, MN 55104, USA

Tariku Ayana Abdi
Department of Psychology, University of Campania, 8100 Caserta, Italy

José M. Peiró
IVIE & IDOCAL, University of Valencia, 46010 Valencia, Spain

Yarid Ayala
Department of Economics and Management, Pontificia Universidad Javeriana, 110111 Bogotá, Colombia

Clas-Håkan Nygård and Heini Huhtala
Faculty of Social Science, Health Unit, University of Tampere, 33014 Tampere, Finland

Salvatore Zappalà
Department of Psychology, University of Bologna, 40126 Bologna, Italy
Department of Human Resource Management and Psychology, Financial University under the Government of the Russian Federation, 125993 Moscow, Russia

Shamona Maharaj, Ty Lees and Sara Lal
Neuroscience Research Unit, School of Life Sciences, University of Technology Sydney, 15 Broadway, Ultimo, Sydney, NSW 2007, Australia

Birgitta Ojala
Faculty of Social Science, Health Unit, University of Tampere, 33014 Tampere, Finland
Tullinkulma Occupational Health Unit, 33100 Tampere, Finland

Philip Bohle
Tasmanian School of Business and Economics, University of Tasmania, Private Bag 84 Hobart, Tasmania 7001, Australia

Seppo T. Nikkari
Tullinkulma Occupational Health Unit, 33100 Tampere, Finland
Faculty of Medicine and Health Technology, Tampere University, 33100 Tampere, Finland

Brian Moore, Stuart Woodcock and Dean Dudley
Department of Educational Studies, Faculty of Human Sciences, Macquarie University, North Ryde, NSW 2109, Australia

Karolina Skonieczna-Z˙ ydecka and Igor Łoniewski
Department of Biochemistry and Human Nutrition, Pomeranian Medical University in Szczecin, 71-460 Szczecin, Poland

Wojciech Marlicz
Department of Gastroenterology, Pomeranian Medical University, 71-252 Szczecin, Poland

AgataMisera
Department of Child and Adolescent Psychiatry, Charité Universitätsmedizin, 13353 Berlin, Germany

Anastasios Koulaouzidis
Endoscopy Unit, The Royal Infirmary of Edinburgh, EH16 4SA Edinburgh, UK

Sarvenaz Esmaeelzadeh, John Moraros and Yelena Bird
School of Public Health, University of Saskatchewan, Saskatoon, SK S7N 2Z4, Canada

Lilian Thorpe
FRCP, Faculty, Community Health and Epidemiology, University of Saskatchewan, Saskatoon, SK S7N 2Z4, Canada

Jennifer Bingham and Nicole Scovis
SinfoníaRx, Tucson, AZ 85701, USA

David R. Axon and Ann M. Taylor
College of Pharmacy, University of Arizona, Tucson, AZ 85721, USA

Index

www.ingramcontent.com/pod-product-compliance
Lightning Source LLC
LaVergne TN
LVHW080927210926
848485LV00004B/741